Artificial Intelligence in Surgery

Ken Masamune • Kaori Kusuda
Hiroyuki Nakamura • Yoshihiro Muragaki
Editors

Artificial Intelligence in Surgery

Recent Advances and Future

Springer

Editors
Ken Masamune
Tokyo Women's Medical University
Tokyo, Japan

Kaori Kusuda
Tokyo Women's Medical University
Tokyo, Japan

Hiroyuki Nakamura
Tokyo Medical University
Tokyo, Japan

Yoshihiro Muragaki
Tokyo Women's Medical University
Tokyo, Japan

ISBN 978-981-96-6634-8 ISBN 978-981-96-6635-5 (eBook)
https://doi.org/10.1007/978-981-96-6635-5

This Springer imprint is published by the registered company Springer Nature Singapore Pte Ltd.
The registered company address is: 152 Beach Road, #21-01/04 Gateway East, Singapore 189721, Singapore

Preface

In recent years, the potential for Artificial Intelligence (AI) to bring about innovations in surgical techniques has garnered significant attention. While there are already some practical applications of AI systems in diagnostic fields, including medical imaging analysis, the utilization of AI in surgical operations remains an ongoing research topic. As this trend progresses, it's increasingly likely that surgeries assisted by AI could become commonplace in future clinical settings.

To implement AI in surgical procedures, there are several challenges and issues that must be addressed. Standardization of the vast amount of medical data, as well as its secure management, is imperative. Moreover, the cybersecurity of Internet of Things (IoT) technologies, which enable integration with medical devices, faces unique and stringent requirements different from those in other industries. Added to these are the complexities unique to the medical field, including personal and genetic data protection and legal regulations.

This book focuses on the intersection of cutting-edge technology and clinical medicine in the surgical field, offering multifaceted discussions on data standardization, legal regulations, and security. In each chapter, experts specializing in related topics provide an in-depth look at the subject matter and offer important insights into the research and development of AI-assisted surgery. Furthermore, practical clinical examples will be presented to illustrate the application of each theme.

The primary audience for this book includes biomedical engineers, students, AI developers, and healthcare professionals interested in AI-assisted surgery. Although the book does not go into detail about the fundamentals of medicine or engineering, it serves as a useful resource for those wishing to deepen their basic knowledge in topics that interest them. Ultimately, we hope that this book will contribute widely to all those involved in the research and development of AI-assisted surgery.

Tokyo, Japan Ken Masamune

Contents

Introduction/Definition of "AI Surgery"

Ken Masamune, Kaori Kusuda, and Yoshihiro Muragaki

Abstract In this chapter introducing AI surgery, the close relationship between medicine and technology is explored, along with the evolution of medical information and the integration of artificial intelligence with peripheral technologies such as IT, IoT, and robotics. Patient-derived biometrics play a critical role in surgical decision-making, highlighting the need for seamless intraoperative information exchange in the future. As a result, research and development efforts for smart cyber ORs and related technologies are ongoing, driving the accumulation of valuable data. In addition, the advancement of innovative technologies, including AI surgery, follows three types of approaches: needs-driven, seed-driven, and concept-driven. The development of novel medical devices requires synergies between emerging technologies and medical expertise, shaping the landscape for the next generation of surgical procedures. The emergence of transformative technologies such as AI and VR, along with the concept of smart therapy devices, will have a profound impact on the trajectory of AI surgery in the future.

Keywords Artificial intelligence · Regulation · Software as a medical device · Computer-aided diagnosis · Computer-aided surgery

1 Introduction

1.1 Quality of Medical Care and the Relation of Science and Technology

The quality of medical care will improve with the development of science, engineering, and technology. In particular, X-ray imaging technology, which was invented in the latter half of the nineteenth century, has made a big leap forward in

K. Masamune (✉) · K. Kusuda · Y. Muragaki
Tokyo Women's Medical University, Tokyo, Japan
e-mail: masamune.ken@twmu.ac.jp

K. Masamune et al. (eds.), *Artificial Intelligence in Surgery*,
https://doi.org/10.1007/978-981-96-6635-5_1

medical care, and many medical devices have been developed for the measurement of biological information such as blood pressure, electrocardiogram, CT, MRI, ultrasound imaging, and so on. In the latter half of the twentieth century, the digitization of information progressed, and IT, IoT, and robot technology began to be applied in the medical domain. Furthermore, the convergence of mixed reality and artificial intelligence (AI) is rapidly penetrating the field of medicine.

For example, X-ray images taken with conventional film have migrated to a digital format, allowing information to be stored as digital data. In addition, the traditional paper-based medical records containing patient information have been digitized through the widespread use of personal computers, and network-connected online medical records are becoming more widespread. Furthermore, the widespread availability of the Internet has played a key role in the increasing digitization of information. This, coupled with the miniaturization of information display devices such as mobile phones and smart phones, has been seamlessly integrated into the medical care environment. As a result, it is now easier to transmit medical information to remote health facilities through network connections. Furthermore, the accumulation of digitized medical big data is beginning to open up the possibility of achieving automated image-interpreted diagnosis and AI-driven pathological diagnosis. These developments promise to streamline the diagnostic process and improve accuracy through the use of artificial intelligence. In addition, telemedicine and epoch-making surgery support systems have been developed through the collection and use of medical information by surgery support robots and IoT, and the use of the next-generation communications standard 5G has begun, which is helping to improve the quality of medical care [1–3].

1.2 Information in Medicine

Before looking at the latest developments in the healthcare sector, let's take an overview of what medical information is. Generally, "medical information" refers to a range of data on a patient's health. This includes personal information such as the patient's name, date of birth, address, and contact details, as well as records of interactions with the doctor during the consultation. It also includes medical information such as test results, anesthesia records, and treatments received during surgery. It also includes records of post-operative rehabilitation and progress reports. In diagnosis and treatment, doctors rely on a variety of preoperative and past medical information, as well as information obtained directly from the patient, in order to make informed decisions.

This information will be used as scientific evidence for the next new patient. The doctor's own knowledge, experience, and skill, the patient's values about treatment,

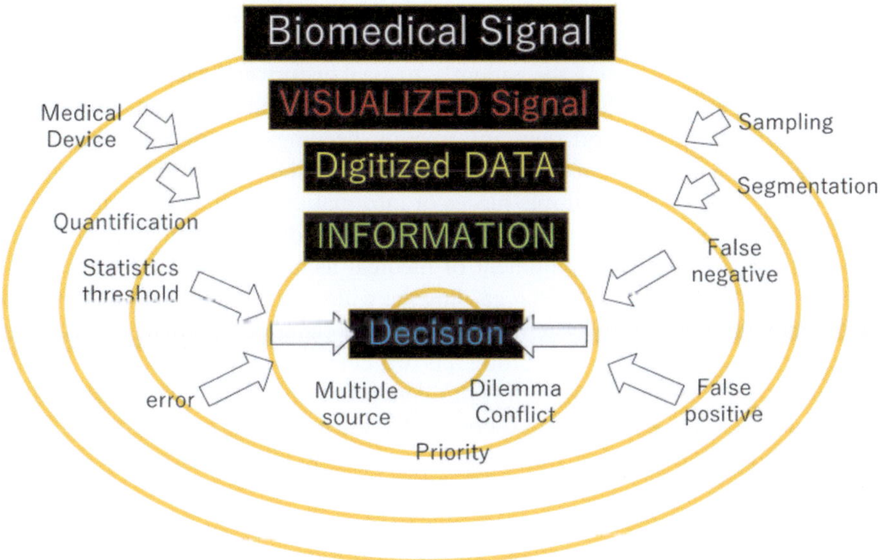

Fig. 1 Data flow of biological signals: continuity from raw biological signals generated by the patient to multiple source data for decision-making by the surgeon

family situation, and quality of life are taken into account when making the final decision. Such informed, scientifically based medicine is one form of evidence-based medicine (EBM) and is an important concept underpinning current healthcare [4].

Medical information includes not only medical information directly related to patients, such as diagnostic support, treatment support, and rehabilitation support, but also nursing and pharmaceutical information, such as dispensing support, nursing admission management, medical equipment inventory and logistics management, and patient services owned by hospitals. It refers to an extremely wide range of information, including electronic medical records for management and administration, medical accounting systems, and booking systems. This publication focuses on the most advanced parts of these, particularly in the perioperative period.

The flow of medical information in the operating theater, from biological signals obtained from the patient to the final information required for diagnostic and therapeutic decisions, is summarized in Fig. 1.

The patient, or human body, is composed of living tissue from which various biological signals are generated. The distribution of each organ in the body, as well as biological signals such as heartbeat, blood pressure, respiration, etc., is sampled and quantified by medical equipment. The quantified measurement signals are digitized, but are themselves mere data and have no clinical usefulness or other significance. Meaningful information can only be obtained through statistical analysis and threshold setting using the patient's medical history and data accumulated in the past from patients with the same disease. This is called "informatization," and only through informatization does information become meaningful information. Final decisions and judgments are not made solely on the basis of information, but by the physician based on multiple pieces of information and his experience.

In "informatization," data connectivity and standardization of data formats are important for the further development of medical technology. This is because, as mentioned in the previous section regarding the wide scope of medical information, data is often closed to each system or hospital and cannot be used across different software that stores the data. Therefore, it is difficult to share data processed for different purposes. One way to solve this problem is to implement a smart cyber operating room (SCOT), which is the focus of this document [5, 6]. A smart OR can network medical information from each device in the OR and store the data in a common time-synchronous format.

If data is standardized, it will be possible to share data not only between specific hospitals but also between hospitals around the world, and statistics, learning, and prediction with more information may lead to more accurate treatment. Of course, legislation for the protection of personal data is being developed in many countries, and adequate measures need to be taken for information management and information security of the data to be collected. You will also read in this book that the Society 5.0 [7] initiative will make a significant contribution to healthcare.

1.3 Surgeon's New "Hands," "Eyes," and "Brain"

Not limited to information technology, advanced technologies in multiple fields are being researched and developed to support diagnosis and treatment. Here, the functional classification of technologies to assist surgeons can be broadly divided into "new hands," "new eyes," and "new brain." "The new eyes" is the technology for the information acquisition/presentation for the surgeon. New brains are rapid information processing and learning predictive technologies for decision making. And new hands are the machines, robots, and other technologies that augment and improve the ability of the surgeon's hands [8]. For each technology, advanced information technology including AI will be used in the future, resulting in some level of autonomous surgery.

1.4 Needs-Driven/Seeds-Driven (Tech-Push)/Concept-Driven Medical Device Development

Research and development in medical devices have received a great deal of attention, and, as this publication shows, a great deal of research is being carried out with excellent state-of-the-art technology and technological development capabilities.

On the other hand, one output of research and development is marketing as a medical device product. There are not many cases that start with basic research in academia and end up in commercialization. Medical device development differs from mere manufacturing in its peculiarities, which involve examination and licensing. The key to the future development of this field is the training of personnel who can promote research and development based on a bird's eye view of the manufacturing and marketing system for medical devices, including clinical trials, approval procedures, insurance reimbursement, distribution, and sales. Pharmaceutical and medical device regulations and standardization of medical devices using AI are also currently being actively discussed [9, 10].

Medical device development, which explores medical needs and considers commercialization based on these needs, is known as "needs-driven." Stanford University's "Biodesign" program, which systematizes a needs-driven approach to medical device development, is well known [11], where, for example, new catheters are developed and commercialized. On the other hand, it is also important to develop "seeds-driven" where new technologies and ideas such as robots and AI lead to new medical treatment, and medical treatment using the latest technology covered in this book will continue in the future.

Yet another approach is "concept-driven medical device development," in which a major treatment concept is set, and various R&D efforts are directed toward it, leading to a future medical revolution. For example, in cancer treatment, the concept of double-targeting therapy, which combines a highly tumor-accumulating drug with a physical force that acts only within the tumor, has been proposed. One solution is sonodynamic therapy (SDT), a concept-driven approach that combines drug delivery system (DDS) drugs and focused ultrasound (HIFU) to control cancer and tumors deep within the body. The resulting treatment is expected to reduce systemic side effects due to tumor accumulation and increase anti-tumor efficacy, which is not possible before [12].

AI technology will become increasingly necessary to realize these new development concepts.

1.5 Summary

This book summarizes the latest medical innovation trends focusing on medical big data, AI technology, AR/VR technology, and high-speed mobile communication technology, which are particularly important in the progress of medical care by the latest technology as mentioned above. The smart cyber operating theater was also discussed as a current status and trend in information infrastructure technology contributing to high-risk treatment in AI surgery.

The intended audience for this publication is the following:

- Engineers and researchers considering the application of AI, image processing technology, and AR/VR technology to the medical field.
- Technicians, researchers, or medical professionals who handle medical big data.
- Management level of hospitals with operating theaters.

This publication is a collection of topics on the use of AI, which is currently being increasingly used, in high-risk surgical procedures. In addition, generative AI, such as ChatGPT, has begun to evolve in recent years. For example, the research of [13] presents its performance on surgical knowledge questions and assessed the stability of this performance on repeat queries. And more, each of these AI technologies will be linked by generative AI and further linked to robotics and other technologies, leading to more advanced AI surgery. It is greatly hoped that this publication will help in new research and development.

References

1. Levin M, McKechnie T, Kruse CC, Aldrich K, Grantcharov TP, Langerman A. Surgical data recording in the operating room: a systematic review of modalities and metrics. Br J Surg. 2021;108(6):613–21. https://doi.org/10.1093/bjs/znab016.
2. Ushimaru Y, Takahashi T, Souma Y, et al. Innovation in surgery/operating room driven by internet of things on medical devices. Surg Endosc. 2019;33:3469–77. https://doi.org/10.1007/s00464-018-06651-4.
3. Bravo N, Paredes I, Loyola L, Vargas G. Use of 5G technology for oncological surgery streaming. Data Metadata [Internet]. 2023;2:126. [cited 2024 Mar. 9]. Available from: https://dm.saludcyt.ar/index.php/dm/article/view/126
4. Sackett DL, Rosenberg WM, Gray JA, Haynes RB, Richardson WS. Evidence based medicine: what it is and what it isn't. BMJ. 1996;312:71–2.
5. Okamoto J, Masamune K, Iseki H, Muragaki Y. Development concepts of a Smart Cyber Operating Theater (SCOT) using ORiN technology. Biomed Eng/Biomed Tech. 2018;63:31–7. https://doi.org/10.1515/bmt-2017-0006.
6. Masamune K, Nishikawa A, Kawai T, Horise Y, Iwamoto N. The development of Smart Cyber Operating Theater (SCOT), an innovative medical robot architecture that can allow surgeons to freely select and connect master and slave telesurgical robots. Impact. 2018;2018:35–7. https://doi.org/10.21820/23987073.2018.3.35.
7. Hitachi-UTokyo Laboratory(H-Utokyo Lab.). Society 5.0 a people-centric super-smart society. Singapore: Springer; 2020. https://doi.org/10.1007/978-981-15-2989-4.
8. Sun X, Okamoto J, Masamune K, et al. Robotic technology in operating rooms: a review. Curr Robot Rep. 2021;2:333–41. https://doi.org/10.1007/s43154-021-00055-4.
9. FDA. Proposed regulatory framework for modifications to artificial intelligence/machine learning (AI/ML)-based software as a medical device (SaMD). Discussion paper and request for feedback. https://www.fda.gov/media/122535/download; 2019.
10. Gerke S, Babic B, Evgeniou T, et al. The need for a system view to regulate artificial intelligence/machine learning-based software as medical device. NPJ Digit Med. 2020;3:53. https://doi.org/10.1038/s41746-020-0262-2.

11. Stanford BIODESIGN, https://biodesignguide.stanford.edu/. Accessed Jan 2024.
12. Horise Y, et al. Sonodynamic therapy with anticancer micelles and high intensity focused ultrasound in treatment of canine cancer. Front Pharmacol. 2019;10:Article 545.
13. Beaulieu-Jones BR, et al. Evaluating capabilities of large language models: performance of GPT-4 on surgical knowledge assessments. Surgery. 2024;175:936–42.

Development of AI Analysis Platform—Smart Cyber Operating Theater (SCOT)—For Medical Information in Neurosurgery

Kaori Kusuda, Jun Okamoto, Yoshihiro Muragaki, and Ken Masamune

Abstract Most medical data are stored in electronic medical records and recorded as text because there are individual differences in patients and pathological conditions. AI researchers decipher the information necessary for research from these data to create a dataset manually. Tokyo Women's Medical University has built a surgical prognosis management system, the Clinical Information Analyzer (CIA). This system consists of three functions: cleansing and accumulating medical data, analyzing data, and feeding back the analysis results to doctors. Additionally, the prognosis of patients who have undergone brain tumor resection will be proposed using AI and data of CIA system. Two models, "survival prognosis" and "functional prognosis," will be developed as prognosis prediction models. In the future, we would like to use this follow-up information to improve the accuracy of prognostic prediction.

Keywords Medical informatics · Neurosurgery · Electronic medical record · Prediction model

1 Introduction

In recent medical AI research, topics involving the use of medical images have become mainstream. Recently published studies have explored AI-based detection of lung lesions from X-ray [1] images and segmentation of brain tumors from magnetic resonance imaging (MRI) images [2]. Additionally, an automatic extraction model was developed to locate cerebral aneurysms from MRI images [3]. A feature of image-based AI studies is that the size and imaging methods are almost uniform; therefore, it is possible to obtain standardized images. Owing to the large number of

K. Kusuda (✉) · J. Okamoto · Y. Muragaki · K. Masamune
Tokyo Women's Medical University, Tokyo, Japan
e-mail: kusuda.kaori@twmu.ac.jp

K. Masamune et al. (eds.), *Artificial Intelligence in Surgery*,
https://doi.org/10.1007/978-981-96-6635-5_2

training images that can be created, the accuracy of this model tends to be as high as 90%.

On the other hand, models created by AI studies using medical data tend to be inferior in accuracy to medical image-based models. This can be attributed to the presence of various data defects and the unstructured nature of data [4, 5]. Most medical data are stored in electronic medical records and recorded as text because there are individual differences in patients and pathological conditions. AI researchers decipher the information necessary for research from these data to create a dataset manually.

Recently, blood test values and digital data from medical devices have been structured and stored in various databases. However, many items that require the professional judgment of medical staff (doctors, nurses, laboratory technicians) have not yet been structured, mainly because the purpose of electronic medical records is practical, and not meant for research. Since electronic medical records are created for the purpose of medical support, recording detailed items necessary for research, even in daily workflow, may be burdensome and time-consuming. To accelerate medical AI research, gathering the knowledge of medical staff and accumulating it as structured data is necessary.

2 Neurosurgery with AI

Tokyo Women's Medical University has built a surgical prognosis management system and has accumulated clinical information on over 2000 cases of brain tumor surgery since 2000. This system facilitates the management of inpatient data in the clinical workflow. In addition, basic patient information, such as surgery date, presence or absence of recurrence, pathology (WHO classification, genotype), and follow-up data, such as survival days, have been recorded. Our group has used these structured data in clinical research.

Saito et al. evaluated whether the results of motor evoked potentials (MEP) and intraoperative voluntary movement (IVM) during surgery could help predict postoperative motor function [6]. Awake surgery was performed to remove tumors around the motor and verbal areas. In this surgical method, the patient is awakened after craniotomy, and the motor and language functions are confirmed. The tumor is removed while checking MEP and IVM to determine the occurrence of functional site damage. As a result, it was found that the magnitude of the rate of decrease in these values is related to the level of decrease in motor function after surgery.

Shibahara et al. considered the predictive potential of blood cell count in the myelosuppression process caused by ACNU, using machine learning and basic patient and medical data before treatment as learning data in chemotherapy for glioma (ACNU therapy) [7]. Traditionally, doctors predict myelosuppression, which is a side effect of ACNU, and change medication dose according to the rule of thumb. Based on the results of this study, appropriate drug administration can be performed according to the clinical data of the patient before treatment.

Matsui et al. developed a model for predicting pathological diagnoses using positron emission tomography (PET) and computed tomography (CT) images and basic patient information on a surgical prognosis management system [8]. Conventionally, invasive sample acquisition, such as biopsy and surgery, is indispensable for the definitive diagnosis of tumor grade and genotype. Based on the results of this study, pathological results can be predicted from preoperative images, and invasive medical practices can be reduced. Furthermore, in cases where tumors adjacent to the speech and motor areas are removed, dysfunction can be prevented, and the patient's quality of life is thought to improve.

In addition, we developed a flow cytometry system to enable rapid pathological prediction in the operating room [9]. Clinical efficacy was evaluated by comparing the malignancy calculated from the sample using the system with malignancy based on pathological diagnosis.

3 Clinical Information Analyzer System

Currently, the information generated in the operating room is stored independently on each device. However, this information is not routinely extracted. In other words, IT in the operating room is limited to the visualization and digitization of data obtained from each medical device.

Therefore, we aimed to perform AI-assisted surgery. A smart cyber operating theater (SCOT), as shown in Fig. 1, has been built as a platform for the integrated management and analysis of various types of information gathered during the perioperative period [10]. To achieve information-guided surgery, the system establishes a network with basic surgical equipment, such as MRI and various medical devices. The data from these medical devices can then be time-synchronized and stored.

Furthermore, by analyzing a huge amount of information, including not only SCOT data but also electronic medical records and surgical records, it is possible to examine the prognosis information of patients. This enhances its clinical significance. Intraoperative statistical prediction of the effects of surgical procedures is useful for deciding whether to remove or preserve residual tumors. For instance, this can be used to predict how many months of survival will be extended by increasing the intraoperative removal rate by 10% during surgery. As a challenge, medical information used for models such as AI is scattered in the hospital and in each system and is recorded in a unique format.

At Tokyo Women's Medical University, the Clinical Information Analyzer (CIA), as shown in Fig. 2, was developed as a basic system for handling data. This system consists of three functions: cleansing and accumulating medical data, analyzing data, and feeding back the analysis results to doctors. The target is electronic medical record system information such as basic patient information/physical characteristics, blood test information, and prescription information. Furthermore, intraoperative medical information is assumed to be medical device information, such as biological monitor information gathered via SCOT.

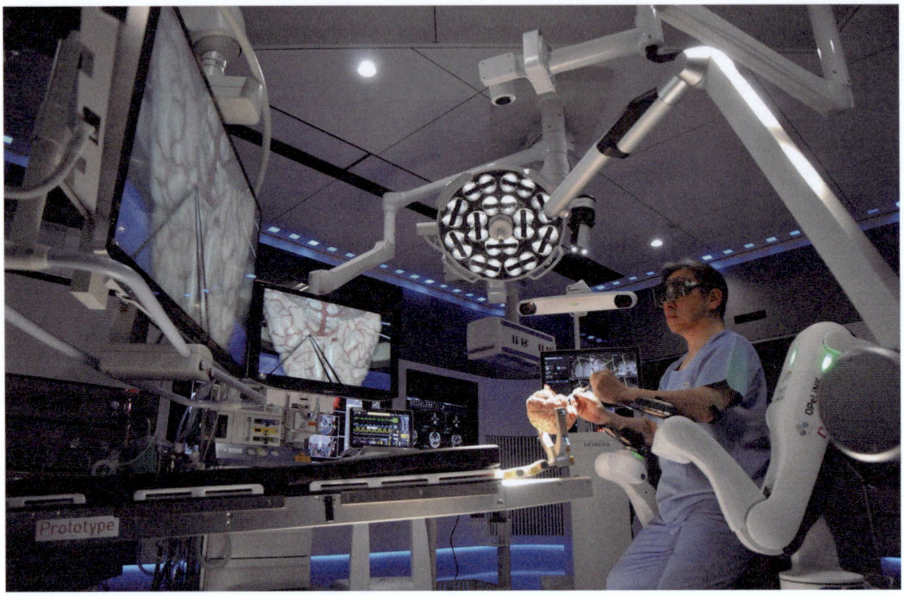

Fig. 1 SCOT operation room

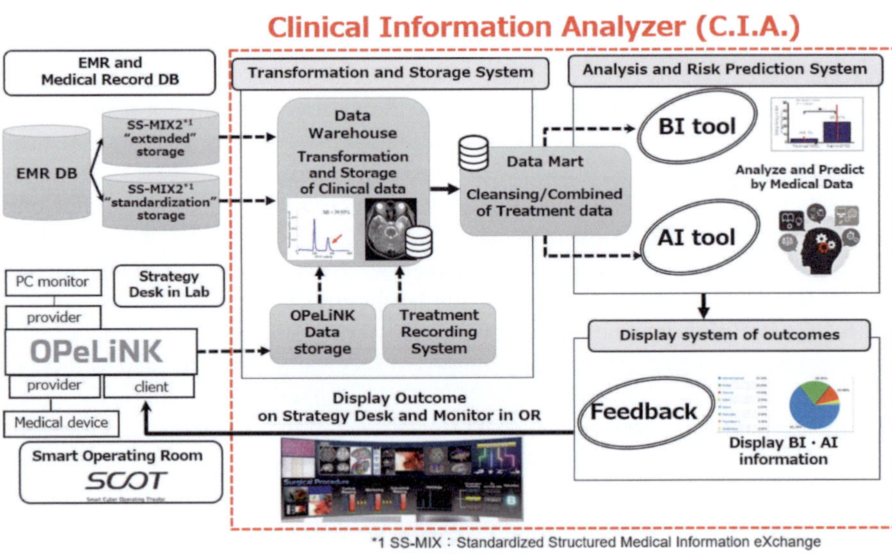

Fig. 2 Clinical Information Analyzer (CIA)

In this project, the prognosis of patients who have undergone brain tumor resection will be proposed using AI. Two models, "survival prognosis" and "functional prognosis," will be developed as prognosis prediction models.

"Survival prognosis" indicates the number of days a patient survives after surgery and has been established as an index for clinical evaluation for all surgeries, not limited to brain tumor resection. Currently, doctors use empirical rules to predict survival and present these rules to patients at the time of informed consent. "Functional prognosis" refers to new functional complications that may occur after surgery. Paralysis and aphasia are two examples, which occur when the brain and nerves (cranial nerves, motor nerves, arcuate fasciculus, etc.) are damaged. At present, functional sites are identified during awake surgery by brain function mapping.

AI (machine learning) using Python was used to develop the prognosis prediction model. As explanatory variables, the parameters considered in the prediction of survival prognosis and functional prognosis in clinical diagnosis performed by a doctor were adopted. Specifically, the pathological results, age, presence or absence of radiation therapy, and excision rate were selected. The excision rate, maximum tumor diameter, and age were selected as explanatory variables for functional prognosis. As a result, in the survival prognosis prediction model, an accuracy of 90% was obtained in two classifications, and 62% in four classifications. Additionally, in the functional prognosis prediction model, results with an accuracy of 94% were obtained for the two classifications.

Engineers should minimize the number of classifications because multiple objective variables generally reduce accuracy. However, from the standpoint of doctors and patients, it is thought that knowing the probability of every 1, 3, or 5 years rather than the probability of survival after 1 year will increase the patient's motivation for treatment. Therefore, more accurate results can be obtained for the two classifications, but their clinical importance diminishes. In the future, we would like to set the variables according to a bedside operation to improve the prediction accuracy of the model.

4 Future Study in CIA

Collecting prognostic information is an issue for the entire research field. In our study, follow-up information was collected to create survival and functional prognosis models. Since patients after discharge do not report their health condition to the hospital visited in the past, it is necessary to actively ask the hospital for follow-up information. This process requires a lot of time and the cooperation from doctors, and it is difficult to investigate all patients, so we collected information for a limited period.

However, in addition to long-term follow-up information after discharge, there are issues in collecting short-term follow-up information during hospitalization. Functional deterioration that occurs during surgery (such as decreased MEP) is divided into disorders that recover immediately after surgery, those that recover every few months, and those that are difficult to recover. It is desirable to predict where these functional deteriorations should be classified before or during surgery. Past short-term follow-up information can be extracted from rehabilitation records using a model. To quantitatively and accurately evaluate the level of functional recovery, evaluation over time by a rehabilitation therapist is required. However, this information is recorded in electronic medical records in text format. Additionally, because the recording method differs depending on the therapist, manual structuring is required to create an AI dataset.

In our study, two projects were launched to collect follow-up information. First, to gather long-term follow-up information, a chatbot-style interview system using an SNS was developed. Patients registered on this SNS can collect progress information by answering interviews that are delivered regularly. Next, to gather short-term follow-up information, we are trying to structure the data in collaboration with a rehabilitation therapist. We will expand the complete data by improving the efficiency of data entry. In the future, we would like to use this follow-up information to improve the accuracy of prognostic prediction.

Acknowledgments This research was supported by AMED under Grant Number 21he1602003h0005 and JSPS KAKENHI Grant Number JP 20 K19942. Members of HITACHI, Ltd., Waseda University, and Future University Hakodate support to develop the CIA system.

References

1. Lakhani P, Sundaram B. Deep learning at chest radiography: automated classification of pulmonary tuberculosis by using convolutional neural networks. Radiology. 2017;284(2):574–82. https://doi.org/10.1148/radiol.2017162326. Epub 2017 Apr 24
2. Lao J, Chen Y, Li ZC, Li Q, Zhang J, Liu J, Zhai G. A deep learning-based radiomics model for prediction of survival in glioblastoma multiforme. Sci Rep. 2017;7(1):10353. https://doi.org/10.1038/s41598-017-10649-8. PMID: 28871110; PMCID: PMC5583361
3. Ueda D, Yamamoto A, Nishimori M, Shimono T, Doishita S, Shimazaki A, Katayama Y, Fukumoto S, Choppin A, Shimahara Y, Miki Y. Deep learning for MR angiography: automated detection of cerebral aneurysms. Radiology. 2019;290(1):187–94. https://doi.org/10.1148/radiol.2018180901. Epub 2018 Oct 23
4. Chen Y, Qiu Z, Kamruzzaman A, Snodgrass T, Scarfe A, Bryant HE. Survival of metastatic colorectal cancer patients treated with chemotherapy in Alberta (1995–2004). Support Care Cancer. 2010;18(2):217–24. https://doi.org/10.1007/s00520-009-0647-x. Epub 2009 May 15. PMID: 19440737; PMCID: PMC2795864
5. Chambless LB, Kistka HM, Parker SL, Hassam-Malani L, McGirt MJ, Thompson RC. The relative value of postoperative versus preoperative Karnofsky performance scale scores as a predictor of survival after surgical resection of glioblastoma multiforme. J Neuro-Oncol. 2015;121(2):359–64. https://doi.org/10.1007/s11060-014-1640-x. Epub 2014 Oct 26
6. Saito T, Muragaki Y, Tamura M, Maruyama T, Nitta M, Tsuzuki S, Fukuchi S, Ohashi M, Kawamata T. Awake craniotomy with transcortical motor evoked potential monitoring for resection of gliomas in the precentral gyrus: utility for predicting motor function. J Neurosurg. 2019;132(4):987–97. https://doi.org/10.3171/2018.11.JNS182609.

7. Shibahara T, Ikuta S, Muragaki Y. Machine-learning approach for modeling myelosuppression attributed to nimustine hydrochloride. JCO Clin Cancer Inform. 2018;2:1–21. https://doi.org/10.1200/CCI.17.00022.
8. Matsui Y, Maruyama T, Nitta M, Saito T, Tsuzuki S, Tamura M, Kusuda K, Fukuya Y, Asano H, Kawamata T, Masamune K, Muragaki Y. Prediction of lower-grade glioma molecular subtypes using deep learning. J Neuro-Oncol. 2020;146(2):321–7. https://doi.org/10.1007/s11060-019-03376-9. Epub 2019 Dec 21
9. Suzuki A, Maruyama T, Nitta M, Komori T, Ikuta S, Chernov M, Tamura M, Kawamata T, Muragaki Y. Evaluation of DNA ploidy with intraoperative flow cytometry may predict long-term survival of patients with supratentorial low-grade gliomas: Analysis of 102 cases. Clin Neurol Neurosurg. 2018;168:46–53. https://doi.org/10.1016/j.clineuro.2018.02.027. Epub 2018 Feb 21
10. Okamoto J, Masamune K, Iseki H, Muragaki Y. Development concepts of a smart cyber operating theater (SCOT) using ORiN technology. Biomed Tech (Berl). 2018;63(1):31–7. https://doi.org/10.1515/bmt-2017-0006.

Deployment of Smart Cyber Operating Theater-Based Digital Operating Room to a Mobile Operating Theater

Kitaro Yoshimitsu, Yuki Horise, Jun Okamoto, Ken Masamune, and Yoshihiro Muragaki

Abstract Information-guided surgery performed using digital technology provides better treatment results for patients and advanced skills for surgeons and clinical teams managing perioperative patients. Precise guided surgical digital transformation (DX) therapeutic goals connect all information and test data from admission to discharge to all devices via the Internet of Things (IoT). It is aggregated, used, and fed back as objectively visualized digital information. The smart cyber operating theater (SCOT) is a place for performing precision-guided surgery using this ultimate digitization. SCOT becomes a digitized treatment unit with all input-> analysis-> output schemes, and the entire operating room performs accurate guided treatment as a single medical device. Medical devices are networked to OPeLiNK, and aggregated data is used as valuable information necessary for intraoperative decision-making. Tokyo Women's Medical University Hyper SCOT has introduced intraoperative MRI and MR-compatible equipment as an intraoperative diagnostic imaging device for malignant brain tumor resection, which is a package in a sense. SCOT for IoT is headed for new development. We conducted a demonstration experiment of a mobile treatment room that simulates remote-surgery support using technology (5G). The idea of moving between the hospital and operating room will sooner or later permeate society. Therefore, we proposed a mechanism to spread advanced medical care to the surrounding area by operating SCOT in combination with SCOT and 5G and touring the surrounding area. Assuming a diagnosis using an ultrasound imaging device in a mobile SCOT, an onsite cardiologist received remote support from a gynecologist in front of a strategic desk. The image of the ultrasonic diagnostic imaging device, remote-control signal of the device, operation image at hand when operating the echo probe, and communi-

K. Yoshimitsu (✉) · Y. Horise · J. Okamoto · K. Masamune · Y. Muragaki
Tokyo Women's Medical University, Tokyo, Japan
e-mail: yoshimitsu.kitaro@twmu.ac.jp

K. Masamune et al. (eds.), *Artificial Intelligence in Surgery*,
https://doi.org/10.1007/978-981-96-6635-5_3

cation call were transmitted and received by 5G communication in this demonstration experiment. Both physicians in charge of the demonstration experiment commented that they could communicate as if they were present and without information delay or discomfort in conversation, demonstrating low latency and wide bandwidth of 5G.

Keyword Smart cyber operating theater (SCOT) · Internet of Things (IoT) · Precise guided surgery · Mobile SCOT · 5G

1 Digital Operating Theater

As of 2022, digitization has been accelerating with technologies, such as video/imaging, artificial intelligence (AI), energy devices, and robotics. Information-guided surgery performed using digital technology provides better treatment results for patients and advanced skills for surgeons and clinical teams managing perioperative patients. Digital technology combines images and anatomical information to capture visual information, drawing nerve fascicles behind tissues, unknown to the surgeon, and creating milliorder mechanisms from the fingertips. Precise control enables surgery on inaccessible tissue, significantly increasing the likelihood of surgery. Robotic surgery using these augmented reality (AR), surgical robot da Vinci and Hinotori is a representative example of digital technology in the operating room. Numerous surgeries cannot be performed without these digital surgery support solutions. However, with a rigorous understanding of the system, it is possible that only the inputs are digital (imaging) and only the outputs are digital (surgical robots) and are not fully or partially digitized. Most systems are analog mixtures.

Moreover, this mixed analog information hinders the maximum efficiency improvement that end users need. Precise guided surgical digital transformation (DX) therapeutic goals connect all information and test data from admission to discharge to all devices via the Internet of Things (IoT). It is aggregated, used, and fed back as objectively visualized digital information.

Consequently, quality medical care for individuals, which was limited to skilled doctors and certain specialists, has become widespread and highly reproducible and enables ultra-minimally invasive diagnosis and immediate treatment. The smart cyber operating theater (SCOT) is a place for performing precision-guided surgery using this ultimate digitization. This section introduces the high-performance smart treatment room (Hyper SCOT) as the DX of the operating room (Fig. 1) and the mobile SCOT, which is a portable SCOT under development for future remote treatment.

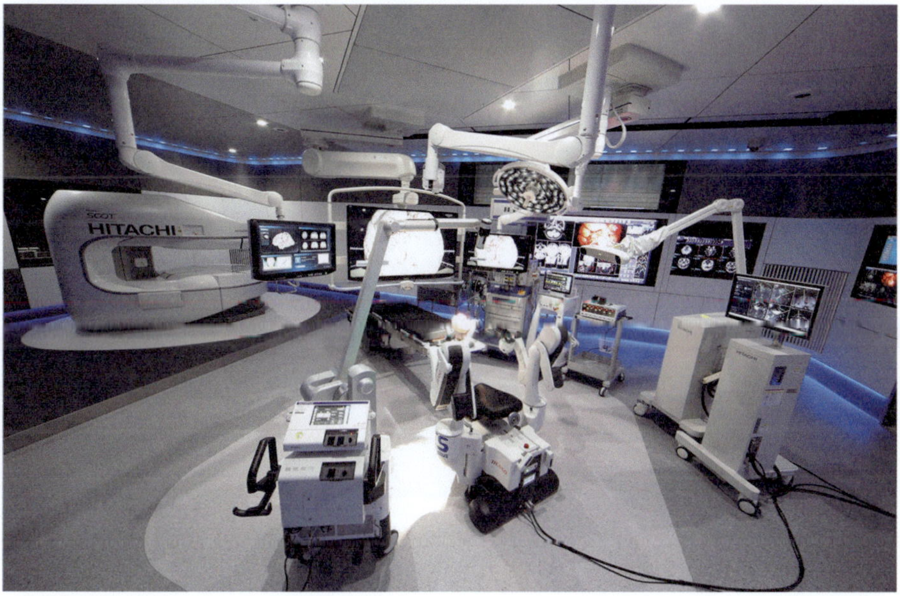

Fig. 1 The high-end version of smart cyber operating theater (SCOT) of Tokyo Women's Medical University

2 Smart Cyber Operating Theater (SCOT)

Digital data aggregated by organically linked devices in SCOT is used by AI to predict prognosis and support ultra-high levels of decision-making with intraoperative feedback. Intraoperative feedback supports the judgment of the surgical team and is reused as an input signal for surgical support systems and robotics to achieve highly functional and optimal treatment. Consequently, SCOT becomes a digitized treatment unit with all input- > analysis- > output schemes, and the entire operating room performs accurate guided treatment as a single medical device.

Specifically, devices that acquire information, such as intraoperative monitoring devices and intraoperative diagnostic imaging devices and basic infrastructure devices, such as operating tables and surgical lights, are grouped (packaged) as their respective basic devices. Medical devices are networked to OPeLiNK and aggregated on the OPeLiNK server (network) (Fig. 2). The aggregated data is used as valuable information necessary for intraoperative decision-making (information conversion). Although several approaches for leveraging aggregated data exist, in critical situations, AI offers multiple treatment options by comparing treatment results with similar cases that are visited several times during surgery. Surgeons are expected to consult AI and make decisions (AI conversion).

Surgical robots would be miniaturized in the future; however, reproducible inputs, such as intraoperative monitoring, imaging, and pathological diagnosis, would enable the removal and treatment of ultra-minimally invasive cells at the cellular level. This is

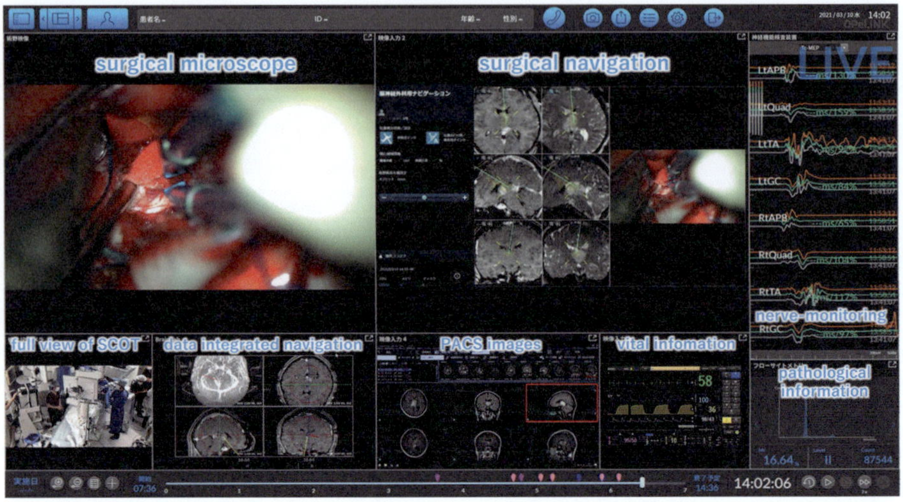

Fig. 2 The strategy desk. The information-integration application integrates the video and renders the data retrieved from each device in time synchronization on the screen

the future image of a precision-guided munition for robot engineering. Specifically, in a quantitative assessment of surgical safety, the average number of "errors" in a single procedure is 15.55, of which 23.5% are equipment or technology malfunctions or failures. This is because 37% do not have the necessary equipment and 43% have the wrong combination or setting. To solve this problem, the device must be pre-packaged from the surgeon-case combination pattern as a risk measure.

Tokyo Women's Medical University Hyper SCOT has introduced intraoperative MRI and MR-compatible equipment as an intraoperative diagnostic imaging device for malignant brain tumor resection, which is a package in a sense. Intraoperative MRI began operation at Shiga University of Medical Science and Tokyo Women's Medical University in 2000, and the coil and operating table are designed exclusively for surgery as MRI dedicated to surgery, and not MRI for diagnosis. Fujifilm Holdings Corp. has been commercializing and insuring since December 2021. Intraoperative MRI has been introduced at more than 30 institutions in Japan, and intraoperative images are often used in combination with surgical navigation systems [1, 2].

3 IoT of Equipment in SCOT

Previously, packaged devices were not linked to each other; it worked alone. Circulating medical staff would monitor the display information of each device and notify surgeons of any abnormality. Additionally, if the surgeon asks for information, medial staff confirm the information by oral contact from the field of surgery. Therefore, for surgeons who must make a comprehensive judgment of information, the information cannot be obtained unless it is fragmented and actively obtained. Thus, they are always "hungry for information."

Conversely, SCOT deploys OPeLiNK (made by OPExPARK) to aggregate information about each device on the server over the network and display it in a single application. OPeLiNK is middleware that aggregates device data to a server by connecting more than 40 medical devices, regardless of the type of device used in the operating room, manufacturer, and operating system. OPeLiNK has been used in studies and development at SCOT; however, it would be located in the operating room and intensive care unit (ICU) and ward in the next step [3].

The information-integration application integrates the video and renders the data retrieved from each device in time synchronization on the screen. For example, in SCOT, the center of the displayed image changes in real time by linking with the surgical navigation system centered on the image taken by intraoperative MRI, based on the surgical position of the surgeon. Nerve-monitoring information related to the actual surgical position and intraoperative pathological information are linked and displayed because spatial information can be added and displayed besides surgical position information. Simultaneously, this integrated information is centrally displayed on the surgical strategy desk to an expert surgeon, who helps the surgeon to make decisions based on what is happening in the field.

Furthermore, OPeLiNK has been introduced in the standard SCOT of Shinshu University School of Medicine (Fig. 3) and is widely used in glioma and other neurosurgical cases, such as pituitary adenoma. In future surgery, specifically minimally invasive therapy, surgical techniques are expected to be robotized and replaced by new treatments, some of which are beginning to be realized in the SCOT demonstration room: robotics-operating table and microscope, fertilizer image viewer that can be viewed freely by hand action without touching [4], and hand-assist robot that prevents operator's arm fatigue [5, 6].

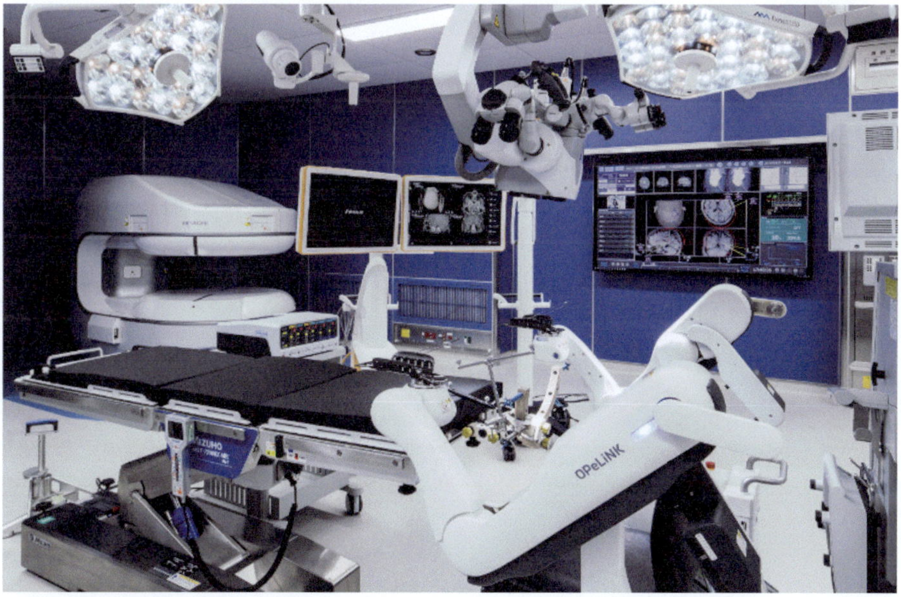

Fig. 3 The standard SCOT of Shinshu University School of Medicine. OPeLiNK has been introduced in this operating theater

4 SCOT × 5G = Mobile SCOT

SCOT for IoT is headed for new development. In October 2020, we made SCOT portable, changed the patient's traditional social wisdom to "go to the hospital," and realized the idea that "the hospital comes to the patient." We conducted a demonstration experiment of a mobile treatment room that simulates remote-surgery support using technology (5G).

Several things around us are becoming smaller with the advancement of technology, medical devices inclusive. Therefore, the idea of carrying items will naturally change, and the idea of moving between the hospital and operating room will sooner or later permeate society. Furthermore, when comparing regions and cities, the differences in medical care are remarkable; however, there are several economic disadvantages, such as the challenges associated with introducing the latest diagnostic and treatment equipment to regional hospitals.

Therefore, we proposed a mechanism to spread advanced medical care to the surrounding area by operating SCOT in combination with SCOT and 5G and touring the surrounding area. As a concept model, we developed a vehicle (Isuzu Giga vehicle size: length = 11.88 m, height = 3.7 m, width = 2.49 m, total load capacity = 18.33 t) equipped with a generator and a loading platform that can be expanded to the left and right. The vehicle is equipped with ultrasound diagnostics, a biological information monitor, an operating table, a mobile surgical light, four large wall-mounted displays, and 5G communications equipment (Fig. 4). The concept car is not equipped with air-conditioning equipment, such as medical gas and negative pressure equipment.

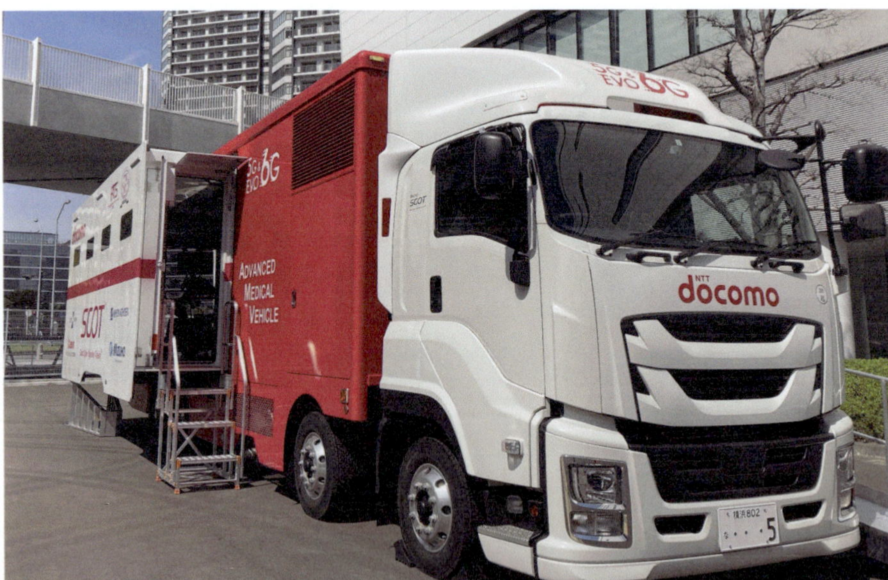

Fig. 4 The concept model of mobile smart cyber operating theater (mobile SCOT). This mobile SCOT has demonstrated experiment of remote ultrasonic diagnostic imaging via commercial 5G

5 Demonstration Experiment of Remote Ultrasonic Diagnosis Using 5G in Mobile SCOT

Assuming a diagnosis using an ultrasound imaging device (Fujifilm Holdings Corp.) for pregnant women housed in a mobile SCOT, an onsite cardiologist received remote support from a gynecologist in front of a strategic desk. The simulation was performed using a fetal model. The frequencies of commercial 5G used are 3.7GHz and 4.5GHz bands as sub 6 and 28GHz band as millimeter wave. The obstetrician and gynecologist remotely guide the doctor in the vehicle on how to apply the convex probe and, simultaneously, remotely control the device while observing the image transmitted from the ultrasonic diagnostic imaging device to support the treatment of the patient. Thus, the image of the ultrasonic diagnostic imaging device, remote-control signal of the device, operation image at hand when operating the echo probe, and communication call were transmitted and received by 5G communication in this demonstration experiment. The doctor in the car operated the echo probe based on the instructions on the remote control. The amount of data of the video information on the mobile SCOT side and the control information of the ultra sonic diagnostic imaging device was 20 Mbps and 0.2 Mbps, respectively. Conversely, the amount of data of the strategic desk remote controller on the strategic desk side of the clinic and the remote controller of the ultrasonic diagnostic imaging device were 5 Mbps and 20 Mbps, respectively.

Both physicians in charge of the demonstration experiment commented that they could communicate as if they were present and without information delay or discomfort in conversation, demonstrating low latency and wide bandwidth of 5G. In the future, the mobile SCOT would bridge the medical gap between urban and rural areas. Furthermore, we plan to conduct and develop a demonstration experiment assuming that specialists will support remote treatment at disaster/accident sites and dispatch vehicles for treatment.

Additionally, if the 5G area expands in the future, mobile strategy desk would be able to support decision-making using 5G smartphones and tablet devices even at academic conferences or external workplaces. It could be used as a mobile strategy desk that can accurately send the information collected in the operating room. Further stabilization of communications and expansions of 5G areas are considered essential to solving the technical problems associated with the social implementation of mobile SCOT.

6 Conclusion

SCOT is being developed as a single medical device that must be used for all invasive procedures, procedures, and treatments, not only surgery. The SCOT network system extends beyond the operating room to perioperative patients, outpatients, ICUs, wards, and long-term care facilities and homes. It is a future in which tailor-made treatments tailored to the characteristics and needs of individual patients will be possible.

Additionally, advanced surgical robots and fully automated treatment robots will perform ultra-minimally invasive treatments. In the future, surgery other than large-scale surgery may be performed in various places where mobile SCOT is deployed. In an age, where a wide range of medical services can be enjoyed through digital transformation, we believe that it is expedient for society as a whole to develop social infrastructure and comply with laws and regulations to aim for a better future.

Acknowledgments We thank Hiroshima University; Tohoku University; Tottori University; Denso Corporation; OPExPARK Inc.; Nihon Kohden Corporation; Mizuho Corporation; Pioneer Corporation; Canon Medical Systems Corporation; Hitachi, Ltd.; Solize Corporation; Central Uni Co.; Green Hospital Supply, Inc.; Air Water Inc.; and Air Water Safety Service Inc. We would also like to thank Masayasu Takahashi from Nihon Sekkei, Inc., and Medicaroid Corporation for their invaluable assistance.

Declaration of Interests In relation to this paper, JP6188612B2 has been patented, and WO2018105467A1 has been filed. SCOT and Smart Cyber Operating Theater are registered trademarks at Tokyo Women's Medical University. OPeLiNK is a registered trademark from OPExPARK, Inc. JO and YM are consultants for OPExPARK, Inc. There are no further conflicts of interest to declare.

Funding This research was conducted under the Japan Agency for Medical Research and Development Project "Research and development of advanced medical devices and systems to achieve the future of medicine/Development of a smart treatment chamber for the improvement of both medical safety and efficiency (Grant number: 18he0202263h0005)" and the Japan Society for the Promotion of Science Bilateral Exchange Project "Evolutionary fusion of SCOT and OR.net for the next generation intraoperative smart cyber operating theater."

References

1. Muragaki Y, Iseki H, Maruyama T, et al. Information-guided surgical management of gliomas using low-field-strength intraoperative MRI. Acta Neurochir Suppl. 2011;109:67–72.
2. Muragaki Y, Iseki H, Maruyama T, et al. Usefulness of intraoperative magnetic resonance imaging for glioma surgery. Acta Neurochir Suppl. 2006;98:67–75.
3. Okamoto J, Masamune K, Iseki H. Development concepts of a smart cyber operating theater(SCOT) using ORiN technology. Biomed Tech. 2018;63(1):31–7.
4. Yoshimitsu K, Muragaki Y, Maruyama T, Yamato M, Iseki H. Development and initial clinical testing of "OPECT": an innovative device for fully intangible control of the intraoperative image-displaying monitor by the surgeon. Operative Neurosurgery. 2014;10(1):46–50.
5. Okuda H, Okamoto J, Takumi Y. The iArmS robotic arm rest prolongs endoscope lens-wiping intervals in endoscopic sinus surgery. Surg Innov. 2020;27(5):515–22.
6. Goto T, Hongo K, Ogiwara T, et al. Intelligent surgeon's arm supporting system iArmS in microscopic neurosurgery utilizing robotic technology. World Neurosurg. 2018;119:e661–5.

Surgical Processing Models

Ikuma Sato

Abstract The introduction of novel technologies in the medical field has enabled the treatment of previously untreatable conditions. However, the introduction of novel technologies in the surgical field has made surgical procedures more sophisticated and specialized and, thus, more complex. Thus, the complexity of surgical procedures owing to their sophistication and specialization requires optimization and efficiency through visualization and the analysis of surgical procedures using surgical processing models (SPMs). This chapter introduces SPMs and surgical process visualization based on their application to awake surgery in gliomas.

Keywords Surgical process · Machine learning · Modeling · Awake tumor resection · Neurosurgery

1 Introduction

The introduction of novel technologies in the medical field has facilitated the treatment of previously untreatable conditions because of novel diagnostic devices, improved performance of diagnostic devices, and novel surgical devices. The information obtained from these devices is used for treatment. In the surgical field, surgeons can make a detailed preoperative plan using information from the diagnostic instruments. Preoperative planning and the use of surgical instruments have enabled minimally invasive and safe treatment. Consequently, the quality of life in patients has improved, and errors have been prevented. Overall, this advancement represents a highly positive development.

Novel technologies in the surgical field include the development of surgical devices, such as endoscopes and laser therapy, and the emergence of novel concepts

I. Sato (✉)
Faculty of System Information Science Engineering, Future University Hakodate, Hakodate, Hokkaido, Japan
e-mail: ikuma-is@fun.ac.jp

K. Masamune et al. (eds.), *Artificial Intelligence in Surgery*,
https://doi.org/10.1007/978-981-96-6635-5_4

in the operating room. Surgical instruments include endoscopes and navigation systems. Minimally invasive endoscopic surgery is performed using endoscopes to minimize the risk of wounds. Navigation systems are of two types as follows: (i) that use preoperative images and (ii) that use intraoperative images. Some systems use intraoperative images obtained by magnetic resonance imaging (MRI) or computed tomography (CT) at each stage of surgical procedures, whereas others use real-time images obtained by diagnostic equipment. Furthermore, image-guided surgery using surgical instruments and navigation is available. Laser and photodynamic therapies have also been used to treat cancers. A new operating room (OR), namely, the Smart Treatment Room, is now available. In a Smart OR, a medical device is connected to a network, and intraoperative data from these devices can be collected in a time-synchronized manner. Because intraoperative information can be obtained as digital data, artificial intelligence (AI) therapy using these data is desired.

In addition to surgical instruments, surgical robots are an emerging technology in this field. Researchers have reported on several types of surgical robots; however, endoscopic surgical robots are the most common. The master-slave types da Vinci and Hinotori are examples of endoscopic surgical robots. The slave robot has multiple arms and is equipped with a stereoscopic endoscope and forceps with multiple degrees of freedom. The master robot is a control panel. The master side is the operating table, where the surgeon observes the surgical field with a 3D viewer and influences the manipulators to perform the surgical procedure. The manipulator enables a more precise surgical procedure by using the "scaling function" and "anti-shake function." Thus, the use of a robot dramatically increases the number of degrees of freedom in difficult laparoscopic surgical procedures. In addition, it can increase the accuracy of the surgical procedure and reduce the burden on the surgeon. Furthermore, the robot has several advantages, such as enabling surgical procedures in cases that are difficult to perform with conventional surgical procedures, for example, when the area around the affected part is excessively narrow. In addition, because the surgical robot can record endoscopic images and operation logs, AI medicine is expected to use this information.

With the introduction of novel technologies in the surgical field, surgical procedures have become more sophisticated, specialized, and complex. Two key reasons contribute to this increase in surgical complexity. First, the operating room has become a complex environment owing to the introduction of advanced medical devices using technologies, such as medical engineering and ICT. Therefore, surgeons and surgical staff are required to possess knowledge of and skills in advanced treatment using these devices. Second, the growing sophistication and specialization of the field have increased the amount of required surgical knowledge, thus increasing the number of surgical procedures, methods, and techniques that surgeons must learn, memorize, and practice. In addition, owing to the increasing sophistication and complexity of surgical procedures, only the surgeon discerns the exact progress of the procedure.

Surgical procedures, which are becoming more complex owing to increasing sophistication and specialization, should be optimized and made more efficient through visualization and analysis using surgical processing models (SPMs). Several studies on SPMs have been reported in general reviews [1]. SPMs are used to construct a surgical model from intraoperative information, such as endoscopic and intraoperative video images of the surgical field. Using this model and the acquired intraoperative information, SPMs can visualize and optimize the surgical process by discriminating and analyzing it through machine learning, including deep learning. Furthermore, we reported on a surgical process identification system for awake tumor resection in neurosurgery [2]. In the following sections, we introduce our SPMs for awake tumor resection in neurosurgery and the surgical process identification system using these SPMs.

2 Introduction of a Surgical Process Identification System Using SPMs

Brain tumor resection surgery requires maximal tumor removal and minimal postoperative complications. Maximum tumor removal is ideal for brain tumors, particularly gliomas, because of a correlation between the removal rate and postoperative survival time [3]. However, aggressive removal of tumors adjacent to the eloquent area may lead to postoperative complications. For example, if brain functions, such as speech and motor areas, are adjacent to the tumor, aphasia and motor functions may be impaired because of damage to normal tissues. Therefore, while considering patient prognosis, surgeons should identify the location and size of the tumor as well as the location of brain structures and functions, which vary among patients, to maximize tumor removal and minimize postoperative complications. To this end, we have constructed an intelligent operating room (IOR) with advanced medical equipment to maximize tumor removal; we performed awake brain tumor resection to understand brain functions intraoperatively [4]. Currently, IOR has been improved into a smart OR termed a smart cyber operating theater (SCOT).

Awake brain tumor resection in the IOR and SCOT is an advanced surgical procedure that allows visualization of the brain structure, residual tumor, and functional localization of the brain in different patients during surgical procedures for maximal tumor removal and minimal postoperative complications. Intraoperative MRI after a brain shift in open MRI in these ORs enables accurate tumor localization. During tumor removal, a real-time updating navigation system visualizes the surgical position on intraoperative MRI, allowing the surgeon to confirm the tumor location and normal brain area at any time [5]. Intraoperative MRI is repeated after tumor removal to confirm the presence of a residual tumor and maximize the removal.

In addition, awake surgery, in which the patient is kept conscious by switching to local anesthesia during a surgical procedure, facilitates confirming the localization of brain functions near the speech and motor cortices in real time. Because the localization of brain functions, such as speech and motor functions, varies among patients, the primary surgeon identifies the localization by applying a small amount of electric current to the brain several times during tumor removal to determine the line for removal. Thus, awake brain tumor resection is performed with the identification of brain function interspersed during tumor removal to maximize the removal and minimize postoperative complications. Therefore, the surgical procedure involves multiple transitions and repetitions, and the primary surgeon must be aware of these processes and their flow. In addition, a skilled physician should confirm these situations and those in which the surgeon is at a loss to make a decision. Simultaneously, it is difficult for junior surgeons and surgical staff to grasp and predict surgical flow owing to multiple and repetitive surgical transitions.

Awake surgery involves numerous surgical transitions and repetitions; therefore, primary surgeons, junior surgeons, and surgical staff require assistance in understanding the flow of surgical procedures. To optimize complex surgical procedures, primary surgeons vary the order of the surgical processes and procedures on a case-by-case basis. However, the complexity of the surgical procedure poses a risk of skipping the necessary steps. In addition, postoperative review of the surgical procedure is cumbersome because it is necessary to reconfirm its course using a long video image. Therefore, the primary surgeon should have a system that allows understanding of the progress of the surgical procedure and easy analysis of it later. Therefore, although the primary surgeon can able to assist by advice of a remote location expert surgeon, a system that automatically captures the surgical process is required because it requires significant human labor.

In addition, it is difficult for young doctors and surgical staff to understand and predict the surgical flow during awake surgery. Particularly, they encounter difficulties in understanding the surgical process from craniotomy to actual tumor removal because the order of the surgical procedures and techniques varies among patients. An experienced surgical staff, such as instrumentation nurses, assesses the monitor displaying the surgical field, prepares the necessary instruments, and provides them to the primary surgeon, who generally anticipates the intraoperative situation. Thus, veteran staff members understand the intraoperative situation through video images and perform smooth surgical procedures. However, it is difficult for young and inexperienced surgeons to understand the surgical flow and predict the next procedure by viewing images of the surgical field on a monitor. However, it is not feasible for young primary surgeons and surgical staff to communicate with each other or continuously watch videos to understand the intraoperative situation. Therefore, it is necessary to develop a system that automatically captures and presents the surgical flow in real time, without requiring the work of all surgical staff, including the primary surgeon. This necessitates a surgical process identification system that automatically captures the process during and after the surgical procedure and presents information that enables the prediction of the current and subsequent surgical process for optimal and efficient surgical procedures.

Aizawa et al. developed a process analysis system using surgical navigation system logs for brain tumor resection to achieve efficient surgical planning [6].

This system automatically monitors the surgical progress and predicts the completion time based on the navigation system log and depth/shade information of the tumor segmented from intraoperative MR images. Aksamentov et al. reported on a machine learning method for predicting the end time of endoscopic surgery using endoscopic camera images. Lalys et al. reported on a process identification method for hypothalamic surgery to automatically identify surgical processes and provide tailored support [7]. This method can automatically identify six surgical processes from surgical microscopic images using a support vector machine (SVM) and the Hidden Markov Model (HMM) (machine learning) [8]. In the case of awake brain tumor resection, the surgical process involves complex transitions and repetitions of these processes; therefore, a novel method for highly accurate process identification is required.

For accurate process identification during awake surgery, surgeons should combine information from multiple medical devices. Previously, the types of surgical instruments used were extracted from medical devices for process identification. In awake surgery, the surgical process depends on the type of surgical instrument and the location of the procedure; therefore, it is necessary to extract this information. However, it is difficult to obtain information from a single medical device or system using the current equipment and environment. Particularly, while using only information from the logs of surgical navigation systems, it is difficult to identify surgical procedures using instruments that do not have position measurement markers or missing logs because of shielding the markers of surgical instruments. Particularly, because the patient's head is immobilized for cortical/white matter mapping and tumor removal, the surgeon is in the most comfortable position to perform the procedure; most information is lost from the surgical navigation system log because the surgeon shields the surgical instruments. Therefore, the information needed to identify the surgical process can be interpolated and determined by video estimation using surgical microscope images when a log is missing or upon using surgical instruments without a position measurement marker. Thus, the surgical process of awake brain tumor resection can be identified using information from multiple medical devices.

We aimed to develop a system for identifying the process of awake surgery using information from medical devices in the OR. The patient's brain structure, the location of the tumor, and the location of the procedure can be extracted using MR images and information from the surgical navigation system logs. The types of surgical instruments used in each procedure can be extracted from the surgical navigation system logs and surgical microscope images. Thus, using information from multiple medical devices, a large amount of information about the surgical procedure can be obtained. In addition, it is possible to complement individual data by obtaining similar information from the surgical microscope images as well as from the logs missing because of the shielding problem while using surgical navigation system logs.

3 SPMs for Awake Surgery Using Information from Multiple Medical Devices

Target Surgical Procedure and Information Used for Process Identification.

In this method, awake surgery is the target procedure for surgical process identification. Awake surgery is used to remove tumors in eloquent areas, such as the speech and motor cortices. It can be performed considering brain function; however, this advanced and complex surgical procedure requires techniques and judgment that depend on the knowledge and experience of the primary surgeon [9]. Therefore, awake surgery was selected as the target procedure because it is difficult to understand the surgical flow. In addition, the process depends on the tumor grade. Therefore, we selected patients with World Health Organization grade II and III tumors who underwent awake surgery [10].

To identify the surgical procedure, we obtained information from several medical devices in the OR. Using information about the patient's brain structure and on surgical instruments used by the primary surgeon during the surgical procedure (types of instruments and positions of surgical procedures) facilitates identifying the surgical process [8, 11]. Therefore, we identified the process using information about the patient's brain structure, the types of surgical instruments used by the surgeon, and their position. Thus, we used intraoperative MR images, surgical navigation system logs, and surgical microscope images from medical equipment in the OR. The reasons for this selection and the obtained information are described below.

3.1 *Intraoperative MR Images*

Intraoperative MRI is useful for obtaining information about the patient's brain structure during surgical procedures. Intraoperative MR images are the patient's brain image data after the brain shift and can therefore provide information on the intraoperative tumor location and brain structure (brain surface and normal brain regions). These two types of images differ in their representation of normal brain tissues and tumors. This method uses T1-weighted MR images, which enables determining the brain structure.

3.2 *Surgical Navigation System Log*

The surgical navigation system log is useful for obtaining information about the surgical procedure. It provides information on the types of surgical instruments used by the surgeon (bipolar, electrical stimulation probe) and 3D position information (surgical instrument tip position). Furthermore, the combination of this log with intraoperative MR images allows for accurate and real-time acquisition of the surgical site, which serves as a process identification element during surgical procedures. Therefore, the type of surgical instrument used by the primary surgeon and the location of the procedure can be determined from the surgical navigation system log.

3.3 Surgical Microscope Images

Surgical microscope images are useful for determining the type of surgical instrument used by the primary surgeon. Images from the surgical microscope are equivalent to the surgical field of the primary surgeon and demonstrate surgical instruments that cannot be identified from the surgical navigation system log. Therefore, it is possible to obtain the types of surgical instruments used in operating microscope images. In this method, we use surgical microscope images to detect three surgical instruments primarily handled by the lead surgeon: bipolar forceps, an electrostimulation probe, and scissors. Furthermore, the bipolar and the electrostimulation probe are acquired surgical instrument information by surgical microscope images when the type of instruments cannot be obtained from the surgical navigation system log owing to the shielding problem.

3.4 Construction of SPMs for Awake Surgery

We constructed a surgical process model that enabled junior doctors and surgical staff to understand the current process and predict the subsequent process during surgical procedures, other skilled doctors to assess the surgical status during surgical procedures, and the primary surgeon to efficiently review the procedures later. Each surgeon optimizes different surgical processes; therefore, the order of the processes often changes depending on the patient's condition and other factors, which complicate the transition points of the process. Therefore, it is necessary to visualize the complicated surgical process logically and present it to young doctors, surgical staff, and primary surgeons during and after surgical procedures. This model was designed to identify the surgical process every second.

The scope of the surgical process model encompasses the process followed by the primary surgeon, beginning from the preoperative procedure after MRI, which is a complicated procedure in awake surgery, to the time before repeating MRI after tumor removal. Therefore, the constructed model is a part of the process performed by a skilled surgeon and excludes craniotomy. We excluded craniotomy because it was considered less necessary to support the understanding of the process. This is because it is a typical surgical procedure and the process transitions have few branches.

Surgical process modeling can be divided into the top-down approach and the bottom-up approach. The top-down approach models the surgical process based on knowledge and experience, whereas the bottom-up approach models the surgical process based on recorded data. This recorded data identification method identifies surgical processes based on information from multiple medical devices. Therefore, we adopted a bottom-up approach using actual surgical record data. In conventional research methods using the bottom-up approach, surgical process models are constructed on the basis of interviews with surgeons, information about the types of surgical instruments used from video recordings during surgical procedures, and data from manual records of instrument exchanges [12–14]. Here, we constructed a surgical process model using intraoperative MR images, surgical navigation system logs, and surgical microscope images that could be obtained intraoperatively.

We defined the process as an element of the model and eventually constructed the model. The surgical process is defined together with the clinician using clinical data (preoperative and intraoperative MRI images, surgical navigation system logs, and surgical microscope images) that have been acquired in the past for grades II and III. First, the surgical process was defined by the following elements: "which" surgical instruments were used by the surgeon, "what" part of the surgical process occurred, and "when" did the process occur. Next, we obtained specific information on the surgical procedure elements. Using clinical data, we manually recorded the type of surgical tool used during the procedure (bipolar, electrostimulation probe, scissors) and its position (on the brain surface, inside the tumor, in normal tissue, or the surgical field) every second along the time axis. The recording involved loading intraoperative MR images and surgical navigation system logs into a 3D Slicer, which determined the surgical position from the position of the surgical instrument tip on the intraoperative MR image. Simultaneously, the type of surgical instrument (bipolar, electrostimulation probe, or scissors) was visually confirmed and recorded from the surgical microscope images. Finally, based on the recorded information, the surgeon and clinician defined the surgical process from the time of the MRI to the end of tumor removal. Table 1 summarizes the surgical process defined by the primary surgeon and clinician.

The surgical process model was based on a defined surgical process, and a hierarchical state transition model was constructed by considering the goal of the process transition from a clinical perspective. In conventional research, the transition of a surgical process is often a left-to-right type of model that moves in a constant direction without looping, which is unsuitable for cases where the surgical process has multiple transition destinations, such as awake surgery. Therefore, we modeled the surgical process in a hierarchical structure to abstract multiple processes as a single process and simplify its transition. The first level

Table 1 Definition of surgical processes for awake surgery

1st Layer	2nd Layer	3rd Layer
***P^1*: Pre-tumor removal process**	P_1^1 : Preparation	P_{11}^1 : Device setting
		P_{12}^1 : Verification of the tip position of the surgical instruments
	P_2^1 : Cortical mapping and pathology diagnosis	P_{21}^1 : Examined on the cortex by electric stimulation probe
		P_{22}^1 : Dealing with convulsive wave and marking of brain functional position during cortical mapping
		P_{23}^1 : Coagulation of cortex
		P_{24}^1 : Meninges incision and sampling lesion of glioma
***P^2*: Tumor removal process**	P_1^2 : Tumor approach	P_{11}^2 : Venous and sulcus detachment
		P_{12}^2 : Incision of cortex and clipping of arterial
		P_{13}^2 : White matter incision, suction tumor and removal tumor
	P_2^2 : White mapping and pathology diagnosis	P_{21}^2 : White mapping to the cavity of resection
		P_{22}^2 : Dealing with convulsive wave and marking of brain functional position during white mapping
		P_{23}^2 : Sampling lesion to the cavity of resection
***P^{Id}*: Idling**		

of the surgical process model was divided into two classes, namely, procedures performed before tumor resection or tumor resection. The second level consisted of four classes of intraoperative procedures (preoperative preparation, intraoperative rapid diagnosis, tumor removal, and brain function tests during removal). These four classes were constructed at one level of the first hierarchy. At the third level, 12 processes were constructed under one of the four classes. Specifically, "arachnoid incision and pathological section collection," one of the surgical processes, is a part of "intraoperative rapid diagnosis" performed "before tumor removal." Finally, the possible transitions between each class and each of the 12 processes were associated based on manually recorded information to determine the destination of the transition. Thus, we constructed a surgical process model consisting of 12 processes in three layers (Fig. 1).

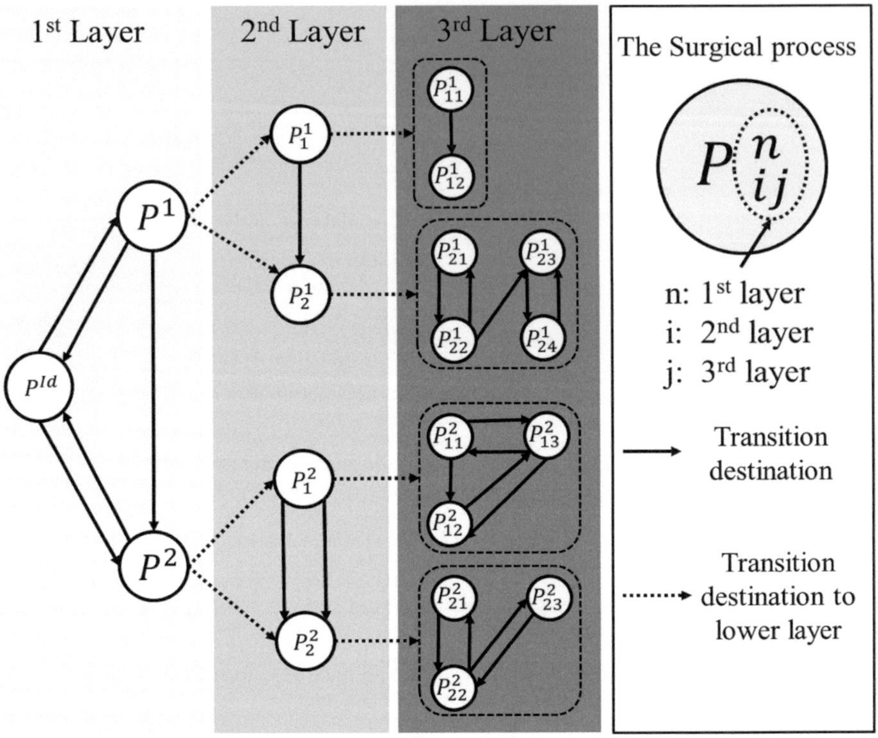

Fig. 1 Construction of SPMs for awake surgery

4 Surgical Process Identification System for Awake Surgery

The surgical process identification system consists of a personal computer, which receives information from multiple medical devices and automatically identifies the surgical process during and after surgical procedures, and a monitor, which displays the identification results to the primary surgeon, residents, and surgical staff (Fig. 2). The system was connected to each medical device, and each piece of information was sent via the internal network of the OR. The system performed multithreaded processing to calculate the process identification results. The user interface (UI) design allowed the user to assess the surgical process identification results during and after surgical procedures (Fig. 3). Intraoperatively, the system displayed the identification results based on the input information obtained from the surgical navigation system and surgical microscope images. In the postoperative stage, an intuitive UI was designed by displaying the surgical flow as a graph based on information similar to that in the intraoperative stage. In addition, the surgical process can be identified by switching the UI during surgical procedures, and the process and videos can be viewed in a way similar to the postoperative function.

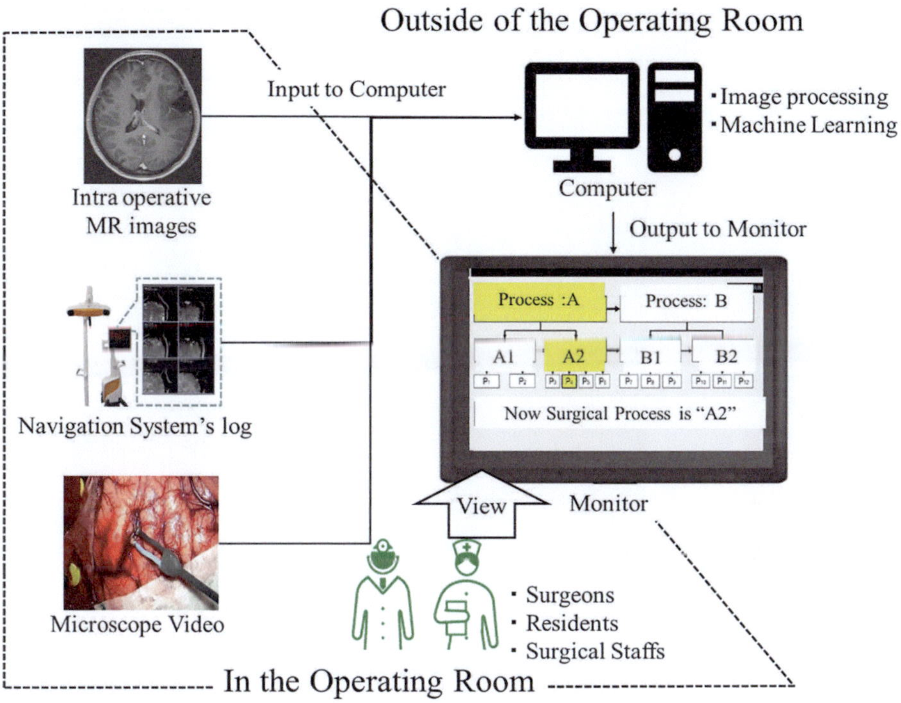

Fig. 2 Overview of the surgical process identification system

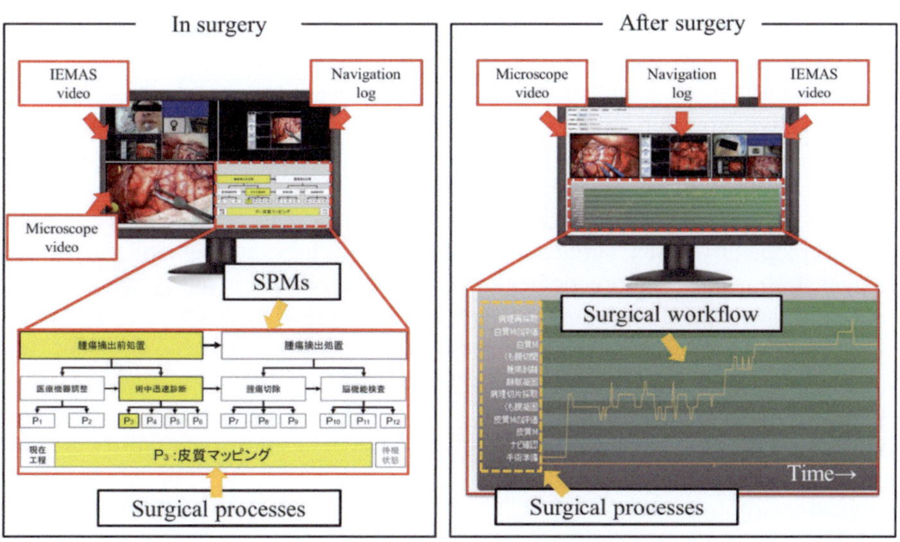

Fig. 3 User interface of the surgical process identification system

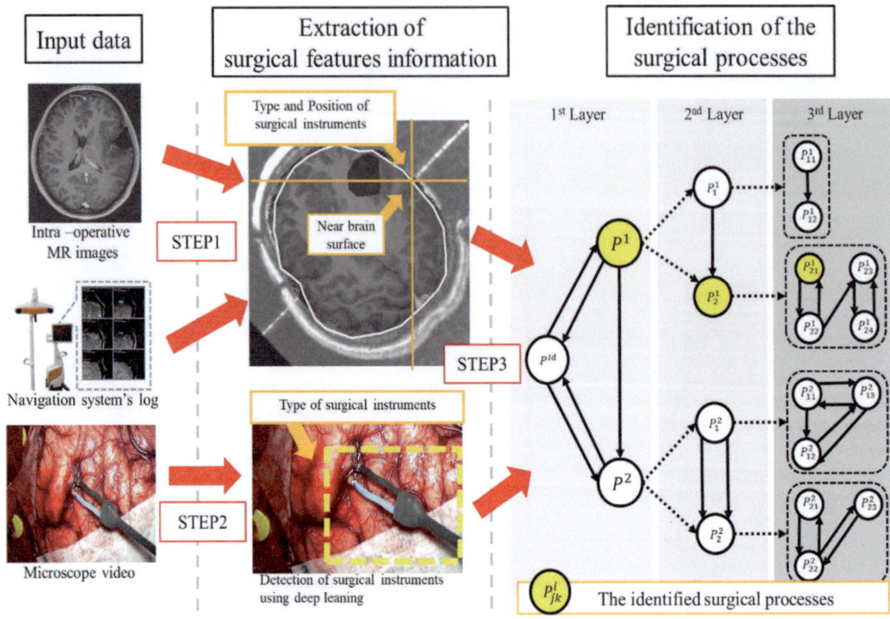

Fig. 4 Surgical process identification using surgical processing models

The surgical process was identified using information processing techniques, including machine learning, based on multiple pieces of medical information. We used three types of information, namely, intraoperative MRI, surgical navigation systems, and microscope images. Elements of the surgical process were extracted and identified from these sources. Two elements of the surgical process were obtained through image processing and deep learning as follows: the location of the intraoperative procedure performed by the primary surgeon and the type of surgical instruments to be used. Surgical process identification was performed using machine learning based on the surgical process model.

Here, we describe the data acquisition before launching the system. The system used intraoperative MRI, surgical navigation system logs, and surgical microscope images. Immediately before the beginning of tumor resection, the system was connected to the surgical navigation system and the surgical microscope to enable the acquisition of intraoperative MR images, log data from each medical device, and video information. Intraoperative MR images were imported into the system using a surgical navigation system.

Here, we describe the identification process flow and time synchronization of the system (Fig. 4). The process consists of three steps: step 1, determining the type of surgical instruments and the location of intraoperative procedures using intraoperative MRI and surgical navigation system logs; step 2, determining the type of surgical instruments using surgical microscope images; step 3, identifying the surgical process using the obtained information. During tumor removal, the data were

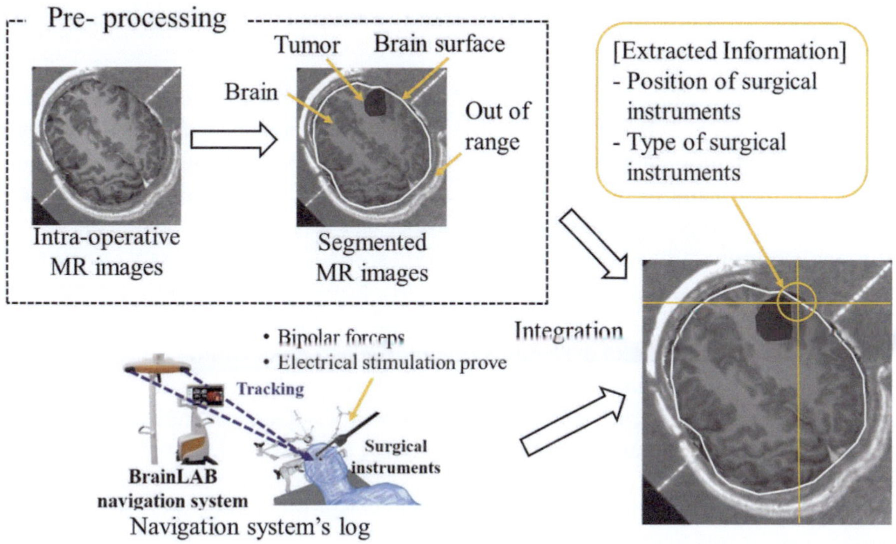

Fig. 5 Extracted information: position and types of surgical instruments using intraoperative magnetic resonance imaging and the navigation system's log

stacked in the system upon obtaining information from the surgical navigation system log and operating microscope. The identification process was performed every second, and steps 1 and 2 were processed in a multi-threaded method using the initially stacked data. If a log was missing, the data were stacked 1 s before the missing log was used. Step 3 was not processed until both steps 1 and 2 were completed, and the results were displayed on the monitor after processing.

Step 1: Determining the type of surgical instruments and the location of intraoperative procedures using intraoperative MRI and surgical navigation system logs.

In step 1, the types of surgical instruments used by the primary surgeon and the location of this procedure were captured by image processing. The types of surgical instruments consisted of bipolar and electrical stimulation probes. The four definitions of the treatment points were "brain surface," "inside the tumor," "near normal brain tissue," and "open surgical field." Prior to acquisition, the brain regions were segmented from the intraoperative MR images and labeled to clarify the regions. Using the labeled data and logs from the surgical navigation system, we determined the types of surgical instruments and the location of the procedure at each time point based on 3D image processing (Fig. 5). First, we determined the log of the coordinates of the surgical instrument tip from the surgical navigation system. Subsequently, we identified the location of the surgical tool by searching for the label value of the tool tip coordinates on the segmented image of the brain region during surgical procedures. If the log of the tool pointed outside the brain region, it was assumed to be in the surgical field; if the log was absent, it was recorded as a missing log.

Step 2: Determining the type of surgical instruments using surgical microscope images.

In step 2, we determined the types of surgical instruments used by the primary surgeon through deep learning. This step served as an interpolation in case of missing log information of the surgical navigation system or upon using a surgical instrument not listed in the log information. Therefore, we acquired three surgical instruments (bipolar, electrostimulation probe, and scissors) primarily used by the surgeon's dominant hand. To identify the types of surgical instruments to be used from the video information, we used You Only Look Ones (YOLO), a supervised deep learning method that is highly accurate and fast in object detection [15]. Upon obtaining an image, YOLO determined the region and object name if the previously learned object is reflected in the image. Therefore, the system used a pre-created training dataset to generate a YOLO neural network capable of detecting the three surgical instruments. During surgical procedures, the system captured images from the surgical microscope at each frame and used YOLO to detect the types of surgical instruments (Fig. 6). If the YOLO neural network determined that no surgical instruments were visible in the image, we assumed that there were no surgical instruments in the image.

Step 3: Identifying the surgical process using the obtained information.

Surgical process identification was based on a surgical process model using machine learning. It estimated the current process from time series data, and machine learning methods, such as SVM, Bayesian inference, long short-term memory (LSTM), and HMM, were used for this purpose. In this method, HMM, which could compute the results rapidly, was used to consider both process identification based on time series transition and real-time performance. Nakamura et al. reported on a Bayesian method for identifying the extraction process using information from a surgical navigation system log for brain tumor resection [6]. The Bayesian method is characterized by features independent at each time and unaffected by the past time series. However, in awake surgery, the feature values of each period are events determined by the past surgical process. Therefore, identification without using time series-related features, such as an SVM or Bayesian estimation, is not optimal. In addition, Panzner et al. reported that LSTM can compute highly accurate results owing to training data and cost, whereas HMM is useful for fast results [16]. Therefore, we improved the machine learning method reported in a previous study and used an HMM capable of Markovianity estimation.

In this method, we used the Hierarchical Hidden Markov Model (HHMM), which is an HMM method adapted to hierarchical models that possess Markovian properties and consider real-time performance. First, the information obtained in steps 1 and 2 was integrated into a single feature, and the values were stored as time series feature data for each second. Subsequently, we identified the surgical process with the HHMM using time series feature data as input information. The identification process was performed sequentially, beginning from the first level defined in the surgical process model and ending at the third level. We used the Viterbi

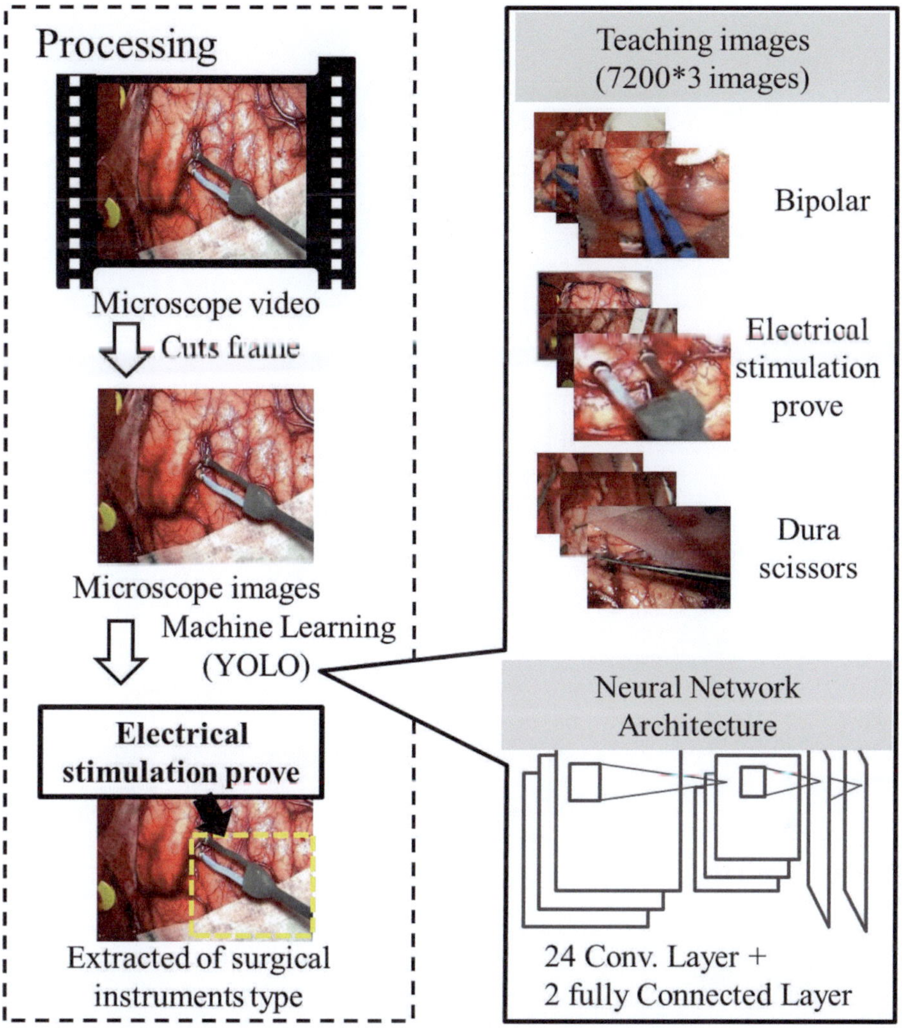

Fig. 6 Extracted information: types of surgical instruments using microscope video

algorithm to reduce the computational complexity and calculated the surgical process with the highest probability as the result.

4.1 Results of Surgical Process Identification

In the hierarchical surgical process model constructed using this method and the developed system, the identification results using clinical data from three cases were 96.3 ± 0.47%, 95.4 ± 0.73%, and 92.2 ± 1.62% for the first, second, and third

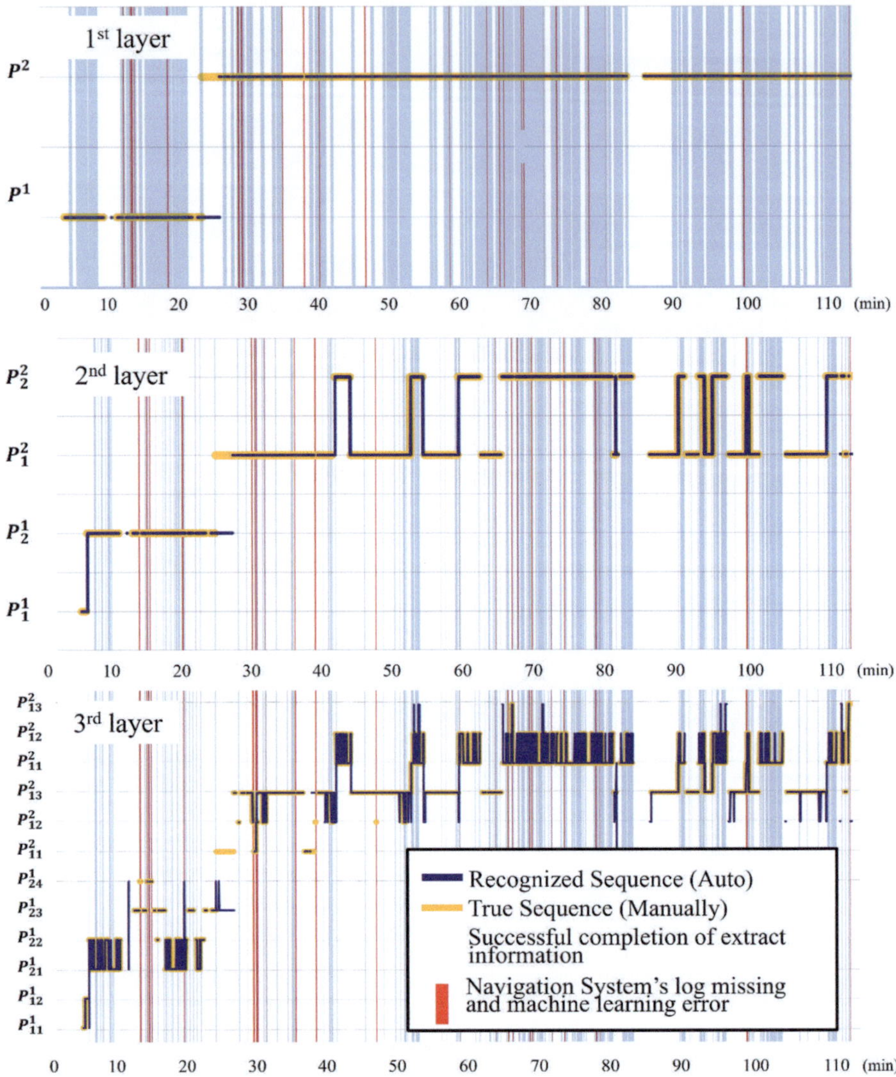

Fig. 7 Results of surgical process identification

levels, respectively. Figure 7 depicts the results for one case. This method possibly facilitates an understanding of the surgical process by using existing medical equipment. However, errors in identifying the surgical instruments from the surgical microscope images contributed to the low identification accuracy. Therefore, it is necessary to reconsider image processing and learning methods in the machine learning process.

5 Conclusion

In this chapter, we describe the background of SPMs and introduced our surgical process identification method using SPMs and a machine learning-based surgical process identification system with multiple pieces of information. The method achieved >90% accuracy in surgical process identification using a 12-procedure surgical process model based on three cases. Our results demonstrated the possibility of facilitating an understanding of the surgical process using the existing medical equipment. In addition, surgeons could easily recognize the surgical process by logically visualizing the surgical flow after surgical procedures. However, the accuracy of the machine learning system decreased owing to errors in the detection of surgical instruments, and it is necessary to reexamine the image processing and learning methods in the machine learning process. In the future, we intend to improve the accuracy of surgical process identification by refining accuracy of surgical process identification and developing a surgical process analysis system to evaluate the process and technique for actual clinical use. Furthermore, we aim to visualize the knowledge of expert surgeons by improving this method to identify detailed surgical processes and analyze numerous surgical cases.

Acknowledgments These research results were obtained from the commissioned research by the National Institute of Information and Communications Technology (NICT) and JSPS Grant-in-Aid for Scientific Research (grant number B-22H03443), Japan.

References

1. Neumuth T. Surgical process modeling. Innov Surg Sci. 2017;2(3):123–37.
2. Nagai T, Sato I, Fujino Y, Horise Y, Kusuda K, Tamura M, Muragaki Y, Masamune K. Surgical process identification system in awake surgery for glioma. J Japan Soc Comput Aid Surg. 2020;22(2):87–101.
3. Nitta M, Muragaki Y, Maruyama T, Ikuta S, Komori T, Maebayashi K, Iseki H, Tamura M, Saito T, Okamoto S, Chernov M, Hayashi M, Okada Y. Proposed therapeutic strategy for adult low-grade glioma based on aggressive tumor resection. Neurosurg Focus. 2015;38(1):E7–E10.
4. Iseki H, Nakamura R, Muragaki Y, Suzuki T, Chernov M, Hori T, Takakura K. Advanced computer-aided intraoperative technologies for information-guided surgical management of gliomas: Tokyo women's medical university experience. Minim Invasive Neurosurg. 2008;51(5):285–91.
5. Hong J, Muragaki Y, Nakamura R, Hashizume M, Iseki H. A neurosurgical navigation system based on intraoperative tumour remnant estimation. J Robot Surg. 2007;1(1):91–7.
6. Nakamura R, Aizawa T, Muragaki Y, Maruyama T, Iseki H. Automatic surgical workflow estimation method for brain tumor resection using surgical navigation information. J Robot Mechatron. 2012;24(5):791–801.
7. Aksamentov I, Twinanda AP, Mutter D, Marescaux J, Padoy N. Deep neural networks predict remaining surgery duration from cholecystectomy videos. Medical Image Computing and Computer-Assisted Intervention—MICCAI. 2017;2017(10434):586–93.

8. Lalys F, Riffaud L, Morandi X, Jannin P. Surgical phases detection from microscope videos by combining SVM and HMM. Medical Computer Vision. Recognition Techniques and Applications in Medical Imaging—MCV. 2010;6533:54–62.
9. Takamasa K. The guidelines for awake craniotomy guidelines committee of the Japan awake surgery conference. Neurol Med Chir. 2012;52(3):119–41.
10. Louis DN, Perry A, Reifenberger G, Deimling A, Figarella-Branger D, Cavenee WK, Ohgaki H, Wiestler OD, Kleihues P, Ellison DW. The 2016 World Health Organization classification of tumors of the central nervous system: a summary. Acta Neuropathol. 2016;131(6):803–20.
11. Jakob EB, Afsaneh D, Rune MJ, Poul ML, Kristian LGN, Søren T. Phase recognition during surgical procedures using embedded and body-worn sensors. 2011 IEEE International Conference on Pervasive Computing and Communications. 2011;1:45–53.
12. Jannin P, Morandi X. Surgical models for computer-assisted neurosurgery. NeuroImage. 2007;37(3):783–91.
13. Neumuth T, Strauß G, Meixensberger J, Lemke HU, Burgert O. Acquisition of process descriptions from surgical interventions. International Conference on Database and Expert Systems Applications. 2006;4080:602–11.
14. Padoy N, Blum T, Ahmadi SA, Feussner H, Berger MO, Navab N. Statistical modeling and recognition of surgical workflow. Med Image Anal. 2012;16(3):632–41.
15. Redmon J, Divvala SK, Girshick RB, Farhadi A. You only look once: unified, real-time object detection. CoRR. 2015:1–10.
16. Panzner M, Cimiano P. Comparing hidden Markov models and long short term memory neural networks for learning action representations. Intl Workshop Mach Learn Optimizat Big Data. 2016;10122:99–105.

Semantic Data Modeling

Hideo Suzuki

Abstract To perform surgery, sufficient knowledge and experience based on clinical information are required. Also, AI-aided surgery that is expected to become widely practiced in the near future requires vast amounts of high-quality training data to continually improve accuracy. A database that stores clinical data using a real-world model is needed to meet these requirements. This chapter explains the semantic data model (SDM), an extension of semantic data modeling, which is a method for translating real-world data into a relational database. The SDM extracts clinical data from different database models in hospital information systems, transforms them into the SDM's logical schema, and loads them into the SDM database. The features of the SDM, especially its logical schema, are described. The SDM will be a component of the information infrastructure for AI-aided surgery.

Keywords Semantic data modeling · Relational database · Clinical information · Hospital information systems · Entity-relationship diagram · SDM · EMR

1 Introduction

Databases are among the most important information infrastructure components in all application systems. Hospital information systems (HISs) are application systems, and clinical information generated by medical practice is encoded into clinical data and stored in databases. By decoding this data with the same application, it can be reproduced as clinical information. Each hospital information system consists of many applications such as electronic medical records (EMRs), order entry, and department systems. Each application uses a local area network (LAN) to exchange clinical information by messaging. One of the standards for this communication is Health Level Seven (HL7) [1]. In addition to HL7, Fast Healthcare

H. Suzuki (✉)
CEO of MoDeL Inc, Yokohama, Japan
e-mail: hszk@model-jp.com

K. Masamune et al. (eds.), *Artificial Intelligence in Surgery*,
https://doi.org/10.1007/978-981-96-6635-5_5

Interoperability Resource (FHIR) uses the application program interface (API) method to get clinical data from EMR applications. In radiology, applications such as Picture Archiving and Communication Systems (PACS) and the Digital Imaging And Communications In Medicine (DICOM) standards are well-known [2]. Medical Waveform Format Encoding Rules (MFER) is a standard format. For waveforms of electrocardiogram (ECG), electroencephalograph (EEG), etc. However these standards are not provided for data archiving but message exchanges. Therefore, HIS application providers must define different database systems and different data models.

For example, in the case of surgery, many procedures are performed under time pressure; therefore, a surgery team needs copious clinical information quickly to make a judgment. Generally, the approach is to collect and prepare the necessary clinical information before surgery. However, if the unexpected occurs during surgery, sometimes the optimal treatment cannot be performed because the prepared clinical information is inadequate. Therefore, it is critical to prepare a database previously that can decode, search, and visualize all clinical data in real time. To solve this problem, the clinical data stored in separate databases by each application are combined into one database as a unified data model and should be saved for use in all searches. That makes medical professionals to search for the necessary information and rapidly perform visualizations to facilitate diagnoses.

Currently, many HISs use relational databases (RDBs) for which there are many products of database management systems (DBMSs). It is, therefore, possible to integrate the clinical data stored for each application into the same RDB. In particular, PostgreSQL, which is an open-source RDB, is suitable as a migration destination because there are many examples of migration from other RDBs. However, in a relational database model, anyone can design a logical scheme in an original manner by using table name, entity name, and entity-relationship, of design elements. For example, even if the entity has the same meaning, the entity-name can be defined by different notations, such as PATIENT_ID, PT_ID, and ITEM1. Even in the same HIS, entity-name can be defined by different notations in different tables, for example, PATIENT_ID is defined in one table and PT_ID is used in another table. That is, different names may have the same meaning, or the same name may have different meanings. No conversion from clinical data to clinical information can be done without the definition document such as "both PATIENT_ID and PT_ID are defined as the unique patient identification." This definition of a logical scheme is called a data model, and it differs for each HIS, even if it is integrated into one RDB. The required information cannot be found without each definition of the logical scheme. The data lake function can store many different logical schemes in one archive; the data warehouse (DWH) function can convert all data to the same logical scheme for one archive.

Semantic data modeling is one of the modeling for RDBs that unifies different logical schemes. Using the method, real-world data is converted to a logical scheme via a conceptual scheme. Integrating the data of different applications into one logical scheme easily converts data to information that all users can search for and visualize quickly. The SDM further extends this semantic data modeling can build

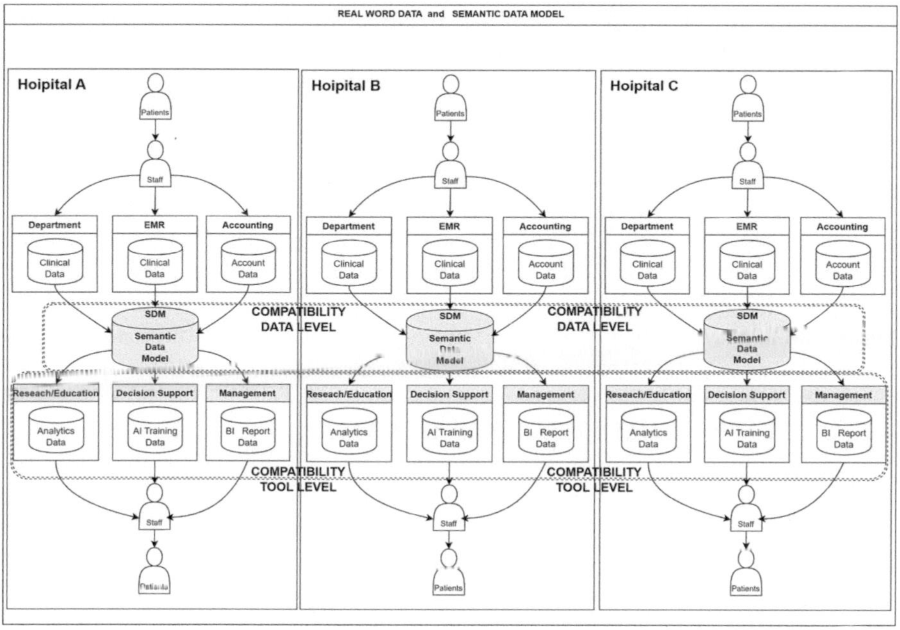

Fig. 1 Compatibility model using an SDM that shares a common data model

DWH, which was developed as a common data model by MoDeL, Inc., in 2014 and is managed by the SDM Consortium (General Incorporated Association, Japan).

Currently, hospitals at medical universities that use the SDM have migrated clinical data that has been stored for more than 10 years to the SDM. Using business intelligence (BI) software connected to the SDM through the open database connectivity (ODBC) protocol, big data analysis is being done. Migrating clinical data to a unified data model reduces the cost of developing unique extraction transformation load (ETL) software for different data models and reduces the migration cost when the HIS provider changes. Other advantages of a unified data model include wide-area data collection, shared analytical methods, and improved AI accuracy using the same data format between training and input data (Fig. 1) [3].

2 The SDM Overview

2.1 Entity-Relationship Model and Semantic Data Model

In relational databases parlance, entity-relationship modeling means establishing a relationship between two tables by entities. Using the common entity of each table as the mutual external key, two tables can be joined. The relationship also has cardinality between the two tables. In the case of table-A and table-B containing the same entity, cardinality represents the relationship of table-B seen from table-A and the relationship of table-A seen from table-B. For example, for a common entity, Table-A:Table-B is expressed as 1:N when there are multiple records in table-B for the record of table-A. The cardinality has variations such as 1:1, 1:N, N:1, and N:N. This relationship is used to join table-A and table-B with a cardinality. By joining these tables, it is possible to treat any entity of table-A and any entity of table-B as if they are the entities of the same table. For example, a clinical database has two tables, which are PATIENT and LABORATORY. The PATIENT table has PATIENT_ID and BIRTHDATE as entities, and the LABORATORY table has PATIENT_ID and VALUE as entities. In this case, "PATIENT_ID" is a common entity, and it becomes the mutual external key. In the PATIENT table, PATIENT_ID is the primary key; therefore, each patient has only one record in the table. For the LABORATORY table, each patient may have no or plural data entered as VALUE, so the cardinality of PATIENT:LABORATORY is 1(mandatory):N(optional). In this cardinality, optional indicates including a case of no record in the table, and mandatory indicates at least one record in the table. For example, the cardinality of PATIENT:VISIT_HISTORY shows 1(mandatory):N(mandatory). This is because the PATIENT table has no records for patients who have never visited the hospital.

Semantic data modeling applies the common sense of the industry such as terminology, work-flow, literacy, etc. to design a logical schema. In the clinical world, if a logical schema is designed using medical terminology, clinical process flow, and clinical literacy, then clinical professionals can convert clinical data to clinical information without needing a database definition document. The SDM employs the semantic data model to design the tables' and entities' names. The SDM is a common data model developed by referring to the semantic data modeling methodology. Its features are described below.

2.2 Common Entities in the SDM

In each table, SDM defines universal elements as common entities that can be understood by non-clinical professionals. These are elements that represent actions and are entities related to the When, Who, Where, What, and How order of presentation. In the general EMR, entity names in a table are defined as required, e.g., ORDER_DATE, DOCTOR_ID, and DEPARTMENT_CODE. In other tables, different entity names are set, e.g., RECORD_DATE, NURSE_ID, WARD_CODE, etc. In this case, these two tables, finding no common entity name, cannot be joined. In the SDM, common entities are defined in each table, such as KEY_DATE, AUTHOR, PERSONAL_ID, DEPARTMENT/SECTION, ACTION_TYPE, etc. Since a universal and common entity name that does not depend on the type of business or occupation is defined in each table, table joining is possible by using a common entity. Also, regarding AUTHOR, since AUTHOR_TYPE and AUTHOR_OCCUPATION are defined to specify a role, the AUTHOR entity can use "doctor" or any other professional title. It is designed for the same entity name

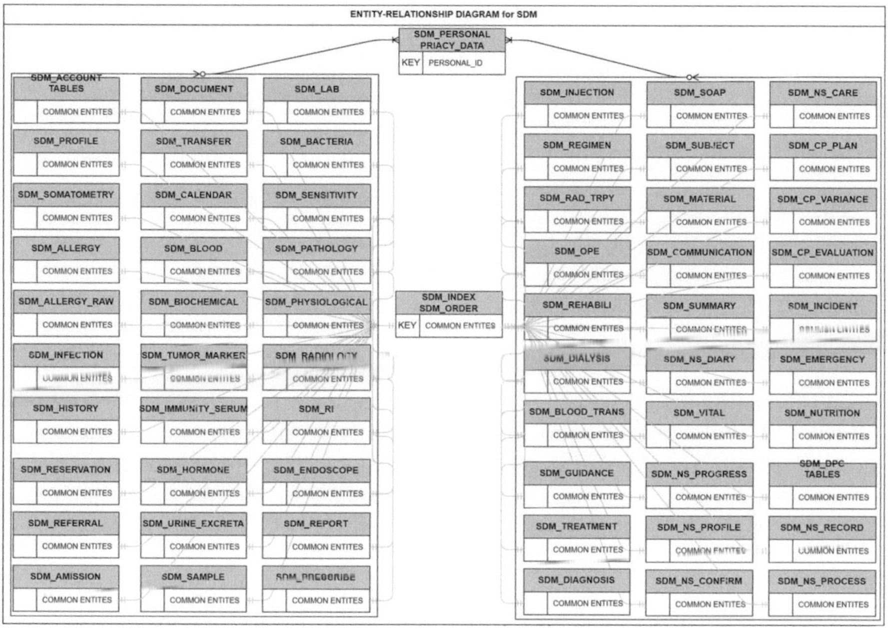

Fig. 2 The ER (entity-relationship) diagram for the SDM, with universal entities

to accommodate the differences in roles and occupations, and by using these common entities, table joins can be effected for all table combinations (Fig. 2) [4].

2.3 Primary Key

Since the primary key of the SDM table is RECORD_ID, which is based on the primary keys of the extraction source main table, a user can search for and confirm the record in the extraction source table. When the data of the extraction source is updated or deleted, it can be compared with the data of the extraction source, and then the SDM data can be updated. By this method, consistency is maintained with the data in the extraction source to establish whether the data of the extraction source has been subject to tampering.

2.4 Data Types

The SDM defines several rules for data types in the logical schema used for the relational database. For the numeric types, INT and REAL are recommended for integral number and real number, respectively. The units of each item should be consistent. For example, the unit of body weight uses Kg even for a newborn. The character types that follow allow for high-speed searching.

- Keys such as ID use CHAR (n) type: Fixed length with blank padding.
- Fixed phrases such as options use VARCHAR (n) type: Variable length with limit.
- Free text such as comments uses TEXT type: Variable unlimited length.

The default value is an empty string ""without using NULL. If NULL is used, the database index will be invalid because there are SQL restrictions since the slow processing speed "IS NULL" or "IS NOT NULL" syntax must be used to determine whether it is a NULL or an empty string. The default of an unassigned entity is N/A (not applicable) to distinguish it from a missing value.

When recording the date and time, if date and time are set to different entities, when calculating the difference between two times, one must always convert to the TIMESTAMP type before calculating. Therefore, regardless of whether the time is recorded or not, it is recorded as a TIMESTAMP type. The date type allows a NULL value, but it will be slow search if there is no data or NULL, so the default is "9999/12/31 23:59:59" for a specific date and time.

2.5 *Normalization*

In the relational database model, normalizing the tables eliminates data duplication. In the EMR, the disease name is often selected on each medical intervention. In that case, the disease name code instead of the disease name is only recorded in the disease history table with a developed date instead of in each EMR table. And the disease master table is created separately and includes the disease name and the attribute information associated with the disease name code. If the disease name or the attribute information are searched on each EMR table, the disease history table will simultaneously be joined to each table and the disease master table. This normalization contributes to saving the amount of data, but multiple tables must always be joined, and then it causes the searching response to slow down. Because SDM uses a denormalization method that includes the code and its conversion results simultaneously, table joins are minimally required, and it achieves high-speed search. The advantage of the method is that it is not affected by master-generation management issues. For example, if a temporary code is assigned to a new disease, the code in the disease master table will be changed when a formal code is assigned. If a record in the disease history table that includes the temporary code would be searched, the disease name would not be found. Also, if the name is changed with the same code, the new name is extracted when searching the medical records. The SDM records both the code and the name simultaneously; thus searching by name can find both past and present records. In addition, the past master table can be reproduced.

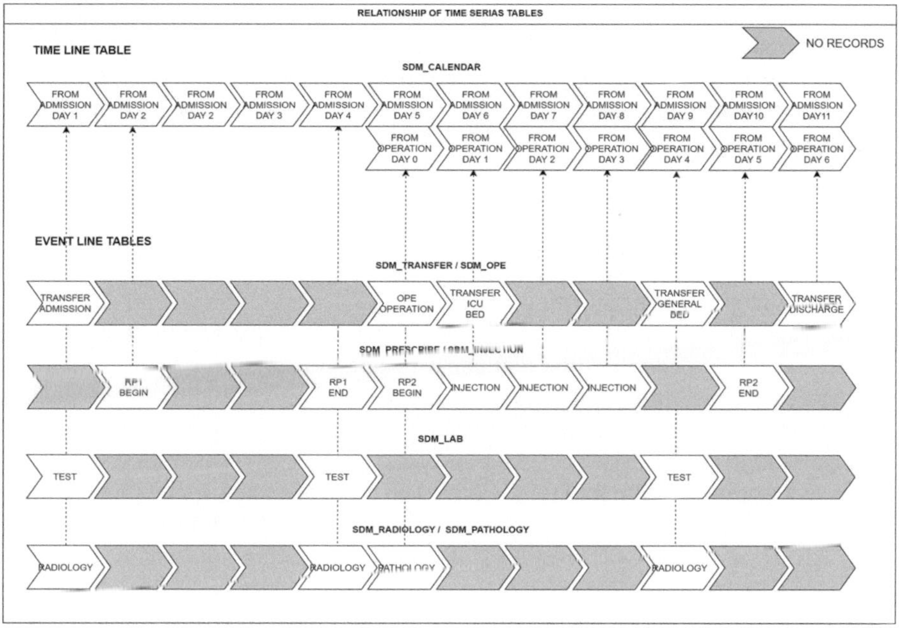

Fig. 3 The calendar-based table of the SDM is useful for comparing entities in transaction tables

2.6 *Time-Series Data*

Almost all HIS databases have separate tables for each of the medical activities. These are recorded in every table along with the date when the clinical actions occurred. Each entity is displayed as time-series data in the same table. However, different tables cannot be joined because the data of the same day may not exist. In the SDM, the calendar table is defined, includes the relative number of days from the date of hospitalization, surgery, etc. and the bed address, as entities, and each data is recorded everyday. By joining each table to the calendar table, entities in different tables can be displayed on a single chart. It is then possible to know the effect of the medication by comparing the date of the medication with the test results thereafter (Fig. 3).

2.7 *Latest Record*

Searching a relational database for the latest record among a significant number of records slows the response time. In the SDM tables, EXPIRE_TIMESTAMP of the common entities allows you to search for the latest record with a specific date 9999/12/31 and time 23:59:59. When a newer record is registered,

EXPIRE_TIMESTAMP of the current record is changed to the registration date and time of the new record, and EXPIRE_TIMESTAMP of the new record is set to the specific date 9999/12/31 and time 23:59:59. By repeating this process, the history of the latest record can be retained. Also, the latest record and the previous record can be searched quickly.

2.8 Duration and Time

In the case of clinical data, the TIMESTAMP type (yyyy/mm/dd hh:mm:ss) is often used to record the time that can be searched. However, every action has its start time, end time, and duration. In consultation cases, the SDM defined the reserved date and time as RESERVED_DATE, the reception date and time as RECEPTED_TIME, the start date and time as OPERATON_BEGIN, and the end date and time as OPERATION_END. The SDM also defines the waiting time against the reserved time as LATENCY_AFTER_RESERVATION is calculated by "OPERATION_BEGIN—RESERVED_DATE," the waiting time against reception as LATENCY_AFTER_RECEPTION is calculated by "OPERATION_BEGIN—RECEPTED_TIME," and consultation time as OPERATION_TIME is calculated by "OPERATION_END—OPERATION_BEGIN." That is, the action has a duration other than time. The TIME type can only be stored until 23:59:59, so the data type must be integral number or real number in the case of over 24 hours. Since the SDM includes BEGIN_TIMESTAMP, END_TIMESTAMP, and DURATION in common entities, extracting each table using the AUTHOR filter helps optimize the operational flow, working volume, traffic line, etc. It can also be used for skill management. If a patient is the search filter, it can also be used for reducing the waiting delay and queueing time. In surgical cases, accurately predicting surgery times would increase the availability of the operating theatre.

2.9 Hierarchy

Each SDM table has a three-layer key. RECORD_ID represents a unique key in the table, and GROUP_ID contains multiple RECORD_IDs, and TRANSACTION_ID defines the included multiple GROUP_ID. These three-layer keys are useful for filtering. For example, in the medication table, there are three levels: drug, recipe, and order. Order contains multiple recipes and recipe contains multiple drugs. If you want to search by order unit, you can use TRANSACTION_ID. If you want to process by recipe unit, search by GROUP_ID, and if you want to extract by drug unit, you can just use RECORD_ID as it is. In the case of radiology, according to the DICOM standard, ACQUISITION, SERIES, and STUDY form three layers; they can be easily aggregated. In other common entities, there are also three layers, RECORDER, AUTHOR, and AUTHORIZER. For example, a resident doctor as the AUTHOR asks a medical clerk as the RECORDER to input the medical record, and an medical instructor as the AUTHORIZER signs the medical record for the resident doctor as the AUTHOR. In this case, three layers are required.

2.10 Key Date and Query Date

In the SDM, the most important date and time in each table are defined as KEY_DATE. For example, in the case of laboratory tests, the most important date is the sampling date. This is because the patient's condition at the time of the test is reflected in the result. In this case, KEY_DATE is the same as SAMPLING_DATE of the table's unique entities. Thereby, the common entity, selected from among the table's unique entities, is recorded in duplicate. Conversely, QUERY_DATE in the common entities does not necessarily have to be the same as KEY_DATE. For example, in the reservation table, the reservation date is KEY_DATE, but there are cases where the reservation is canceled or executed without a reservation. Therefore, the performing date should be recorded as the QUERY_DATE of the reservation table. Since KEY_DATE contains both date and time and QUERY_DATE just the date, QUERY_DATE is used to search by day, and KEY_DATE is used when time is required. For example, if one wants to search data for a specific date (yyyy/mm/dd), "query_date = yyyy/mm/dd" is faster than "yyyy/mm/dd 00:00:00≤key_date<yyyy/mm/dd+1day 00:00:00."

2.11 Patient Privacy

In the SDM, all private information is recorded in the personal table, and the other tables do not include any private information, not even PATIENT_ID. Each table records CASE_ID instead of PATIENT_ID. PATIENT_ID and CASE_ID can be linked in the personal table. Therefore, privacy is protected by ensuring the security of the personal table. This method also allows patients to have multiple IDs. For example, since a patient transported by emergency vehicle may not be conscious, a temporary patient ID is given. If it is later found that the patient has a formal patient ID, then the temporary patient ID is changed to the formal ID later, or the temporary patient ID is registered as the new formal patient ID. In the SDM, assuming such a case, INTEGRATE_ID is set in each table for it to determine later whether they are the same person or not. Also, in the case of patients who visit several hospitals, there are cases where the same patient is counted as a different patient because their data were acquired in multiple locations. INTEGRATE_ID is also useful for avoiding such instances [5].

3 AI in Surgery and the SDM

To predict results quickly, AI learning needs a huge amount of data that interpolates human knowledge and experience. The accuracy of AI output depends on the quality and quantity of the training data. In surgical cases, the situations change from moment to moment; therefore surgeons must make decisions quickly while always predicting the prognosis. At that time, the AI that makes predictions based on past data greatly influences the judgment of the surgeon. However, if the learned data is of poor quality or insufficient, it may lead the surgeon to make an incorrect decision. To avoid these outcomes, the SDM stores all clinical data, including surgical data, into a relational database using the semantic data modeling method. This stored clinical data can be quickly extracted as clinical information when needed. The SDM's clinical data and semantics are learned by the AI as training data, and in real time, the data of surgical patients is corrected and imported into the SDM as AI input data. The quality of such data is assured by using the same data model. Further amounts of data can be obtained by training the AI in other hospitals that use the SDM (Fig. 4).

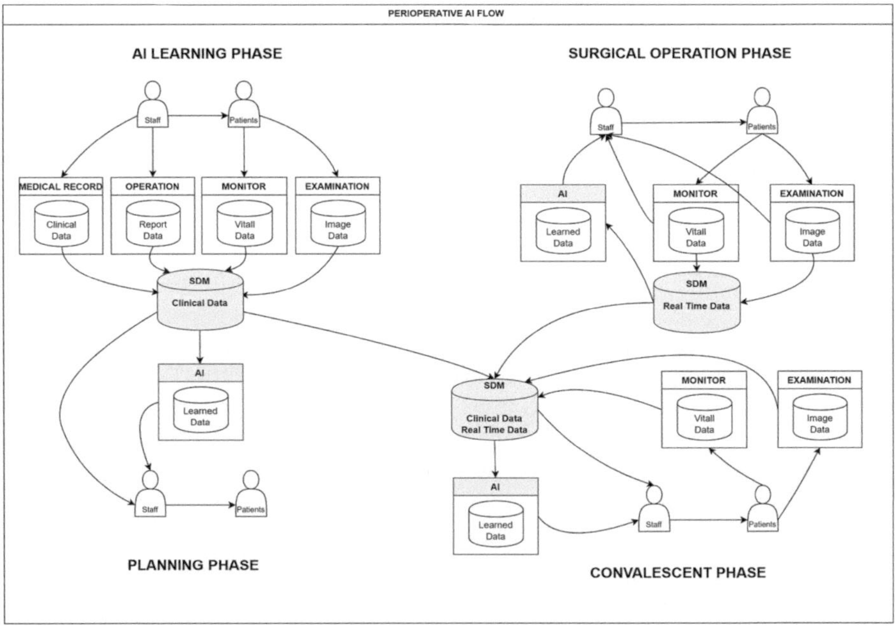

Fig. 4 AI-aided surgery in the perioperative period

References

1. Health Level Seven. International. 1987; https://www.hl7.org/.
2. DICOM Standard. 1983. https://www.dicomstandard.org/
3. Codd EF. The relational model for database management. Addison-Wesley; 1990. p. 371–88.
4. Rishe N. Database design, The semantic modeling approach. McGraw-Hill; 1992. p. 528.
5. Kimura E, Suzuki H. Development of a common data model facilitating clinical decision-making and analyses. In: Proceedings of the 17th world congress on medical and health informatics; 2019. p. 1522–3.

Trends in Regulatory Systems for AI-Based Medical Devices and Issues in Performance Evaluation

Mitsuru Yuba and Yutaka Tomioka

Abstract The development of artificial intelligence (AI)-based medical devices is expanding in scope and accelerating in pace. In order to improve patient access to these innovative medical devices, it is necessary to consider how the views of regulatory authorities have evolved from the early stages of development. This chapter outlines (1) regulatory trends in Japan and the USA regarding AI-based medical devices and (2) issues in performance evaluation. To deal with the constant improvements in performance that are inherent in AI, both Japan and the USA have established systems that allow the submission of improvement plans prior to the application for approval of devices, thereby simplifying subsequent applications. In addition, although there are differences in terms of transparency regarding the applicability of medical devices, the basic concept is the same in both countries. An important factor in the acquisition of data for performance evaluation is the protection of personal information. In Japan, a law has been enacted to allow the commercial use of personal information with opt-out consent. However, to evaluate the performance of a product, it is of major importance to ensure and prove that the data are sufficiently comprehensive to accommodate the diversity of analysis targets. As discussions on these issues continue into the future, medical device companies need to remain cognizant of the changes that occur and ensure that they stay abreast of the latest regulations.

Keywords Artificial intelligence · Regulation · Software as a medical device · Computer-aided diagnosis · Computer-aided surgery

M. Yuba (✉)
Cooperative Major in Advanced Biomedical Sciences, Joint Graduate School of Tokyo Women's Medical University and Waseda University, Waseda University, Tokyo, Japan
e-mail: yuba-mitsuru@aoni.waseda.jp

Y. Tomioka
Project Management Office for Medical Device Innovation, Department of MDI Incubation, Division of Medical Device Innovation, National Cancer Center Hospital East, Chiba, Japan
e-mail: ytomioka@east.ncc.go.jp

K. Masamune et al. (eds.), *Artificial Intelligence in Surgery*,
https://doi.org/10.1007/978-981-96-6635-5_6

1 Introduction

The development of medical devices based on artificial intelligence (AI) has been evolving rapidly. An annual survey by the American College of Radiology revealed that more than 30% of radiologists used AI to improve the accuracy of diagnostic interpretation [1]. This embrace of AI includes computer-aided diagnosis (CAD) as well as computer-assisted surgical systems (CAS). AI-based CAS is expected to improve the safety of surgical procedures because it is associated with increased accuracy of surgical procedures and organ discrimination. The scope of research focused on developing CAS is rapidly expanding.

One consequence of the increasing diversification of AI-based medical devices is the difficulty of making decisions within the conventional regulatory framework. There is a need for regulations that take into account the characteristics of AI in order to prevent medical accidents and the distribution of products whose efficacy is not guaranteed. Therefore, the US Food and Drug Administration (FDA) and the Ministry of Health, Labour and Welfare (MHLW) and the Pharmaceuticals and Medical Devices Agency (PMDA) in Japan are in the process of issuing guidelines for performance evaluation and reforming the regulation system to accommodate the growing presence of AI. In particular, it will be necessary for medical device companies to stay abreast of changes introduced by regulatory authorities; when a particular product is categorized as a medical device, this directly affects the requirements of efficacy and safety imposed on the device.

Based on this background, this chapter outlines the following: (1) regulatory trends in Japan and the USA regarding AI-based medical devices and (2) factors impinging on the evaluation of AI CAS.

2 Regulatory System in the USA

The USA has been a world leader in the regulation of software as a medical device (SaMD) since 1998, when the world's first CAD device named "Image Checker" (R2, now manufactured by Hologic) [2] was introduced to assist in the detection of breast cancer. Furthermore, in order to deal with the continuing development of AI technology, the twenty-first Century Cures Act [3] was enacted in December 2016, also in the USA. This Act describes the policy for the regulation of SaMD and the criteria for software to be regulated. The following year, the Digital Health Innovation Action Plan [4] was released, which included (1) the development of guidance on SaMD, (2) a pilot implementation of the Precertification Program, and (3) a strengthening of the Digital Health Unit at the Center for Devices and Radiological Health (CDRH). Twelve guidance documents on Digital Health were published by the FDA between 2017 and 2020, some of which are still in draft version at the time of writing. The Precertification Program became fully operational in

January 2019. Furthermore, the Digital Health Center of Excellence (DHCoE) was established at CDRH in 2020 [5].

A key feature of the Precertification Program [6] is that the FDA certifies the company rather than the individual products. The reason for certifying companies rather than products is that it is inefficient to evaluate the effectiveness and safety of each individual medical SaMD, since the functionality of a SaMD is constantly updated. The Precertification program envisioned by the FDA entails that the FDA will review a company's process of software design, verification, and maintenance, as well as its transparency as a company, risk management, and other factors, and determine whether the company qualifies as a company of excellence.

In this program, the FDA certifies whether a manufacturer develops high-quality, safe, and effective medical software. Manufacturers that have received such FDA certification will be able to apply for authorization to manufacture new products with simplified submissions and audits.

Furthermore, in April 2019, the FDA published a Discussion Paper [7] on AI/ML-based SaMD and proposed Good Machine Learning Practice (GMLP) to address the characteristics of AI medical devices, which have a short life cycle compared to traditional medical devices. GMLP specifies that the FDA classifies updates to AI/ML based SaMD into three categories: (1) changes in performance as a device, (2) changes in data used, and (3) changes in the intended use. To accommodate these updates, the FDA has defined the SaMD Pre-Specifications (SPS) and the Algorithm Change Protocol (ACP). The SPS indicate the range of possible changes in AI/ML-based SaMD, while the ACP indicates details of machine learning models, data collection, and management methods. If an update is conducted at post-market, the FDA will determine the application category by reviewing what impact the update will have on the SPS and ACP. Public comments on the Discussion Paper were solicited, and the "Artificial Intelligence/Machine Learning [AI/ML]-Based Software as Medical Device [SaMD] Action Plan" [8] was published in January 2021 as a response to the comments received.

3 The Applicability of Software as a Medical Device in the USA

The twenty-first Century Cures Act [3, 9] excludes certain software functions, including those intended for:

A. Administrative support.
B. General wellness.
C. Electronic patient records.
D. Transfer, storage, or format conversion of data or the display of related information.
E. Clinical Decision Support.

Noteworthy as a software function that is not recognized as SaMD is that the products intended for Clinical Decision Support (CDS) fall under this category. The FDA issued guidance on the medical device applicability of CDS in 2019. This guidance describes software classified as CDS as follows: "CDS provides health care professionals (HCPs) and patients with knowledge and person-specific information, intelligently filtered or presented at appropriate times, to enhance health and health care." It further specifies four conditions as criteria for determining that a device does not fall under the category of a medical device (Table 1). Among them, a product developed using AI deviates from condition 4, "health care professional can independently review the basis for such recommendations that such software presents," due to the black-box nature of AI. As a result, a product developed using AI qualifies as a medical device. In addition, in a guidance issued in 2019 and beyond, the FDA will primarily focus on software as either CDS (Clinical Decision Support) [10], OTS (Off-The-Shelf) [11], GW (General Wellness) [12], MDDS (Medical Device Data System) [13], Mobile Medical Application (MMA) [14], or Medical Device Accessories (MDA) [15]. The concept of medical device applicability for each of these categories is explained with specific examples (Table 1).

Table 1 List of guidance for applicability of SaMD, as published by FDA

Guidance title	Overview
Clinical decision support (CDS) software	Definition of CDS: Provides healthcare professionals and patients with knowledge and person-specific information, intelligently filtered or presented at appropriate times, to enhance health and healthcare. However, software that meets all the following four conditions does not constitute a medical device: (1) not intended to acquire, process, or analyze a medical image or a signal from an in vitro diagnostic device or a pattern or signal from a signal acquisition system (2) intended for the purpose of displaying, analyzing, or printing medical information about a patient or other medical information (such as peer-reviewed clinical studies and clinical practice guidelines) (3) intended for the purpose of supporting or providing recommendations to a healthcare professional about prevention, diagnosis, or treatment of a disease or condition (4) intended for the purpose of enabling such healthcare professional to independently review the basis for such recommendations that such software presents so that it is not the intent that such healthcare professional relies primarily on any of such recommendations to make a clinical diagnosis or treatment decision regarding an individual patient

(continued)

Table 1 (continued)

Guidance title	Overview
Off-the-shelf (OTS) software used in medical device	Definition of OTS: A generally available software component, used by a medical device manufacturer for which the manufacturer cannot claim complete software life cycle control Although it does not fall under the category of medical devices, it is necessary to have a concept regarding safety evaluation as a medical device, taking compatibility with OTS into consideration
General wellness (GW) products	Definition of GW: (i) are intended for only general wellness use, (ii) present a low risk to the safety of users and other persons GW categories Category 1: An intended use that relates to maintaining or encouraging a general State of health or a healthy activity Category 2: An intended use that relates the role of healthy lifestyle with helping To reduce the risk or impact of certain chronic diseases or conditions And where it is well understood and accepted that healthy lifestyle Choices may play an important role in health outcomes For the disease or condition
Medical device data system (MDDS)	Definition of MDDS: Devices that transfer, store, convert formats, and display medical device data or medical imaging data Software that merely monitors patients or stores data is not considered a medical device. However, software that analyzes patient data in an active manner, such as that used in mammography and radiotherapy, is categorized as a medical device
Mobile medical application (MMA)	Definition of MMA: ①those used as an accessory to a regulated medical device, ②to transform a mobile platform into a regulated medical device The app that encourages patients to change their behavior, but merely to lose weight or manage their daily diet, is not a medical device. However, an application that informs patients when it is time to take their medications is a medical device This guidance provides specific examples of what is not a medical device (Appendix A), what can be a medical device (Appendix B), and what is a medical device (Appendix C)
Medical device accessories (MDA)	Definition of MDA: A finished device that is intended to support, supplement, and/or augment the performance of one or more parent devices Definition of parent device: A finished device whose performance is supported, supplemented, and/or augmented by one or more accessories An accessory is classified as a medical device because it has the function of assisting the parent device

In contrast with the situation with respect to CAD, no guidance on determining the applicability to CAS has been published. However, the concept of CAD may be useful for the functions of CAS, such as organ identification by image analysis. In addition, if a device is used together with CAS and improves the function of CAS, it can be classified under MDA; the guidance discussed in this chapter may be of value in such an instance.

4 Regulatory System in Japan

In Japan, the 2014 amendment of the "Act on Securing Quality, Efficacy and Safety of Products Including Pharmaceuticals and Medical Devices" [16] led to the recognition of stand-alone software products as medical devices.

To address the short life cycle of AI medical devices, the MHLW issued the Improvement Design within Approval for Timely Evaluation and Notice (IDATEN) system in 2019 [17]. Under this system, approved medical devices can be modified by notifying changes in their intended use or effect, shape, structure, principle, raw materials, performance and safety specifications, method of use, storage method, validity period, manufacturing method, and other factors, as long as the ethical, scientific, and reliable nature of the modification is ensured. The prepared change plan can be submitted together with the application materials at the time of initial application.

Furthermore, the Digital Transformation Action Strategies in Healthcare for SaMD (DASH for SaMD) were issued in November 2020 [18]. The DASH for SaMD strategy package includes (1) early identification of budding seeds and announcement of the review approach, (2) centralized consultation services (applicability consultation, development consultation, and medical insurance consultation), (3) a review system based on the characteristics of programmed medical devices (utilization of IDATEN), and (4) strengthening the system for early commercialization of the devices. In March 2021, guidelines on the applicability of programmed medical devices were issued, and in April of the same year, the Programmed Medical Device Review Office was newly established within the MHLW and PMDA.

Under the IDATEN system, it is possible to change the change plan itself. In such cases, the PMDA should be consulted to determine whether an additional quality, efficacy, and safety evaluation is required in comparison with the original change plan and whether an application for confirmation of the change plan or a minor change notification should be filed to implement such a change. In making a change according to the change plan, a comprehensive judgment is made as to whether the change is within the scope of notification according to the scope of change or whether an application for the partial change of approved items should be filed and whether an evaluation of the quality, efficacy, and safety associated with such change is necessary.

5 The Applicability of Software as a Medical Device in Japan

The classification of software as a medical device is based on the following two main considerations:

① The degree of contribution to the treatment and diagnosis of diseases in view of the importance of the results obtained by the programmed medical devices.

② The probability of the overall risk, including the risk of affecting human life and health, in the event of impairment of the functions of the programmed medical device.

Since the amendment of the "Act on Securing Quality, Efficacy and Safety of Products Including Pharmaceuticals and Medical Devices" in 2014, the notice on the applicability of software as a medical device was slightly updated in 2018, but with the increased development of medical devices using artificial intelligence technology. The "Guideline on the Medical Device Applicability of Programs" was issued on March 31, 2021 [19]. This guideline describes how the intended use of software determines whether it is classifiable as a medical device or not, as follows:

<Intended uses of software that qualify the software as a medical device>

① Programs that display disease candidates and disease risks based on input information.
② Programs for diagnosis, treatment, and prevention of diseases (CADe/CADx).
③ Programs used in combination with tangible medical devices.
④ Programs to assist in determining treatment plans and methods including simulations.

<Intended uses of software that do not qualify the software as a medical device>

① Programs to transfer, store, and display data acquired by medical devices for use as medical records.
② Programs for processing and treating data (excluding images and use for diagnosis).
③ Programs for education.
④ Programs for explanation to patients.
⑤ Programs for maintenance.
⑥ Programs to support in-hospital operations.
⑦ Programs for healthcare.
⑧ Programs equivalent to general medical devices that have little risk of affecting human life and health in the event of functional failure.

In terms of the probability of risk, AI functions that simply identify organs intraoperatively can reduce risk when allied with physician experience, but when surgery is performed automatically by AI, strict evaluation is required because the outcome depends on the AI's functions. Therefore, it is important to determine to what extent the functions of AI should be advocated and to what extent interventions in the surgical procedures of physicians should be authorized. The evolution of regulations and guidance related to AI medical devices in Japan and the USA is depicted in Fig. 1.

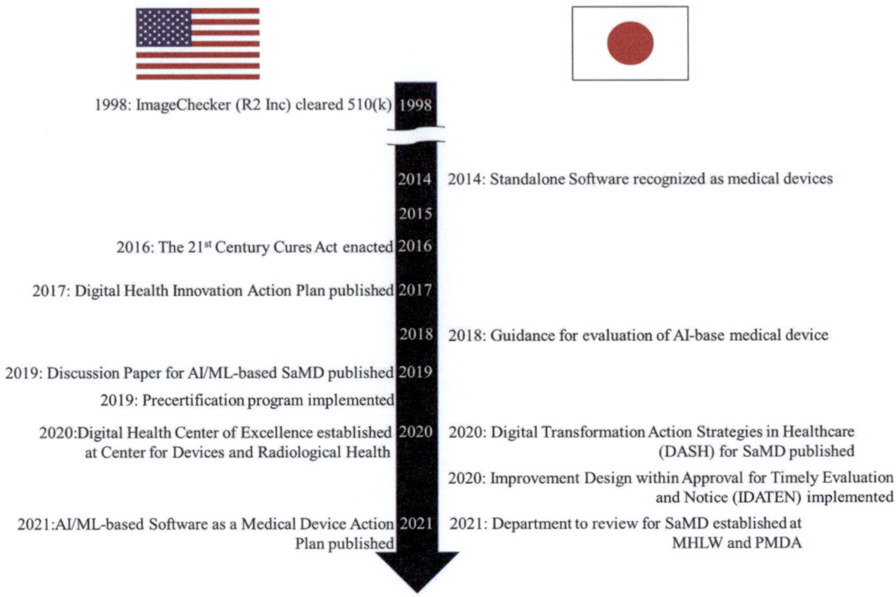

Fig. 1 History of regulatory measures for SaMD in the USA and Japan

6 Challenges in the Evaluation of Medical Devices for Artificial Intelligence Surgery

The concept of AI surgery may be viewed from many perspectives. In order to realize fully automated surgery, the technologies that are needed include robots as hands, scopes as eyes, and image recognition technology as the brain, all of which need to be coordinated by methods for integrating these technologies (Fig. 2). In both Japan and the USA, the introduction of "hand" robots, which are necessary technologies for realizing fully automated surgery, has already been initiated in the form of surgical support robots that are manually operated by surgeons, such as the da Vinci series marketed by Intuitive Surgical Inc. and Hinotori marketed by Medicaroid Corporation. Conversely, object recognition technology in endoscopic images, which is an elemental technology for automatic control and plays the role of the "brain" in fully automated surgery, is being developed as a recognition support tool for surgeons who perform endoscopic surgery. In Japan, the endoscopic realm leads the endoscopic surgical realm in tumor recognition technology implemented in clinical practice. As of March 2022, six SaMD products had been approved to enter the market by the MHLW. These products were intended to support endoscopists by detecting polyps and making a differential diagnosis of tumors in gastrointestinal endoscopy. Japan is a world leader in object detection technology in the field of gastrointestinal endoscopy. On the other hand, although research and development of object recognition technology in endoscopic images for endoscopic

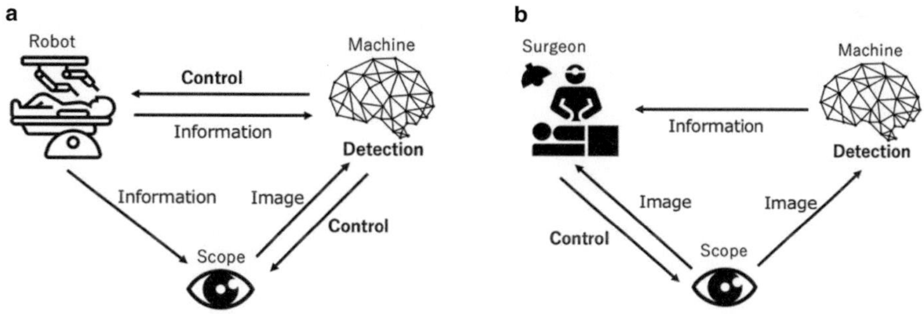

Fig. 2 (**a**) Fully automatic AI surgery (future). (**b**) AI-aided surgery (current)

surgery are in progress, there are no SaMDs on the market at this time, and the technology is still in the development phase.

In parallel with the development of object recognition technology for fully automated surgery, SaMDs are currently being developed to provide object recognition assistance for surgeons and endoscopists performing endoscopic surgery and endoscopic diagnosis.

In the development and evaluation of object recognition technology for endoscopic video, whether for AI surgery or to assist surgeons and endoscopists, the main challenges in obtaining data for evaluation are (1) obtaining consent to use images for development purposes and (2) ensuring a target will be recognized, notwithstanding the large variety of individual patient physiologies.

7 Obtaining Consent to Use Images for Development Purposes

Laws related to the protection of personal information are being developed independently by each advanced country and are being revised as needed when operational problems emerge. Since surgery is a medical procedure performed on a patient with a disease, surgical videos are treated as information that should be handled with special care (personal information requires special consideration under Japan's Personal Information Protection Law), since the video content can be used to identify a person with a disease if it is linked to information that identifies the person. Although there is a way to anonymize the information that identifies an individual and treat the video itself as non-personal information, details of the patient's background and prognosis may also be necessary depending on the function of the algorithm to be developed. Therefore, a situation may arise in which the information cannot be anonymized and, accordingly, cannot be exempted from being treated as personal information. If the patient's background information is not required, so that only the video is required, it is possible in Japan to use the video with opt-out

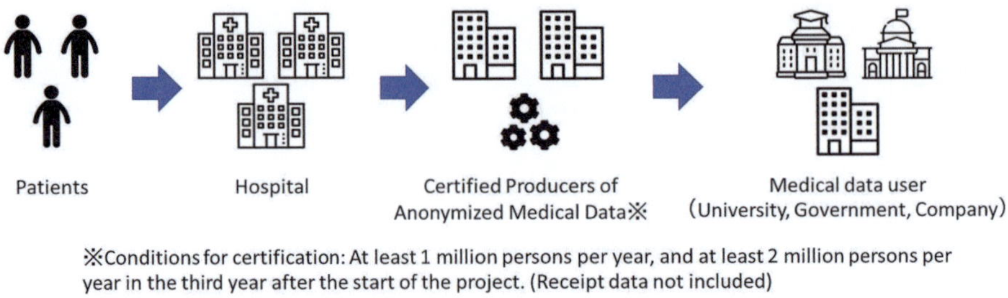

Fig. 3 Information flow in the Next Generation Medical Infrastructure Law

consent for academic research purposes by using the video as anonymized data (the Personal Information Protection Law does not apply in Japan). In addition, a recent amendment to the law in Japan exempts the practitioner from the obligation to obtain consent for the acquisition of personal information requiring special consideration if the video is to be used for academic research purposes. However, even with anonymized image data, individual consent is required to use the data for commercial purposes (including the development of medical devices), and the fact that comprehensive consent for academic research purposes cannot be used for the development of medical devices is a major hurdle in the development process. This is one of the key points that should be taken into consideration when developing a SaMD. In the recent MHLW guidance for SaMD development, it was clarified that GCP does not need to be applied when evaluating SaMD for regulatory submission using images and medical information already obtained in an actual clinical situation. The need to obtain patient consent for the use of patient information for commercial purposes was also reiterated in the guidance [20].

The Next Generation Medical Infrastructure Act enables (1) the provision of medical information from medical institutions to certified providers and (2) the provision of anonymized processed information from certified providers to users by opting out of personal information constraints resorting under the Personal Information Protection Law in Japan, in the manner described in the previous paragraph (Fig. 3). However, in terms of ensuring the quality, quantity, and comprehensiveness of data essential for the development of medical devices using artificial intelligence (AI), data collected under the Next Generation Medical Infrastructure Act are not likely to be organized into the format desired by companies engaged in medical device development. As a result, it may currently be more efficient for companies engaged in AI medical device development to contract with medical institutions on their own and obtain information that matches their needs in an opt-in manner.

8 Ensuring a Target Will Be Recognized, Notwithstanding the Large Variety of Individual Patient Physiologies

Object recognition in endoscopic images viewed by surgeons in endoscopic surgery is not easy because of the wide variety of recognition targets. Object recognition targets in endoscopic surgery images include surgical instruments and anatomy. The difficulties in constructing algorithms for object recognition using AI techniques for surgical tools and anatomy, respectively, are described below.

8.1 Instruments

An argument may be made that it is relatively straightforward to improve the accuracy of object recognition because surgical instruments are easily distinguished from image backgrounds, which consist of body cavities. However, it is necessary to continually relearn such an algorithm in order to adapt it when a new surgical tool that needs to be recognized is launched in the medical field.

8.2 Anatomical Structures

The recognition of anatomical structures presents greater difficulties than the recognition of surgical tools. Surgeons learn anatomy as background knowledge and are eventually able to recognize the anatomical structures relevant to each surgical process in endoscopic images after repeating the same surgical procedure over lengthy periods of time. However, the same types of anatomical structures may appear differently in images corresponding to different patients. Therefore, it is necessary to train AI systems by using images that accommodate the full range of variety of a particular anatomical structure, in order to improve the accuracy of object recognition using AI technology and reduce the risk of false recognition. A similar degree of comprehensiveness is required in the evaluation procedure.

8.2.1 Gender

Because of the differences in abdominal organs between men and women, it is difficult to construct an algorithm to recognize female organs based solely on images of male patients. The reverse is also true.

8.2.2 Physique

Anatomical tissues that are easily visible in thin patients may not be visible in obese patients because of adipose tissue. In machine recognition, it is necessary for both learning and evaluation to cover the variation in the visibility of anatomical tissues that arise because of differences in body size.

8.2.3 History of Medical Treatment

Surgery or radiotherapy may cause adhesions, fibrosis, or other changes in the treated area, resulting in an appearance that differs from normal anatomical tissue. In both learning and evaluation, it is necessary for machine recognition to accommodate the range of variation in the appearance of anatomical tissues that results from treatment histories.

8.2.4 Individual Difference

Vascular tissue such as blood vessels, ureters and urethrae, and nerve runs vary from person to person, and machine recognition is often subject to error. Poor recognition or misrecognition is unacceptable when damage to the tissues can lead to the development of serious complications.

It may be argued that the abovementioned variety in individual patient backgrounds can be accommodated by increasing the number of image data used. This argument is countered by the rise in the number of training images for machine learning that this would entail and the concomitant increase in the difficulty of developing effective algorithms. The number of evaluation data required would also become very large, in order to accommodate the diversity of individual patients' anatomical tissues during the evaluation process. Furthermore, different surgical fields (e.g., esophageal surgery, colorectal surgery, etc.) require different anatomical tissues to be recognized and, therefore, different patient backgrounds and degrees of variety to be considered. In the absence of a reliable method for accommodating the individual differences in anatomical structure, the number of data required for evaluation would become intractable. Combined with the need to obtain individual consent, this constitutes a major hurdle to the development of AI systems and presents a problem that neither regulators nor developers have an answer to at this time.

9 Summary of This Chapter

We have summarized the regulatory trends of AI-based medical devices and the challenges facing the development of AI-based CAS. Both Japan and the USA are strengthening their review systems and exploring new regulatory frameworks to accommodate medical devices using AI technology, which is undergoing rapid technological innovation. Furthermore, both countries are considering shortening the review period and simplifying the required procedures through pro-active evaluation of the change plan for rapidly evolving AI functionality and the evaluation of effectiveness and safety based invoked by the plan even after the product enters the market. However, there is no consensus on the types of changes that should be eligible for preferential treatment, and it is expected that guidance based on accumulated cases will be published in the future.

In addition, the burden of obtaining consent for the use of patient information, which is indispensable for the development of AI medical devices, presents another major hurdle to development. In Japan, there is a movement to deregulate the use of personal information for academic research purposes when the greater public interest would outweigh individual disadvantage. Notwithstanding these developments, there is currently no movement toward deregulation of the requirement for an opt-in consent to obtain prior permission for the use of patients' personal information (which would constitute personal information requiring special consideration). Expectations are high for a review of the operation of the Next Generation Healthcare Infrastructure Law framework, which allows for the provision of patient information to third parties in an opt-out consent clause, to continue stimulating the promotion of the industrial use of patient information. In addition, since discussions are expected to continue toward revising laws and operational methods for handling personal information in the medical field, companies and academic institutions that are developing AI medical devices will need to remain cognizant of ongoing regulatory changes and remain flexible in responding to changes in regulations and operations.

References

1. Allen B, Agarwal S, Coombs L, Wald C, Dreyer K. ACR data science institute artificial intelligence survey. J Am Coll Radiol. 2020;2021 https://doi.org/10.1016/j.jacr.2021.04.002.
2. HOLOGIC. ImageChecker®2D CAD Technology. https://www.3dimensionsmammography.eu/screening-portfolio/imagechecker-2d-cad-technology/#. Accessed Jan 3, 2022.
3. The 21st Century Cures Act. https://www.fda.gov/regulatory-information/selected-amendments-fdc-act/21st-century-cures-act. 2016.
4. FDA. Digital Health Innovation Action Plan. https://www.fda.gov/media/106331/download. 2017.
5. FDA. Digital Health Center of Excellence. https://www.fda.gov/medical-devices/digital-health-center-excellence. Accessed 3 Jan 2022.
6. FDA. Development a software precertification program: a working model https://www.fda.gov/media/119722/download. 2019.
7. FDA. Proposed regulatory framework for modifications to Artificial Intelligence/Machine Learning [AI/ML]-Based Software as a Medical Device [SaMD]. Discussion Paper and Request for Feedback. https://www.fda.gov/media/122535/download. 2019.
8. FDA. Artificial Intelligence/Machine Learning [AI/ML]-Based Software as a Medical Device [SaMD] Action Plan. https://www.fda.gov/media/145022/download. 2021.

9. FDA. Changes to Existing Medical Software Policies Resulting from Section 3060 of the 21st Century Cures Act Guidance for Industry and Food and Drug Administration Staff. https://www.fda.gov/media/109622/download. 2019.
10. FDA. Clinical Decision Support Software Draft Guidance for Industry and Food and Drug Administration Staff. https://www.fda.gov/media/109618/download. 2019.
11. FDA. Off-The-Shelf Software Use in Medical Devices Guidance for Industry and Food and Drug Administration Staff. https://www.fda.gov/media/71794/download. 2019.
12. FDA. General Wellness: Policy for Low Risk Devices Guidance for industry and Food and Drug Administration Staff. https://www.fda.gov/media/90652/download. 2019.
13. FDA. Medical Device Data Systems Medical Image Storage Devices and Medical Image Communications Devices Guidance for Industry and Food and Drug Administration Staff. https://www.fda.gov/media/88572/download. 2019.
14. FDA. Policy for Device Software Functions and Mobile Medical Applications Guidance for Industry and Food and Drug Administration Staff. https://www.fda.gov/media/80958/download. 2019.
15. FDA. Medical Device Accessories Describing Accessories and Classification Pathways Guidance for Industry and FDA Staff. https://www.fda.gov/media/90647/download. 2017.
16. MHLW. Notification for basic concept regarding the applicability of program as medical devices. (in Japanese) https://www.pmda.go.jp/files/000159993.pdf. 2014.
17. MHLW. Notification for Improvement Design within Approval for Timely Evaluation and Notice (in Japanese). https://www.pmda.go.jp/files/000236900.pdf. 2020.
18. MHLW. Digital Transformation Action Strategies in Healthcare for SaMD. (in Japanese) https://www.mhlw.go.jp/content/11124500/000737470.pdf. 2020.
19. MHLW. Notification for Guidelines on the applicability of the program as medical devices. (in Japanese) https://www.pmda.go.jp/files/000240364.pdf. 2021.
20. MHLW. Notification for handling of performance evaluation tests for diagnostic medical devices using existing medical imaging data without additional invasion or intervention (in Japanese). https://www.pmda.go.jp/files/000243109.pdf. 2021.

Cybersecurity

Kento Hasegawa and Nozomu Togawa

Abstract Cybersecurity has become a critical issue in medical systems. To defend the medical system from threats in cyberspace, understanding the major technical factors of security mechanisms is critical. This chapter presents a brief introduction of security mechanisms in terms of secure data management, malicious traffic detection, and supply chain risks.

Keywords Cybersecurity · Cryptography · Anomaly detection · Machine learning · Supply chain

1 Introduction

Because electronic devices and computers are widely used in medical equipment, *cybersecurity* risks must be considered to provide a secure and reliable medical system. The ISO/IEC 27000 series [1] provides best practices and recommendations on information security management, which cover a wide range of cybersecurity issues. According to the series, information security should ensure the *confidentiality*, *availability*, and *integrity* of information. *Confidentiality* ensures that information should not be made available or disclosed to unauthorized individuals, entities, or processes. *Availability* ensures that a property should be accessible and usable on demand by an authorized entity. *Integrity* ensures that a property should be accurate and complete. Introducing this concept to medical equipment that stores sensitive information is natural. Inherently, medical equipment is expected to be highly reliable, and thus, availability and integrity must be ensured. However, if adversaries

K. Hasegawa (✉)
KDDI Research, Inc., Saitama, Japan
e-mail: kt-hasegawa@kddi.com

N. Togawa
Waseda University, Tokyo, Japan
e-mail: ntogawa@waseda.jp

K. Masamune et al. (eds.), *Artificial Intelligence in Surgery*,
https://doi.org/10.1007/978-981-96-6635-5_7

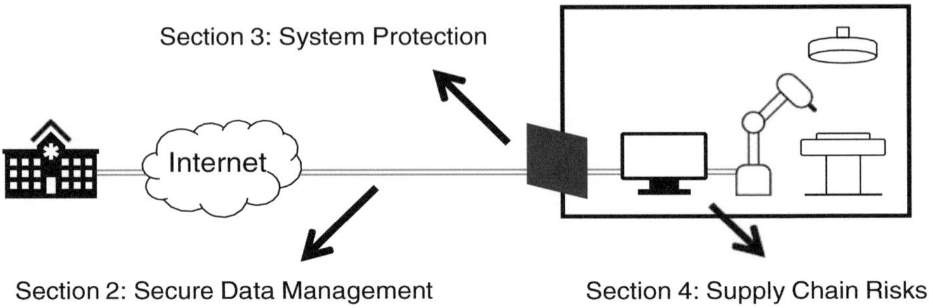

Fig. 1 Overview of cybersecurity described in this chapter

can invade the medical system, they may disturb the original functionalities of the equipment or suspend the system, resulting in the failure of availability. Protecting the medical system from the perspective of cybersecurity is thus important.

Figure 1 shows an overview of the cybersecurity concerns addressed in this chapter. This chapter targets developers and managers of medical system and provides fundamental approaches and methods to implement secure mechanisms and knowledge of security-related issues in medical systems. The following sections present cybersecurity in terms of the following topics: secure data management, system protection, and supply chain risks. Section 2 presents secure data management to protect message exchanges. Section 3 presents system protection to guard against invaders. Section 4 presents the risks in the supply chain of medical equipment. Finally, Section 5 concludes this chapter.

2 Secure Data Management

Medical systems handle sensitive information, including patients' personal information and medical history. When such information is shared with other equipment or systems, it must not be exposed. Properly encrypted data will not be exposed to third persons. This section describes the principles of encryption.

There are two categories of cryptographic algorithms: symmetric and asymmetric [2]. Symmetric cryptographic algorithms use the same key for encryption and decryption. In general, symmetric cryptographic algorithms are faster than asymmetric algorithms with respect to computation time, but the key must be unique for each communication channel. Conversely, asymmetric cryptographic algorithms use different keys for encryption and decryption. Although asymmetric cryptographic algorithms require more computation time than symmetric cryptographic algorithms, they require only one key pair for each receiver.

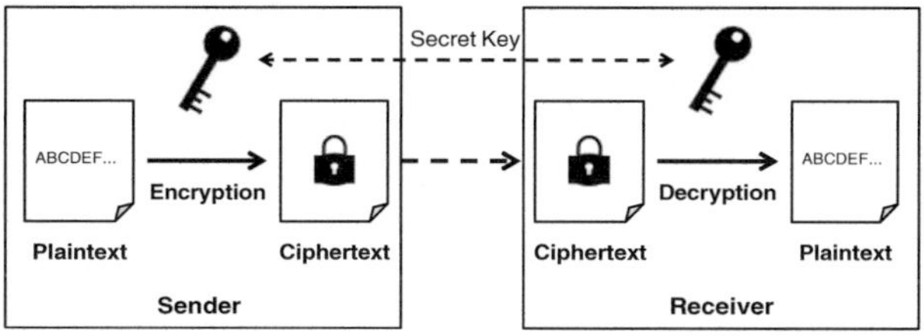

Fig. 2 Symmetric encryption and decryption

2.1 *Symmetric Cryptography*

A secret key is used for both encryption and decryption in a symmetric cryptographic algorithm. AES[1] is a common symmetric cryptographic algorithm that was specified as a standard symmetric-key algorithm by the US National Institute of Standards and Technology (NIST) in 2001 [3]. Symmetric cryptographic algorithms can be classified into two categories: a block cipher and a stream cipher. A block cipher algorithm processes on a fixed length of bits, while a stream cipher algorithm processes a given piece of plaintext sequentially.

Figure 2 shows encryption and decryption with a symmetric cryptographic algorithm. The sender and receiver share the same secret key. The sender encrypts a piece of plaintext using a secret key and sends it to the receiver. The receiver decrypts the ciphertext using the same secret key and obtains the plaintext.

Symmetric cryptography allows for fast encryption and decryption, and its mechanism is simple compared to asymmetric cryptography; thus, the associated algorithms can be easily implemented in a small hardware chip. The weakness of symmetric cryptography is the difficulty of managing secret keys, which must be different from each other. When there are n computers and they can communicate with each other, $n(n - 1)/2$ secret keys are required. The number of required secret keys also rapidly increases as the number of computers increases. If the secret key is leaked, the ciphertexts will be disclosed to those who can access the secret key. Therefore, secure management of the secret keys is critical.

2.2 *Asymmetric Cryptography*

An asymmetric cryptographic algorithm uses a pair of keys: a public key and a private key. RSA[2] is a common asymmetric cryptographic algorithm.

Figure 3 shows the encryption and decryption with an asymmetric cryptographic algorithm. The receiver first generates a key pair: a public key and a private key. The public key is distributed to those who will send something to the receiver, and the private key is hidden. The sender encrypts the piece of plaintext with the public key

[1] AES stands for Advanced Encryption Standard.

[2] RSA comes from the surnames of the designers Ron Rivest, Adi Shamir, and Leonard Adleman.

Fig. 3 Asymmetric encryption and decryption

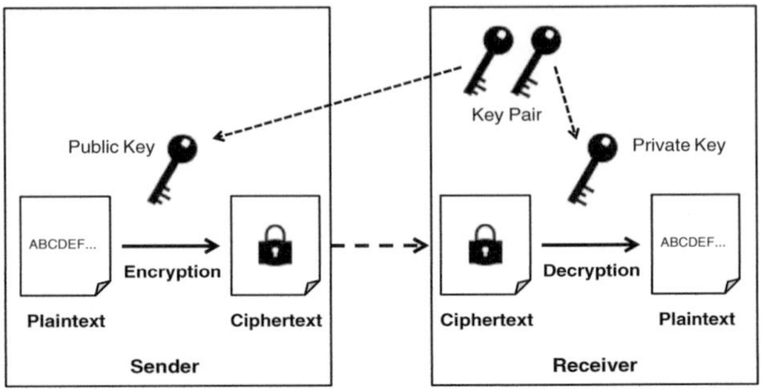

and then sends the ciphertext to the receiver. The receiver decrypts the ciphertext with the private key and obtains the plaintext. Once a plaintext is encrypted with a public key, only the private key that corresponds to the public key used for encryption can decrypt the ciphertext. An asymmetric cryptographic algorithm is established based on the computational difficulty of the inverse function of a certain function. For example, the RSA algorithm uses the computational difficulty of prime factorization. The key feature of asymmetric cryptography is the public key. Due to this feature, the asymmetric cryptography is also called public-key cryptography. Unlike symmetric cryptographic algorithms, unique secret keys for each communication channel are not required; only one public key is used for each receiver. Asymmetric cryptography is suitable for communication between a server and numerous unspecified clients. However, the weakness of this method is its computational complexity. In general, the mechanism of an asymmetric cryptographic algorithm is complex and requires more computation time compared to symmetric cryptographic algorithms. Asymmetric cryptographic algorithms are thus not suitable for processing large data. In practical applications, asymmetric cryptographic algorithms are used to exchange secret keys in symmetric cryptography. In this scheme, a secret key is encrypted with an asymmetric cryptographic algorithm and is exchanged. Then, payload data are encrypted with a symmetric cryptographic algorithm using the exchanged secret key.

Based on the asymmetric cryptographic algorithm, an electronic signature mechanism is used to ensure that the document is signed by the owner of the associated private key and that the document has not been tampered with after the document was signed. When signing a document, a hash value of the document is generated, and a signer encrypts the hash value using her private key and generates a signature. The signature is attached to the original document, and the document is signed digitally. When verifying the signed document, the verifier calculates the hash value of the document. Simultaneously, the signature is decrypted using the signer's public key. If the calculated hash value and the decrypted message are identical, the signature is valid. Otherwise, the following situations are considered. First, the public key is not associated with the document, and thus, the owner of the public key is not the signer of the document. Second, the document has been tampered with by someone after the document was signed. The new signature thus cannot be generated by the person who has not own the original private key.

Asymmetric cryptography has the difficulty in determining the owner of the public keys. For seamless operation using asymmetric cryptography, an infrastructure for managing public keys is critical and is known as the Public Key Infrastructure (PKI) [4]. PKI registers, distributes, and invalidates digital certificates that are used to verify that a public key belongs to a certain entity. For simplicity, we present a partial operation of PKI. In PKI, certificate authorities (CAs) certify requested public keys and issue digital certificates for each public key. The digital certificate contains several piece of information, such as a public key, the owner of the public key, and the issuer of the certificate, and is signed using an electronic signature. CAs might be certified by other CAs recursively; thus, a parent CA certifies a child CA, and the child CA certifies a public key. Several CAs are registered as root CAs and are initially registered as trusted CAs in operating systems and web browsers. When verifying a digital certificate, the CAs that certified the digital certificate are recursively traversed. If a CA is registered as a root CA, the digital certificate can be trusted. In general, the administrator of the system can register or remove root CAs.

2.3 Use Case for EHR

Recently, cloud systems have become widely used and are becoming more reliable and useful. Conventional systems that provide online services require a constantly running computer to be installed on the premises. Managing such a conventional system (i.e., "on-premise") requires several inputs, such as human resources and physical space for the computers. Using cloud services, users prepare their applications, and off-site server machines are shared with other users. When the service for EHR is deployed on a cloud service, protecting data is necessary.

As reviewed in [5], several methods of securely managing e-health data on cloud services were proposed in a few years. To develop a secure service, security and usability must be balanced. For example, if all data are encrypted, then all of the data are secure. However, the computation time for encryption and decryption increases. In addition, searching the data that partially match a given phrase is difficult. Therefore, effective data management frameworks are required to develop a convenient service.

As a new scheme to manage encrypted data, homomorphic encryption has been studied and applied to medical systems [6]. Using homomorphic encryption, the computation for encrypted data can be performed without decrypting the data, thus creating a more secure and convenient system. The problem of homomorphic encryption is that the computation time is particularly high. Further research is expected with regard to the implementation of homomorphic encryption in real-world application.

3 System Protection from Malicious Traffic

This section presents the system protection mechanism against malicious traffic. Intrusion detection systems (IDS) or firewall services protect internal networks and machines from adversaries.

3.1 Data Structure in a Communication Channel

As a preliminary for detection methods, the data structure in the communication channel is introduced. Only the transmitted data do not include information about the communication opponent. To transfer the data to the designated opponent, several piece of information are attached to the data. In this subsection, the TCP/IP protocol stack is presented as a representative architecture of communication data forms.

The TCP/IP protocol stack is a common protocol architecture for electronic communication, which is used in local computer networks and on the Internet. There are four layers in the protocol stack: application, transport, Internet, and link. In this section, the procedure to transmit data is considered. First, transmitted data are generated by an application in the application layer. Second, these data are processed in the transport layer, which splits the data into several chunks. The port number, which indicates the application running on a computer, and the order of the chunks are attached to the data as a header. Third, the data are processed in the Internet layer. The IP address, which shows the opponent in an IP network, is attached to the beginning of the data. The composed data are called a packet. Fourth, the packet is processed in the link layer. The MAC address, which is the address of the directly connected machine, is attached to the beginning of the packet. The composed data are then called a frame, which is transmitted to the designated MAC address via a communication channel, such as a metal cable or Wi-Fi. The receiver processes the received data in the reverse order of the above process.

The key point of the communicated data is that additional information such as the port number, which shows the application to be processed, and several addresses are attached to the data.

3.2 Signature-Based Approach

Pattern matching is the simplest implementation that can be used to examine traffic data and can determine whether the exchanged data match the signatures registered in a list. In general, there are two pattern-matching approaches: whitelist and blacklist [7]. A whitelist-based approach examines whether the traffic signature is acceptable. If the data match the signature that is registered in the list, traffic is allowed;

otherwise, the traffic is dropped. A blacklist-based approach examines whether the traffic signature is unacceptable. If the data match the signature that is registered in the list, the traffic is denied; otherwise, the traffic is allowed.

Selecting a whitelist- or blacklist-based approach depends on the type of connected clients. When only reliable clients are connected, such as the system in an operation room or a closed system in a hospital, a whitelist-based approach is suitable. Conversely, when numerous clients may be connected, such as a public web service, a blacklist-based approach is suitable.

Another aspect is the computation time required for detection. Both whitelist- and blacklist-based approaches intuitively investigate whether an entry is registered in the list. The computation time to search the list is linearly proportional to the number of entries in the list on average. For example, if the number of entries in the list is doubled, the computation time also doubles on average.

3.2.1 Data Investigation

There are several types of content that can be included in a whitelist or blacklist. The communication data consist of a header and body. The header contains information about the source or destination of the data, and the body contains the actual data.

A simple detection approach investigates the header because the format of the header is determined by the protocol specification. Specifically, the source and destination addresses, which are described in the header, are often investigated for signature-based detection. The address is used to identify the communication opponent and varies depending on the communication channel. In an IP network, a set of the IP address and the port number is the representative identifier, which generally differs from the applications running on devices.

An IP address[3] is used to identify each machine connected to an IP network, and the port number identifies the application running on a machine. Specifically, web browser and video-communication applications use different ports on a computer but use the same IP address.

A more sophisticated detection approach investigates the body of the data. The body is typically not formatted, and thus, investigating the body is difficult for general-purpose applications. Investigating the body of the data is often used with data for a specific application. For example, web application firewalls investigate the body of web communications and drop malicious traffic [8]. Although investigating the body of data requires more computational resources, more precise detection is achieved.

Investigating only the header is an effective defense. However, recent adversaries have used sophisticated methods to invade internal networks. If an adversary spoofs

[3]There are generally two types of IP addresses: a private IP address and a public IP address. A private IP address is used on a local area network, and a public IP address is used to communicate with computers outside the local area network (i.e., on the Internet).

the header information using legitimate information, the data pass the investigation of the header. In this case, investigating the body is more effective.

3.2.2 Representation of Signatures

There are several ways to represent patterns in the whitelist or blacklist: exact match, wild-card match, and regular expression.

Exact match investigates whether the target value exactly matches any entry in the list. This approach is simple and fast to process. However, each entry corresponds to only one case. If there are too many cases to be registered in the list, the maintenance cost is increased.

Wild-card match investigates whether the target value matches any entry with wild-card characters. The character "?" represents any one character, and the character "*" represents several characters. This approach is useful to indicate a group of entries. In general, the machines in a group are assigned to partially identical addresses. Such a case can be expressed as one entry using the wild-card approach. Regular expression investigates whether the target value matches any *regular expression* patterns in the list. Regular expression is a powerful method to express the specific pattern of strings and is used in more recent network IDSs [9]. The weakness of regular expression is its computation time. A complex regular expression might take a long time to determine whether the pattern is matched.

Supported representation patterns depend on the detection service. The goal is to select the most suitable method for a given system in terms of maintainability, detection performance, and computation cost.

3.3 Anomaly Detection

In anomaly detection, abnormal traffic, which is unseen or uncommon compared to known benign traffic, is identified by an anomaly detector. In conventional methods, anomalies can be quantified statistically, such as median absolute deviation or Mahalanobis distance [10]. Recently, machine learning has been used to effectively learn traffic trends. Machine learning algorithms can roughly be categorized into two detection approaches: supervised learning and unsupervised learning [11].

3.3.1 Supervised Learning

In supervised learning, the classifier model trains a training dataset that contains training samples and corresponding class labels. In a typical detection method, the labels are categorized as either benign or malicious. The trained model predicts the class label for a given sample. The supervised learning approach works effectively when a training dataset that contains a sufficient number of both benign and malicious classes is prepared. The weakness of this approach is that the malicious samples, which are typically difficult to collect in the real world, are necessary. In addition, an out-of-distribution sample, which is far from any sample in the training dataset, is difficult to predict.

A support vector machine (SVM), a decision tree (DT), and a neural network (NN) are representative supervised learning algorithms. An SVM constructs a hyperplane that separates two classes of training samples with the maximum margin. A DT classifies a given sample based on a set of conditions for each feature of a sample. An NN is composed of multiple layers that consist of multiple calculation units. The suitable algorithms and hyperparameters depend on the downstream task and training dataset. To construct an effective model for detection, carefully selecting the algorithms and tuning the hyperparameters is critical.

3.3.2 Unsupervised Learning

In unsupervised learning, the classifier model learns a training dataset that contains only benign class samples and does not contain any other class labels. The classifier model determines a given sample as benign when the sample is within the distribution of the training samples. Otherwise, the model identifies the sample as an outlier. The strength of the unsupervised learning approach is that no training dataset for the malicious class is required, while its weakness is the difficulty of determining what is an outlier. If a model determines that a sample is outside the boundary that is constructed around the training samples with a narrow margin, several benign samples that are marginally outside the distribution of the training samples may be misclassified as outliers. Similar to supervised learning, carefully selecting the algorithms and tuning the hyperparameters is critical.

One-class SVM, isolation forest, and clustering are representative unsupervised algorithms. One-class SVM is an unsupervised version of SVM that constructs the hyperplane around the training samples. The isolation forest is based on the DT method. The clustering algorithm splits the training samples into several classes based on a certain distance metric. Then, the class that contains few samples or the class with low density compared to neighboring classes is determined to be outliers.

Although machine learning is an attractive approach for anomaly detection, there are several problems. First, machine learning algorithms require more computational resources than signature-based methods. To apply machine learning algorithms to anomaly detection for a large and fast communication channel, a high-performance computer is necessary. Second, the machine learning algorithms often produce misclassifications. There are two types of misclassification: false negatives and false positives. A false negative represents the misclassification of malicious samples as benign. False negatives are unacceptable from the perspective of system protection, and thus, false negatives must be reduced. A false positive represents the misclassification of benign samples as malicious. If false positives increase, the number of alerts reported by the detection system increases. Thus, someone must confirm whether the alert is true. False negatives and false positives must be balanced. To seamlessly use machine learning, this balance must be tuned.

3.4 Enhanced Protection and Real-World Threats

To achieve enhanced protection, behavior-based detection methods have been developed. The method monitors user behavior on the system, such as the creation or deletion of a file, installation of an application, and configuration of a system setting. By monitoring behavior on the system, malicious behaviors launched by malware can be detected. Recently, a high-functioning monitoring system called *endpoint detection and response (EDR)* has been developed, which is often integrated with an operating system. The EDR service collects the information about the user's operation and sends the collected information to the security operation center. By combining the IDS based on signatures or anomaly detection and EDR, the security of the internal network is enhanced.

Because adversaries try to defend existing protection methods, a novel attack scheme cannot be detected by the equipped detector. Ransomware has been a critical threat to medical systems for the past few years. Ransomware encrypts the data in the system, making it unusable, and asks the user for a ransom. Such ransomware can be countered by inspecting suspicious attachments in emails, detecting signatures that are specific to ransomware based on executable files, and detecting massive data rewriting operations. However, adversaries attempt to evade such detection mechanisms by marginally changing the internal parameters of the executable file. To protect the system from novel attack scheme, maintaining latest detection rules and signatures is critical.

4 Supply Chain Risks

Most medical systems are implemented across numerous electronic devices, which are assembled through a complex supply chain. This section presents the threats regarding the supply chain of electronic devices from the hardware and software perspective.

4.1 Hardware-Level Risks

One electronic device product is composed of numerous hardware elements, including integrated circuits (ICs), radio-frequency (RF) modules, and other circuit elements. Due to the complex supply chain of electronic devices, the risks of malicious

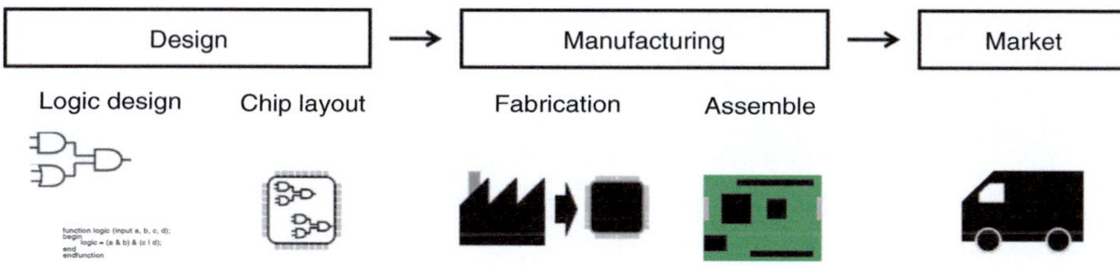

Fig. 4 Overview of the hardware supply chain

hardware have been pointed out [12]. Figure 4 shows an overview of the hardware supply chain, which can be roughly divided into three phases: the design, manufacturing, and marketing phases. Many companies may be involved in the supply chain. In the design phase, the logic design is described in hardware description language (HDL), which is a type of programming language. Frequently used circuits, such as processors and communication interfaces, are provided as a module called intellectual property (IP) by third-party vendors. If the third-party vendor is not trusted, such modules may be infested with malicious circuits called hardware Trojans (HTs). Due to overwhelming price competition, unstable supply of materials, and internationalization of the hardware supply chain, this scenario is somewhat realistic.

An HT is deactivated in an ordinal case to evade testing or to avoid being noticed by users. The malicious function in an HT will be activated when the trigger condition that is configured by an adversary is satisfied. The malicious function of HTs may leak internal information, degrade performance, or suspend IC operation. Adversaries would likely aim to steal confidential information, discredit a target vendor, or disrupt infrastructure facilities.

All components in an electronic device should thus be securely manufactured. Several methods for detecting such malicious circuits have been developed [13]. These detection methods are performed during the design or manufacturing phase. In the design phase, the hardware design is analyzed based on the structural feature of the circuit or simulation using the test inputs. In the manufacturing phase, the manufactured circuit is analyzed using side-channel analysis, including the monitoring method of consuming power or electromagnetic waveform, or is verified in terms of whether the circuit operates correctly according to the specification. Machine learning is often used in these detection methods [14]. Although the detection methods were developed, complete elimination of malicious circuits is impossible. To mitigate the threats of HTs, using products from trusted vendors for security-sensitive systems is recommended.

Security risks in hardware devices have been emphasized in recent years. As discussed above, the detection of malicious functions from a manufactured hardware device is difficult. From the perspective of users of medical system, it is important to carefully verify the reliability of the product vendor and the components used in the product.

4.2 Software-Level Risks

Electronic devices are often controlled by software that can be flexibly configured after manufacturing. There are several levels of software, such as firmware, operating system, and application. The most important process is to ensure that all software has been updated to its latest version.

Software applications often support automatic updating. It is useful for users to maintain the latest application without users' interaction. However, skillful adversaries may exploit the automatic updating scheme and can inject malware into the target system. In this case, traffic may not be dropped by detection systems because the communication channel is registered as benign in an ordinal case. To protect the system from such a case, behavior-based detection scheme effectively works.

Cybersecurity vulnerabilities are reported as common vulnerabilities and exposures (CVEs).[4] The number of reported CVEs is increasing each year. Even if a computer is provided by a reliable vendor, any potential system vulnerabilities due to bugs in development and unintended run-time errors can occur. Thus, most vendors provide software updates that fix security holes if a vulnerability is found and could pose a serious threat to the product. From the perspective of users, it is important to apply the provided update to the relevant product. To ensure that the software version is updated when needed, regular (e.g., monthly) maintenance is effective.

Free software programs and unknown open-source programs should be used carefully. If it is necessary to use them, the sandbox provides a disposable environment that is separated from the host system. Suspicious software can be operated in the sandbox and verified if any harmful behavior occurs. Even if the software maliciously behaves, the operation does not affect the system outside of the sandbox environment.

To protect from software-level risks, it is important to use security protection services, such as a traffic monitoring service and a behavior-monitoring service. Also, regularly maintaining the latest protection service is important.

5 Conclusion

This chapter provides an overview of the cybersecurity surrounding the medical environment. First, the secure data management for protecting the exchanging messages is presented in Sect. 2. There are several cryptographic algorithms, and it is better to choose an appropriate algorithm depending on the required application. Second, anomaly detection to protect from invaders is presented in Sect. 3. There are several detection methods, and machine learning is being applied to detection mechanisms. Finally, the risks in the supply chain of medical equipment are

[4] The website is available in https://www.cve.org/.

presented in Sect. 4. To mitigate security risks, choosing trusted vendors and maintaining the latest software versions are critical.

Security is a continuous game in which adversaries try to defeat defenders with new attack schemes and defenders try to defeat such attacks. From the perspective of developers or managers of medical systems, using products from trusted vendors, monitoring security-related trends, and following security recommendations are important precautions.

References

1. ISO. ISO/IEC 27000:2018. https://www.iso.org/standard/73906.html. 2018.
2. Schneier B. Applied cryptography: protocols, algorithms and source code in C. Wiley; 1996.
3. Dworkin M, Barker E, Nechvatal J, Foti J, Bassham L, Roback E, Dray J. Advanced encryption standard (AES). 2001.
4. Perlman R. An overview of PKI trust models. IEEE Netw. 1999;13:38–43.
5. Chenthara S, Ahmed K, Wang H, Whittaker F. Security and privacy-preserving challenges of e-health solutions in cloud computing. IEEE Access. 2019;7:74361–82.
6. Munjal K, Bhatia R. A systematic review of homomorphic encryption and its contributions in healthcare industry. Complex Intell. Syst. 2023;9:3759–86.
7. Johnson CW. Barriers to the use of intrusion detection systems in safety- critical applications. In: International Conference on Computer Safety, Reliability, and Security; 2015.
8. Prandl S, Lazarescu M, Pham DS. A study of web application fire- wall solutions. In: Jajoda S, Mazumdar C, editors. Information systems security. Cham: Springer; 2015. p. 501–10.
9. Xu C, Chen S, Su J, Yiu SM, Hui LCK. A survey on regular expression matching for deep packet inspection: applications, algorithms, and hardware platforms. IEEE Commun Surv Tutor. 2016;18:2991–3029.
10. Ben-Gal I. Outlier detection. Springer; 2005.
11. Laskov P, Düssel P, Schäfer C, Rieck K. Learning intrusion detection—supervised or unsupervised? In: Image analysis and processing (ICIAP 2005); 2005. p. 50–7.
12. Xiao K, Forte D, Jin Y, Karri R, Bhunia S, Tehranipoor M. Hardware Trojans: lessons learned after one decade of research. ACM Trans Des Autom Electron Syst. 2016;22
13. Jain A, Zhou Z, Guin U. Survey of recent developments for hardware Trojan detection. In: Proceedings of IEEE international symposium on circuits and systems (ISCAS); 2021. p. 1–5.
14. Huang Z, Wang Q, Chen Y, Jiang X. A survey on machine learning against hardware Trojan attacks: recent advances and challenges. IEEE Access. 2020;8:10796–826.

Clinical Case: Neurosurgery

Manabu Tamura, Yutaka Matsui, and Yoshihiro Muragaki

Abstract With the advent of deep learning, the development of artificial intelligence (AI) in the medical field has been rapid. In this chapter, a clinical case in the field of neurosurgery is investigated, i.e., the applications of AI in neurosurgery and image diagnosis are introduced, and prospects for both fields are predicted.

In neurosurgery, navigation systems which project the location of surgical tools to pre- or intraoperative MRI or CT are useful in facilitating tumor removal. In the navigation systems, AI is used for detecting the treatment site and type of surgical tool from the microscopic image and identifying the surgical process in the navigation system.

In the image diagnosis, AI is used for tumor segmentation and predicting molecular diagnosis from preoperative MRI. In glioma resection, treatment strategy is depending on their molecular subtype. However, biopsy or surgery is needed to diagnose them.

Keywords Neurosurgery · Glioma · Deep learning · Brain mapping · Radiogenomics

M. Tamura (✉)
Faculty of Advanced Techno-Surgery, Institute of Advanced Biomedical Engineering and Science, Tokyo Women's Medical University, Tokyo, Japan

Department of Neurosurgery, Tokyo Women's Medical University, Tokyo, Japan
e-mail: tamura.manabu@twmu.ac.jp

Y. Matsui
Faculty of Advanced Techno-Surgery, Institute of Advanced Biomedical Engineering and Science, Tokyo Women's Medical University, Tokyo, Japan

Y. Muragaki
Tokyo Women's Medical University, Tokyo, Japan
e-mail: tamura.manabu@twmu.ac.jp

K. Masamune et al. (eds.), *Artificial Intelligence in Surgery*,
https://doi.org/10.1007/978-981-96-6635-5_8

1 AI-Powered Medical System

The policy of companies to actively engage in research and development in the medical field has been accelerating for the past 10 years. With regard to appealing points in research and development, there are conspicuous proposals to push the use of AI to the forefront and actively utilize it. The government also presented 25 mission target examples in the "Moonshot Research and Development Program" [1], and the "Development of an AI & robot system that autonomously discovers the Nobel Prize by 2050" was nominated. The aim is to research and develop in such a way that the era in which AI and robot systems autonomously discover the Nobel Prize for humans will be reached in 30 years. Many companies in the medical field refer to these trends worldwide.

Regarding the utilization of medical data, the Nihon Keizai Shimbun, on July 9, 2019, is described as follows: "The Next Generation Medical Infrastructure Law was enacted in May 2018, which allows nationally certified businesses to collect and anonymize medical data and provide it to universities and pharmaceutical companies without the refusal of patients. However, there is a shortage of human resources who can collect medical data, anonymize, and analyze big data; therefore, we will develop human resources with the university selected by the Ministry of Education, Culture, Sports, Science, and Technology as leader of the analysis. The most effective treatment methods and drugs may be studied depending on the patient's age, gender, and symptoms. Computed tomography (CT) image data are analyzed using AI to analyze cancer. It is also expected to lead to early detection."

In this way, we introduce the current situation in which research and development that utilize AI have deeply penetrated medical systems and data. In the next section, following the AI classification, we add explain examples of AI utilization initiatives in the field of neurosurgery.

2 Classification and Application of AI

2.1 Artificial General Intelligence (AGI) and Artificial Narrow Intelligence (ANI)

Artificial general intelligence (AGI) is AI that performs intelligent (human-like) processing in all areas. Although it is predicted that it will be created in the distant future, many people think that it is difficult. The reason is that the data that should be the correct answer are not accurate (classification and name may differ depending on the occupation; and, in pathological diagnosis, the result may differ depending on the biopsy site, time, and collection environment). First, the medical diagnosis itself (such as hyperactivity) may be difficult, and big data that should be the basis of AGI do not yet exist. When making a hypothesis that AGI predicts human thoughts, it is an unsolved problem of how to reflect 70% of thoughts that are not verbalized and how the computer predicts AGI. For a medical diagnosis, it is clearly stated that the doctor (human) is responsible for the final diagnosis, and AI assists the diagnosis; thus, the aforementioned AGI is not universal, at least in the medical field.

However, ANI exerts its abilities only in a specific area, and almost all of AI in the world refers to ANI. This chapter is also limited to ANI and explains the AI used in the field of neurosurgery.

2.2 *ANI and Machine Learning (ML)*

To achieve narrow AI, the core technology is machine learning (ML). ML is a data analysis method that allows computers to learn rules and patterns behind the data. It differs from conventional programs in which the rules are written by humans. A computer defines its own rules and processes information, making it appear as if the computer has knowledge. Studies on ML have been conducted for more than 50 years, and various algorithms have been proposed in the meanwhile. Currently, deep learning is the most promising approach.

2.3 *Deep Learning (DL)*

Deep learning (DL) is a ML method that uses a multilayered neural network (deep neural network) model. The key feature of DL is "representation learning," which extracts effective features for performing tasks from higher-dimensional data, such as images, sounds, natural language, and time-series signals. "Representation learning" is expected to enable computers to recognize minute features, which humans cannot do, by processing higher-dimensional signals through neural networks without the need for human knowledge.

In particular, image recognition using DL is promising in the field of medicine, where various images are used, such as radiological, pathological, and endoscopic images. DL, which is widely used in image recognition, is a convolutional neural network (CNN). A CNN repeats the processing that compresses features in local regions of an image with filters, transfers them as feature maps to the next layers, and, finally, extracts features from images. A CNN was first used in LeNet [2] proposed by Yan LeCun in 1999. LeNet is a ML model that consists of three convolutional layers and two fully connected layers; it is a true original CNN. Subsequently, in 2012, AlexNet [3] developed by a University of Toronto team led by Geffery Hinton won the ImageNet Large Scale Visual Recognition Challenge (ILSVRC) by a wide margin over the scale-invariant feature transform (SIFT) + Fisher Vector + Support Vector Machine (SVM) that had been the de facto standard up to that time. This has brought DL into the spotlight. Since the release of AlexNet, studies on DL have progressed rapidly, and ILSVRC scores have continued to be updated annually.

3 Neurosurgery and AI

3.1 Narrow and Deep Microscopic View in Neurosurgery

Taking the case of neurosurgical tumor resection as an example, the dura mater surrounding the brain can finally be visualized by opening a part of the skull; the dura mater and arachnoid incision expose the brain surface. Since the cerebral blood vessels are very thin and it is difficult to distinguish the boundary between the tumor and normal brain tissue with the naked eye, the tumor was identified and removed in a narrow and deep field of view after preparing an operating microscope. The surgeon and his assistant were forced to move their hands in a narrow space for a long time, and other doctors and surgical staff viewed the images on the microscope monitor installed in the operating room to oversee the surgery. It is clear that neurosurgery is backed by the experience of the surgeon, and the doctors and operating room staff around him attempted to overcome the difficulties and smoothly manage the surgery.

An innovative neurosurgical technology developed in recent years is the navigation system, which projects the position of the surgical instrument using magnetic resonance imaging (MRI)/CT performed before or during surgery. Navigation is extremely important for surgeons to facilitate tumor removal, just as it is indispensable for driving a car. A navigation system that promptly updates MR images localizes accurately the surgeon's procedure for tumor removal and helps understand the position of the surgical area has been implemented; thus, it facilitates groundbreaking precision-guided surgery. This technique combined with intraoperative MRI has the potential to provide maximum tumor resection, reduce the intraoperative residual tumor, and prolong the patient survival rate [4]. By applying a navigation system using intraoperative MRI, research using AI is also being conducted for the aforementioned technical learning of skilled neurosurgeons and smooth operation of the operating room, including the operating surgical staff(Fig. 1) [5].

The developed system is for surgical process identification computers to acquire information from MRI images, navigation logs, and microscopic images and to automatically grasp the flow of surgery during and after the process. It consists of a monitor that presents information such as the flow of surgery and the next process for surgeons, young doctors, and surgical staff [5].

In the information sharing system shown in Fig. 1, AI is implemented to identify the surgical process by acquiring elements from multiple medical information (preoperative and intraoperative MRI images, surgical navigation system, and microscopic images) in information processing technology, such as ML. Regarding the elements of the surgical process, the surgeon acquires two points, i.e., the intraoperative treatment site and type of surgical tool used, from image processing and DL, as well as ML that is used to identify the process based on the surgical process model. This method consists of two major processes. First, feature extraction is performed using ML, and then, identification is performed based on the process model from the acquired information.

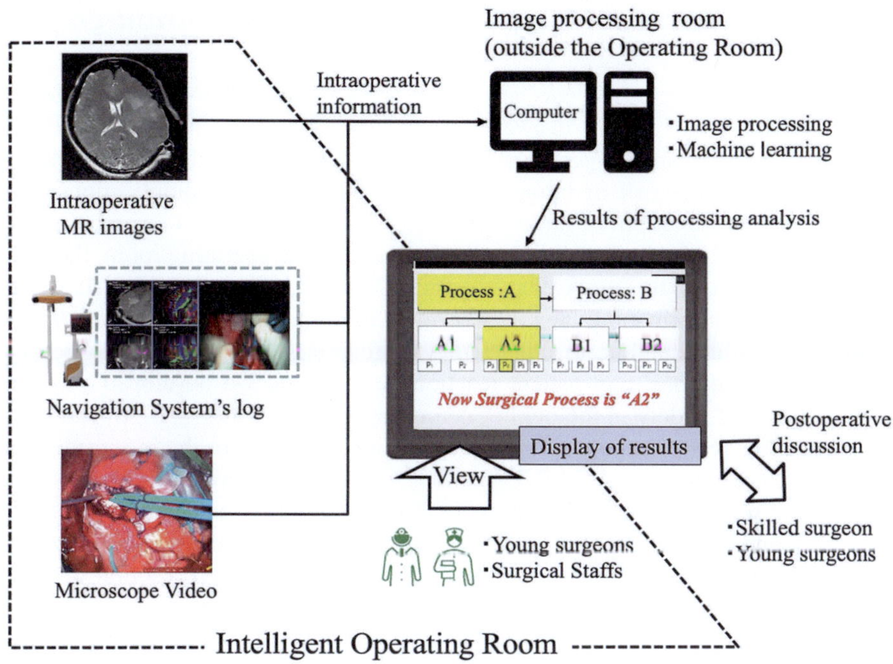

Fig. 1 Information sharing concept of intelligent operating room (neurosurgery)

In feature extraction, the type of surgical instrument used by the surgeon and treatment site are identified by image processing, and the four treatment sites are defined as "brain surface," "inside tumor," "nearby normal tissue," and "outside surgical field." To specify the brain region, a labeled segmentation image was created in image processing. Then the features of the surgical instrument were extracted together with the log information of the surgical instrument tip position data acquired from the surgical navigation system. In addition, the type of surgical instrument is obtained from the microscopic image using the learning dataset created in advance using the DL method You Only Look Once (YOLO) [6].

In identification, the two types of information (position and type of surgical instrument) are integrated and saved as time-series feature data every second for input information; the surgical process is identified by the hierarchical hidden Markov model (HHMM), which is tailored to the hierarchical model. The adopted HHMM is expected to be a high-speed ML method that considers real-time performance [7]. The identification was conducted from the first layer defined in the surgical process model to the third layer in order; the Viterbi algorithm that reduces the amount of calculation was adopted, and the surgical process with the highest probability was calculated as the outcome.

3.2 Brain Functional Mapping Process During Neurosurgery

In the previous section, ANI was used for process identification using a model for awake surgery as an example. In awake surgery, a brain function examination (called brain function mapping) is performed on the brain surface and the area around the tumor to reduce the risk of intraoperative and postoperative complications (language and/or dysfunction) of tumor removal.

From the analog information recorded by video in the operating room, the position information of the probe that electrically stimulated the brain surface was recorded as log information; then, it was stored as digital information consisting of brain function information, together with examination task information, electrical stimulation conditions, and patient reaction information. We developed a system that can be used widely in the field of neurosurgery(shown in Fig. 2). Specifically, an antenna device was attached to the electrical stimulation probe in a navigation system (manufactured by BRAINLAB) that reads intraoperative MR images. The images and position information are read through the image analysis software 3D Slicer [8], and the position of the electrical stimulator is acquired as log information and digitized to create a brain function database. This digitized reaction point on intraoperative MRI (right upper part of Fig. 2) was image-converted and normalized on a normalized brain [9] (left lower part of Fig. 2) using SPM12. Non-rigid registration [10] and SPM12 [11] were used for coordinate transformation of response

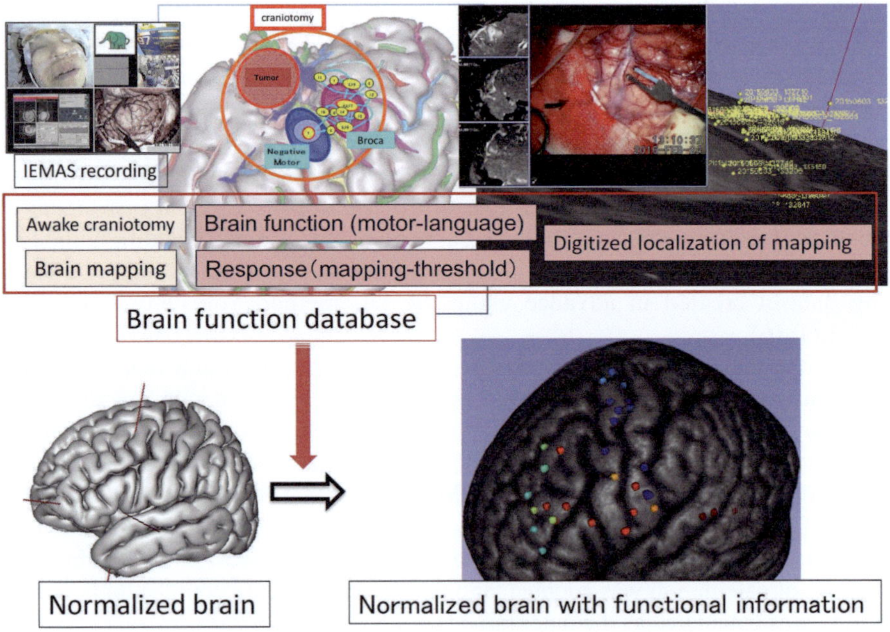

Fig. 2 Digitized brain-mapping data transformation on normalized brain

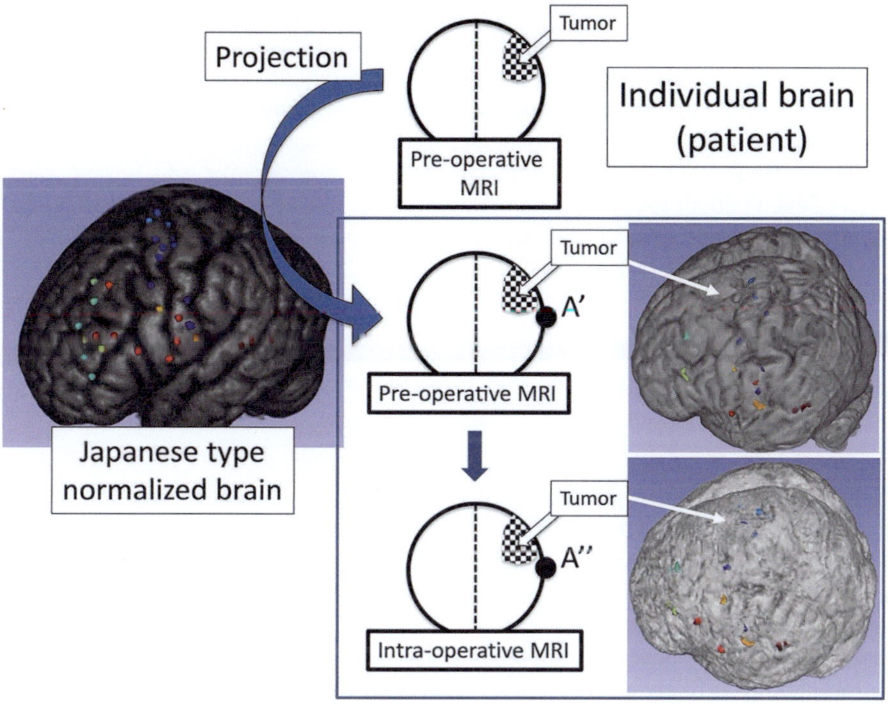

Fig. 3 Projection of brain function onto patient's intraoperative MRI

points. Finally, the brain function response points of multiple cases were aggregated as position information on the normalized brain. These multiple response points provide useful suggestions for estimating brain functions (motor, language, higher brain function, etc.). Thus, a normalized brain with useful information such as tasks presented by the task examiner (picture naming, verb generation, counting, kanji/hiragana reading, calculation), electrical stimulation intensity, threshold value, and so on (right lower part of Fig. 2) is worthy of attention.

The electrical stimulation site during brain function mapping was recorded at the intraoperative MRI position during navigation, and the digitized position information was converted into the standard brain together with the brain function information and stimulation threshold [12].

The normalized brain with the aforementioned brain function information (called the normalized brain function atlas) also adds digital information other than brain function (i.e., pathological findings, postoperative dysfunction, postoperative treatment, treatment results, recurrence rate, and survival rate). Additionally, image conversion (reverse conversion to the procedure in Fig. 2) was likely performed on the patient's MRI, and the brain function of each patient could be predicted preoperatively or intraoperatively (as shown in Fig. 3). After comparing with the mapping results performed in actual surgery, we have investigated the accuracy of this brain function prediction and aimed to develop an application of the normalized brain function atlas. Compared with the normalized brain, individual patient brain information (postoperative brain deformation, movement/plasticity of functional site at tumor recurrence, and temporal change of pathological image due to change in genetic information) was added to create a database. This database is expected to accelerate research and development using ANI as a means of using training data.

The normalized brain was projected onto the preoperative and intraoperative MRI of each patient to predict preoperative and intraoperative functional sites. This information was compared with the actual intraoperative mapping record to verify the accuracy [12].

3.3 *Future of Neurosurgery: Postoperative Prediction Using Intraoperative AI*

In brain tumor treatment, the tumor removal rate, motor/language function complication rate, and higher brain function evaluation that affects rehabilitation impact the patient's postoperative life. When a preoperative image is created by projecting the created normalized brain function atlas onto the brain of each patient according to Fig. 3, it is expected to reflect on the survival curve according to the extent of resection and make postoperative predictions (shown in Fig. 4) [13]. In this case, the brain function is likely arranged in a map such as A to D on the 3D mesh image of the brain surface of the individual patient. The survival rate increases according to

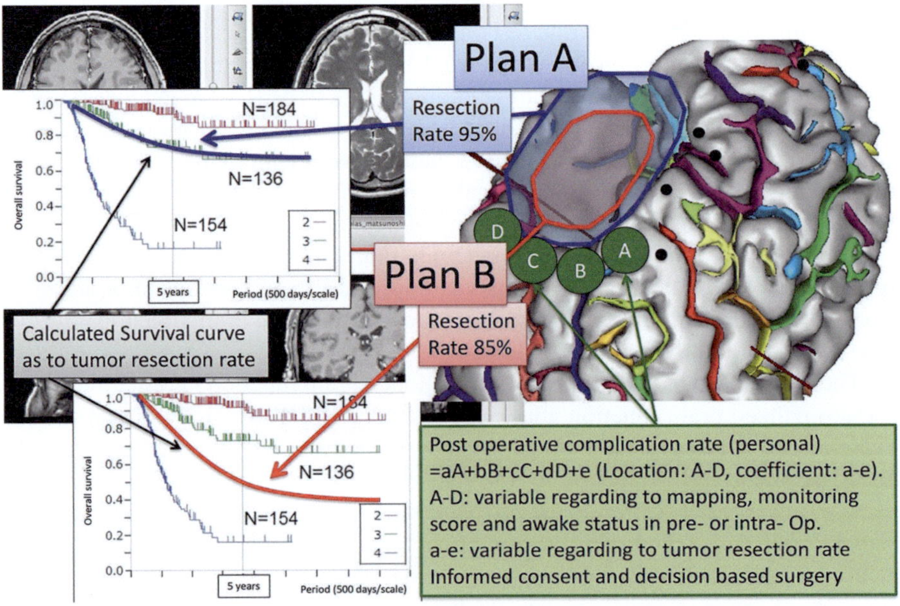

Fig. 4 Predictive neurosurgery

the tumor removal rate, but the probability of postoperative complications increases as well. The survival rate and complication rate of patients are modified based on treatment results of the hospital where the surgery is performed and the malignancy of the removed tumor; further, the malignancy of the removed tumor, treatment results at the hospital facility, and results of postoperative rehabilitation are used as a database. If postoperative predictions by AI analysis become routine, preoperative explanations for individual patients will become considerably more accurate in the future.

If data analysis by ANI develops, it will be possible to revise the intraoperative treatment policy based on intraoperative pathological findings, functional mapping results, tumor resection, and so on while assuming preoperative prediction, as described above. The analysis of electronic medical record data accumulated in hospital facilities and the presentation of information to surgeons based on monitoring results of function mapping updated in real time could provide proposals for advanced intraoperative treatment to minimize postoperative recurrence and prolong life prognosis. Furthermore, it is predicted that the time will come when each patient will be presented in real time, such as proposals for higher brain function recovery and maintenance programs, as well as motor language function recovery and maintenance programs to facilitate postoperative social recovery.

Preoperative survival is estimated from the tumor removal rate, and the probability of postoperative complications predicted from the brain function atlas is estimated. Patients will be provided with specific information while referring to the presentation of similar cases by AI, including postoperative therapy and rehabilitation [13].

4 Glioma Diagnostic Imaging and AI

In the field of neurosurgery, many studies on MRI using DL, such as brain tumor segmentation, prediction of glioma grading according to the World Health Organization (WHO) classification, and molecular diagnosis, have been reported. The glioma grade and molecular subtype provide important information for treatment strategies. However, biopsy or surgery is required to diagnose this condition. Therefore, it is beneficial to predict these factors using MRI before surgery. Many studies have applied other ML methods, such as SVM or random forest to MRI imaging, but this chapter focuses only on DL.

4.1 Dataset

The datasets of the Brain Tumor Segmentation (BraTS) Challenge provided by the Medical Image Computing and Computer Assisted Interventions (MICCAI) society are often used in studies of ML related to gliomas. They consist of four modalities, native (T1), post-contrast T1-weighted (T1Gd), T2-weighted (T2), and T2 fluid-attenuated inversion recovery (FLAIR) volumes, and include hundreds of glioma cases. Furthermore, they have a segmentation mask of tumor regions and labels for grade IV glioblastoma (GBM) in the WHO classification and lower-grade glioma (LGG) of grades II and III. For molecular diagnosis prediction, imaging data from the BraTS or Cancer Imaging Archive (TCIA) are often combined with genomic information from The Cancer Genome Atlas (TCGA), or in-house data are used.

4.2 Evaluation Methodology

The holdout method is used for the evaluation of DL models, where test data are reserved in advance; the model is trained with the remaining data and then evaluated with the test data and cross-validation method, where all data are divided into several groups for training and evaluation. The holdout method is effective in the case of sufficient (tens of thousands) data to save training and evaluation time. However, for datasets of hundreds to thousands of cases, the evaluation results may vary significantly depending on the selection of test data. The cross-validation method, which evaluates all data, is more reliable even for a small dataset because the effect of data selection in each group on the final result is small. Nevertheless, in the case of big data, it takes too long for training and evaluation.

4.3 Brain Tumor Segmentation

In an early study using CNNs for brain tumor segmentation in MR images, Havaei et al. built a CNN-based segmentation model for the BraTS 2013 dataset and achieved Dice scores of 0.88, 0.79, and 0.73 for complete, core, and enhancing regions, respectively [14]. Their model was optimized for brain tumor segmentation using two paths that analyzed the visual details of the region around that pixel and its larger context. Furthermore, as a method to correctly train the model on extremely imbalanced data (where 98% of the pixels were normal tissue), they used two-phase training, i.e., the entire model was trained with label-balanced batches, and then only the output layer was trained with the actual label distribution.

The innovation in the network model for the segmentation task is U-Net [15]. U-Net is a CNN-based network that consists of encoders and decoders; it has the "connection path" that connects the encoders to decoders directly. In the field of neurosurgery, Dong et al. implemented segmentation using a 2D U-Net model and achieved Dice scores of 0.86, 0.86, and 0.65 [16]. U-Net has been the de facto standard of ML models for segmentation and has been used in recent studies [17–19].

4.4 Prediction of Glioma Grading in WHO Classification

In an early study of glioma grading prediction, Yuehao et al. improved the accuracy by 18% in the GBM and LGG classification of the BraTS 2014 dataset with three convolutional layers [20]. Although the BraTS 2014 dataset had 195 cases, the number of LGG cases was less than 15% of the total, making the prediction difficult. Under these circumstances, CNN achieved higher accuracy than conventional neural networks in ML for MRI.

In BraTS2017, the number of cases increased to 285, imbalance of LGGs improved to 25% of the total, and classification of grading using CNN showed rapid development. Ge et al. achieved an accuracy of 90.87% for GBM and LGG classification [21]. In their study, enhanced T1, T2, and FLAIR images were entered into seven-layered CNN models, and feature maps from all models were concatenated and entered into fully connected layers. In comparison with the models by Yuehao et al., the scale of the network became larger (deeper).

Khan et al. adapted the VGGNet base model for GBM and LGG classification and achieved accuracies of 97.8%, 96.9%, and 92.5% in the BraTS 2015, 2017, and 2018 datasets, respectively [22]. In their method, the contrast of MR images was enhanced with edge-based texture histogram equalization, and transfer learning was used with a pre-trained model of VGG16 and VGG19. Furthermore, the features extracted by the CNN were processed using correntropy via mutual learning and extreme ML, which removed redundancy between features and selected only robust features. Their study implicates recent trends in DL in the medical field, which shifted from improving the network structure to developing the pre-and post-processing stages. Although the state-of-the-art models of image recognition have become increasingly deep, such as AlexNet, VGGNet, and residual neural network (ResNet), they were too deep to train with good generalizability in the field where it was difficult to collect a large amount of data. Therefore, recent studies have often used pre-trained models with a moderate number of CNN layers.

4.5 Prediction of Glioma Molecular Diagnosis

LGGs are classified into three molecular subtypes based on the presence of mutations in the isocitrate dehydrogenase (IDH) gene and co-deletion of chromosome arms 1p and 19q (1p/19q). Oligodendrogliomas are defined by the presence of an IDH mutation and a 1p/19q co-deletion. Astrocytomas without 1p/19q co-deletion are classified as IDH-wild-type or IDH-mutant diffuse astrocytomas, depending on the IDH genotype. The prognosis for LGG patients and recurrence patterns vary depending on the molecular subtype; therefore, tumor extraction strategies are different [23, 24].

Matsui et al. achieved an accuracy of 68.7% in the classification of molecular subtypes of LGGs using in-house data [25]. In this study, factors effective in LGG molecular subtype classification, such as T2-FLAIR mismatch [26, 27], the tumor-to-normal ratio of methionine positron emission tomography (PET) [28, 29], and calcification in CT images [30], were entered into fully connected layers in addition to feature maps of image data from CNN outputs. Furthermore, this model classified three molecular subtypes directly to make effective use of model performance; in contrast, conventional studies [31] followed clinical protocols that diagnose IDH mutations and 1p/19q co-deletions.

In a recent study on the classification of molecular subtypes, Li et al. predicted classification of grading (GBM or LGG), IDH mutation of LGG, 1p/19q co-deletion of LGG, and IDH mutation of GBM and achieved accuracies of 89%, 80%, 83%, and 74%, respectively [32]. In their study, the models were designed to predict sequentially from grading to each molecular diagnosis, which was similar to the clinical flow. In particular, IDH mutations should be predicted in GBM and LGG separately because the IDH gene in GBM is biased toward the wild type.

4.6 Prospects of AI Image Diagnosis

In most studies on radiological image analysis of glioma, the state-of-the-art ML model has been implemented with a delay of approximately 3 years. Based on this, it can be predicted that "self-attention" and "contrastive learning" are two of the most important methods in this field.

Self-attention is a DL model that has been proposed for natural language processing and recently been applied to image recognition. In contrast to the CNN process of the relationship between a pixel and a limited area around it, self-attention uses the relationship between a pixel and the entire image to extract features. Furthermore, in contrast to CNNs, where the weights of the weighted sums are fixed, self-attention allows for highly flexible feature extraction because the weights change for each pixel. With regard to the application of self-attention to image recognition, there are many possible models, such as a hybrid of self-attention and CNN, named CoAtNet [33], that has CNN and self-attention blocks.

Contrastive learning is a self-supervised learning method for learning a large amount of data without labeling by comparing and classifying them based on their similarity. In fields such as medical data, where it is difficult to collect a large amount of datasets and specialized knowledge and analysis are required to create correct labels, it is advantageous to make the best use of collected data without labeling. SimCLR [34] is a typical contrastive learning method.

5 AI with Society (Limitations/Future Implications)

Although it is predicted that the AGI mentioned above will be a future story, there is already a society in which ANI surpasses human thinking. Currently, it may be far from the time when AGI can diagnose beyond humans and replace mainstream surgical treatment. Furthermore, the recipients of surgical treatment are humans, and the goals of treatment vary among individuals. People have different values and thoughts in their social lives, and it seems difficult to make treatment decisions based on a uniform rule. Naturally, medical treatment is aimed at treating diseases, and ANI that surpasses human thinking always supports surgical treatment; still, doctors' unwavering diagnosis and treatment, as well as maximum patient satisfaction, are expected.

Acknowledgments This research was supported by JSPS Grant-in-Aid for Scientific Research (grant number C-19 K12845), NICT (National Institute of Information and Communications, grant number 22009), and AMED (grant number JP21he1602003).

References

1. Cabinet Office J: About moonshot research and development program. https://www8.cao.go.jp/cstp/english/moonshot/system_en.html; 2019. Access.
2. LeCun Y, Haffner P, Bottou L, Bengio Y. Object recognition with gradient-based learning. Shape, contour and grouping in computer vision. Springer; 1999. p. 319–45.
3. Krizhevsky A, Sutskever I, Hinton GE. Imagenet classification with deep convolutional neural networks. Adv Neural Inf Proces Syst. 2012;25
4. Nitta M, Muragaki Y, Maruyama T, Ikuta S, Komori T, Maebayashi K, et al. Proposed therapeutic strategy for adult low-grade glioma based on aggressive tumor resection. Neurosurg Focus. 2015;38(1):E7. https://doi.org/10.3171/2014.10.FOCUS14651.
5. Nagai T, Sato I, Fujino Y, Tamura M, Muragaki Y, Masamune K. Surgical process identification system using machine learning in awake surgery for brain tumor. 2019 IEEE 1st Global Conference on Life Sciences and Technologies (LifeTech). 2019;
6. Redmon J, Divvala S, Girshick R, Farhadi A. You only look once: unified, real-time object detection. 2016 IEEE Conference on Computer Vision and Pattern Recognition (CVPR). 2016:779–88.
7. Panzner M, Cimiano P. Comparing hidden Markov models and long short term memory neural networks for learning action representations. Cham: Springer; 2016. p. 94–105.
8. https://www.slicer.org: 3D Slicer. Accessed.
9. http://www.bic.mni.mcgill.ca/ServicesAtlases/ICBM152NLin2009: The McConnell Brain Imaging Centre. Accessed.
10. Liu Y, Kot A, Drakopoulos F, Yao C, Fedorov A, Enquobahrie A, et al. An ITK implementation of a physics-based non-rigid registration method for brain deformation in image-guided neurosurgery. Front Neuroinform. 2014;8:33. https://doi.org/10.3389/fninf.2014.00033.
11. http://www.fil.ion.ucl.ac.uk/spm/: Statistical Parametric Mapping (SPM). Accessed.
12. Tamura M, Sato I, Maruyama T, Ohshima K, Mangin JF, Nitta M, et al. Integrated datasets of normalized brain with functional localization using intra-operative electrical stimulation. Int J Comput Assist Radiol Surg. 2019;14(12):2109–22. https://doi.org/10.1007/s11548-019-01957-7.

13. Tamura M, Mangin J-F, Muragaki Y. New approach of MRI sulci analysis to multidisciplinary computational anatomy. Cell. 2018;50(1):19–23.
14. Havaei M, Davy A, Warde-Farley D, Biard A, Courville A, Bengio Y, et al. Brain tumor segmentation with deep neural networks. Med Image Anal. 2017;35:18–31. https://doi.org/10.1016/j.media.2016.05.004.
15. Ronneberger O, Fischer P, Brox T. U-net: convolutional networks for biomedical image segmentation. Cham: Springer; 2015. p. 234–41.
16. Dong H, Yang G, Liu F, Mo Y, Guo Y. Automatic brain tumor detection and segmentation using U-net based fully convolutional networks. Cham: Springer; 2017. p. 506–17.
17. Ilhan A, Sekeroglu B, Abiyev R. Brain tumor segmentation in MRI images using nonparametric localization and enhancement methods with U-net. Int J Comput Assist Radiol Surg. 2022; https://doi.org/10.1007/s11548-022-02566-7.
18. Qin C, Wu Y, Liao W, Zeng J, Liang S, Zhang X. Improved U-Net3+ with stage residual for brain tumor segmentation. BMC Med Imaging. 2022;22(1):14. https://doi.org/10.1186/s12880-022-00738-0.
19. Chetty G, Yamin M, White M. A low resource 3D U-net based deep learning model for medical image analysis. Int J Inf Technol. 2022; https://doi.org/10.1007/s41870-021-00850-4.
20. Yuehao P, Weimin H, Zhiping L, Wanzheng Z, Jiayin Z, Wong J, et al. Brain tumor grading based on neural networks and convolutional neural networks. Annu Int Conf IEEE Eng Med Biol Soc. 2015;2015:699–702. https://doi.org/10.1109/embc.2015.7318458.
21. Ge C, Gu IY, Jakola AS, Yang J. Deep learning and multi-sensor fusion for glioma classification using multistream 2D convolutional networks. Annu Int Conf IEEE Eng Med Biol Soc. 2018;2018:5894–7. https://doi.org/10.1109/embc.2018.8513556.
22. Khan MA, Ashraf I, Alhaisoni M, Damaševičius R, Scherer R, Rehman A, et al. Multimodal brain tumor classification using deep learning and robust feature selection: a machine learning application for radiologists. Diagnostics. 2020;10(8) https://doi.org/10.3390/diagnostics10080565.
23. Fukuya Y, Ikuta S, Maruyama T, Nitta M, Saito T, Tsuzuki S, et al. Tumor recurrence patterns after surgical resection of intracranial low-grade gliomas. J Neuro-Oncol. 2019;144(3):519–28. https://doi.org/10.1007/s11060-019-03250-8.
24. Koriyama S, Nitta M, Kobayashi T, Muragaki Y, Suzuki A, Maruyama T, et al. A surgical strategy for lower grade gliomas using intraoperative molecular diagnosis. Brain Tumor Pathol. 2018;35(3):159–67. https://doi.org/10.1007/s10014-018-0324-1.
25. Matsui Y, Maruyama T, Nitta M, Saito T, Tsuzuki S, Tamura M, et al. Prediction of lower-grade glioma molecular subtypes using deep learning. J Neuro-Oncol. 2020;146(2):321–7. https://doi.org/10.1007/s11060-019-03376-9.
26. Patel SH, Poisson LM, Brat DJ, Zhou Y, Cooper L, Snuderl M, et al. T2-FLAIR mismatch, an imaging biomarker for IDH and 1p/19q status in lower-grade gliomas: a TCGA/TCIA project. Clin Cancer Res. 2017;23(20):6078–85. https://doi.org/10.1158/1078-0432.Ccr-17-0560.
27. Broen MPG, Smits M, Wijnenga MMJ, Dubbink HJ, Anten M, Schijns O, et al. The T2-FLAIR mismatch sign as an imaging marker for non-enhancing IDH-mutant, 1p/19q-intact lower-grade glioma: a validation study. Neuro-Oncology. 2018;20(10):1393–9. https://doi.org/10.1093/neuonc/noy048.
28. Takei H, Shinoda J, Ikuta S, Maruyama T, Muragaki Y, Kawasaki T, et al. Usefulness of positron emission tomography for differentiating gliomas according to the 2016 World Health Organization classification of tumors of the central nervous system. J Neurosurg. 2019:1–10. https://doi.org/10.3171/2019.5.Jns19780.
29. Kato T, Shinoda J, Oka N, Miwa K, Nakayama N, Yano H, et al. Analysis of 11C-methionine uptake in low-grade gliomas and correlation with proliferative activity. AJNR Am J Neuroradiol. 2008;29(10):1867–71. https://doi.org/10.3174/ajnr.A1242.
30. Saito T, Muragaki Y, Maruyama T, Komori T, Tamura M, Nitta M, et al. Calcification on CT is a simple and valuable preoperative indicator of 1p/19q loss of heterozygosity in

supratentorial brain tumors that are suspected grade II and III gliomas. Brain Tumor Pathol. 2016;33(3):175–82. https://doi.org/10.1007/s10014-016-0249-5.

31. Lu CF, Hsu FT, Hsieh KL, Kao YJ, Cheng SJ, Hsu JB, et al. Machine learning-based radiomics for molecular subtyping of gliomas. Clin Cancer Res. 2018;24(18):4429–36. https://doi.org/10.1158/1078-0432.CCR-17-3445.
32. Li Y, Wei D, Liu X, Fan X, Wang K, Li S, et al. Molecular subtyping of diffuse gliomas using magnetic resonance imaging: comparison and correlation between radiomics and deep learning. Eur Radiol. 2022;32(2):747–58. https://doi.org/10.1007/s00330-021-08237-6.
33. Dai Z, Liu H, Le Q, Tan M. Coatnet: marrying convolution and attention for all data sizes. Adv Neural Inf Proces Syst. 2021;34
34. Chen T, Kornblith S, Norouzi M, Hinton G. A simple framework for contrastive learning of visual representations. International conference on machine learning: PMLR; 2020. p. 1597–607.

Clinical Case: Cardiac Surgery

Naoki Tomii

Abstract Cardiac diseases are the leading cause of death in several countries. They include not only chronic conditions such as arrhythmias and cardiomyopathies but also acute and serious diseases with cardiovascular events such as myocardial infarction. Considering the importance of cardiac function in maintaining life, early detection of cardiovascular diseases and appropriate diagnosis and treatment greatly affect the prognosis of patients.

In many cases, surgical procedures play an important role in the treatment of cardiac diseases, including urgent cases and those that are non-responsive to medication. In addition to highly invasive cardiac surgeries, such as coronary artery bypass surgery and heart transplantation, which are often performed under open chest conditions, minimally invasive cardiac surgery has been expanding in recent years, with an increase in robotic surgeries and percutaneous interventions using catheters and other devices.

Against this background, there is a growing demand for minimally invasive cardiac imaging that can provide preoperative information on the structure and function of the heart and any associated abnormalities. In the cardiovascular field, as in other medical fields, advances in imaging technology are improving evidence-based treatment decision-making and clinical outcomes. Simultaneously, there are growing expectations for artificial intelligence (AI) and machine learning (ML) approaches to properly and efficiently interpret the ever-increasing volume of clinical data. This chapter describes the major classifications of cardiac diseases and their treatment procedures. Next, each diagnostic modality for cardiac disease is outlined, with examples of recent applications of AI technology to these modalities.

Keywords Cardiac disease · Cardiac surgery · Percutaneous intervention · Cardiac imaging · Artificial intelligence · Machine learning · Deep learning

N. Tomii (✉)
School of Engineering, The University of Tokyo, Tokyo, Japan
e-mail: naoki_tomii@bmpe.t.u-tokyo.ac.jp

K. Masamune et al. (eds.), *Artificial Intelligence in Surgery*,
https://doi.org/10.1007/978-981-96-6635-5_9

1 Cardiac Diseases and Procedures

This section describes the classification of major cardiac diseases and associated non-pharmacological treatments, including percutaneous intervention. Figure 1 shows basic anatomy related to cardiac diseases and surgeries.

1.1 Coronary Artery Disease (CAD)

CAD is an ischemic disease where the coronary artery, which is responsible for blood circulation within the heart itself, is narrowed and the blood supply to the myocardium is disrupted. The narrowing is attributed to atherosclerosis, which is caused by the accumulation of cholesterol and other substances in the inner walls of the coronary arteries. This condition is called angina pectoris before the occurrence of complete stenosis and myocardial infarction (MI) after complete stenosis.

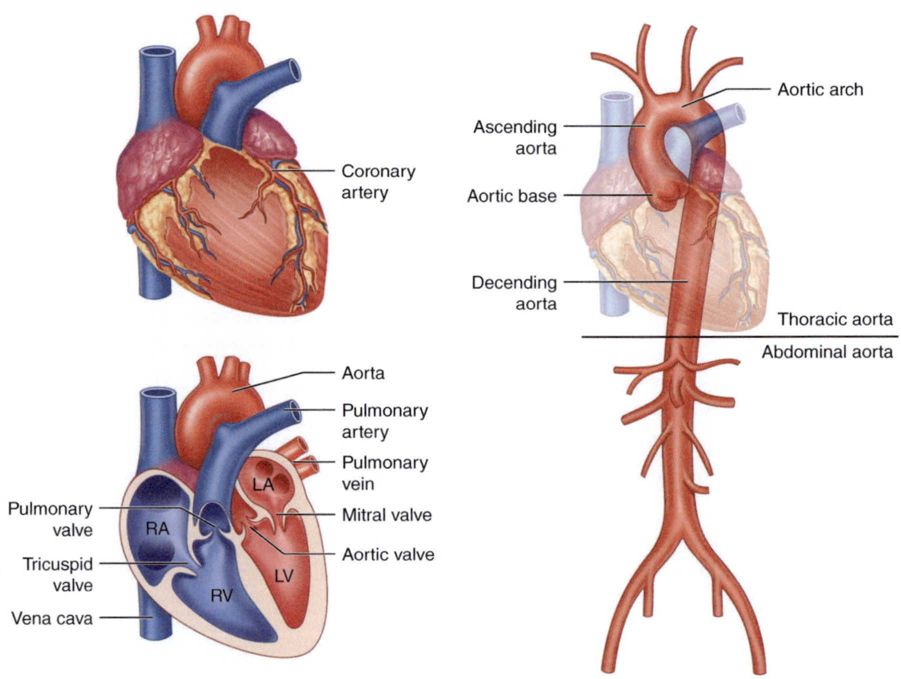

Fig. 1 Basic cardiovascular anatomy

1.1.1 Coronary Artery Bypass Graft (CABG)

CABG is a surgical procedure to bypass blood flow from the aorta to the end of a narrowed coronary artery using grafts obtained from sources such as the great saphenous vein in the leg, internal thoracic artery in the chest, radial artery in the wrist, and gastric aorta in the stomach. Recently, off-pump surgery, which is performed without stopping the heart, and minimally invasive surgery using endoscopes and surgical robots are also being performed.

1.1.2 Percutaneous Coronary Intervention (PCI)

PCI is a treatment to relieve coronary artery stenosis by introducing a catheter into the heart through a blood vessel at the base of the leg, arm, or wrist. A balloon dilatation procedure is performed using a catheter with a balloon attached to its tip to expand the stenosed coronary artery from within. Recently, metal stents have been widely used to prevent postoperative restenosis. The development of drug-eluting stents, in which the surface of the stent is coated with a drug, has reduced the risk of restenosis [1], and PCI has become more widely used in recent years [2, 3].

1.2 Valvular Disease

The heart has four valves: the tricuspid, pulmonary, mitral, and aortic valves, which control blood flow in the heart. Valvular disease is a condition in which these valves malfunction due to congenital (e.g., bicuspid aortic valve) or acquired reasons (e.g., sclerosis and calcification due to aging and infection). Valvular disease is broadly classified as either regurgitation or stenosis. Disorders of the mitral and aortic valves, which are involved in left ventricular blood flow, are more likely surgical targets because of their high risk of causing serious symptoms such as angina pectoris, heart failure, and cerebral infarction due to atrial fibrillation.

1.2.1 Valve Replacement

Replacement of malfunctioning valves with prosthetic valves is a surgical procedure. Prosthetic valves can be broadly classified into mechanical valves made of carbon or other materials and biological valves derived from living tissues. The choice between mechanical and biological valves is based on the safety and durability of blood coagulation.

In the past, most valve replacement procedures were performed under open chest conditions, but recently, transcatheter aortic valve replacement (TAVR), which uses a catheter for minimally invasive replacement of the defective valve with a biological valve, has attracted attention as a minimally invasive valve replacement procedure (also known as transcatheter aortic valve intervention, TAVI) [4].

1.2.2 Valvuloplasty

Prosthetic valves, both biological and mechanical, used in valve replacement surgery have fragility and blood coagulation issues. Valvuloplasty, on the other hand, preserves the patient's valve and restores function by suturing of the valve and surrounding tissue. Valvuloplasty has the advantage of a lower risk of blood coagulation than valve replacement, but also requires a skilled surgeon. The choice of procedure is based on the preoperative and intraoperative diagnosis of the valve.

1.3 Aortic Aneurysm

Aortic aneurysms can be classified into three main types: true aortic aneurysms, in which the arterial wall is normal; dissected aortic aneurysms, in which the arterial wall is detached and a pathway for blood flow called a false lumen is created within the vessel; and pseudoaneurysms, in which the outside of the torn vessel wall undergoes thrombosis and seals the leakage of blood. Aortic aneurysms are primarily caused by atherosclerosis. They are most common in the abdominal and thoracic aortas. Aortic aneurysms due to hereditary Marfan syndrome occur predominantly in the ascending aorta. When an aortic aneurysm ruptures and leaks a large amount of blood, the patient experiences shock and rapidly deterioration leading to death.

1.3.1 Replacement with Vascular Prosthesis

In this procedure, the vessel associated with the aortic aneurysm is replaced with a tubular artificial vessel made of woven chemical fiber. If the aneurysm is at the aortic root and is accompanied by aortic valve regurgitation, in which the aortic valve annulus is enlarged, it may be replaced with an artificial vessel with a valve (Bentall procedure). In most cases, the procedure is performed via open thoracotomy or abdominal surgery.

1.3.2 Endovascular Aortic Repair (EVAR)

EVAR is a procedure used to prevent aortic aneurysm rupture using a stent graft, which is a metal framework attached within an artificial blood vessel. The stent graft is introduced from an artery in the groin to the site of the aortic aneurysm, enlarged, and implanted. The procedure is less invasive than open thoracotomy or open abdominal replacement [5].

1.4 Arrhythmia

In a normal heart, electrical excitation waves generated in the sinus node propagate and disperse regularly through the stimulation conduction system, causing rhythmic contraction and relaxation of the myocardium, thus realizing a pumping function that distributes blood throughout the body. Disruption of this order of excitation causes arrhythmia. Based on electrocardiographic findings, arrhythmias can be broadly classified into extrasystoles, which show excitation at abnormal times; bradyarrhythmia, which shows slow pulses; and tachyarrhythmia, which shows rapid pulses. Bradyarrhythmia is caused by a disturbance of the sinus node or blocked conduction, whereas extrasystoles and tachyarrhythmia are caused by abnormal excitation. Tachyarrhythmia can be further divided into tachycardia, involving periodic excitation with a fast rhythm, and fibrillation, involving chaotic excitation. In fibrillation, the pumping function of the heart is almost completely lost. Ventricular fibrillation can cause sudden cardiac death, whereas atrial fibrillation can cause cardiogenic cerebral infarction due to thrombi.

1.4.1 Maze Procedure

The Maze procedure involves the surgical creation of lesions through incision and sutures to block the pathway of abnormal excitation in atrial fibrillation. Variations of the Maze procedure include electrical isolation of the pulmonary vein through an incision (pulmonary vein isolation, PVI), resection, or preservation of the left or right atrial appendage, which is at high risk for thrombosis, and combination with catheter ablation [6, 7].

1.4.2 Catheter Ablation

During catheter ablation, a percutaneous ablation catheter is introduced into the heart, and lesions are formed to block the pathway of abnormal excitation in the myocardial tissue by radiofrequency energization and cryocoagulation. Catheter ablation has been widely used in recent years, especially for the treatment of atrial fibrillation. Pulmonary vein isolation, which electrically isolates the pulmonary vein via ablation, is effective for atrial fibrillation, and technological innovations for efficient PVI (e.g., cryoballoons) are underway [8].

1.4.3 Stimulation Device Implantation

Stimulation devices are implanted in patients with severe arrhythmias to control the heart rhythm through electrical stimulation. Types of stimulation include pacemaker stimulation for bradycardia, anti-tachycardia pacing (ATP), cardioversion, defibrillation stimulation to prevent and terminate tachyarrhythmia, and cardiac resynchronization therapy to restore cardiac function by simultaneously pacing both ventricles. The CRT-D and ICD have multiple stimulation functions [9].

1.5 Cardiomyopathy

Cardiomyopathy is a cardiac disease in which the structure of the myocardium is altered and cardiac function is impaired. The two most common types of cardiomyopathies are dilated cardiomyopathy (DCM), characterized by thinning of the ventricular walls and reduction of contractility, and hypertrophic cardiomyopathy (HCM), characterized by enlargement of the ventricles and diastolic failure. The decline in cardiac function is accompanied by typical heart failure symptoms, such as palpitations, shortness of breath, swelling, and fatigue. There is also a risk of developing fatal or serious arrhythmias, as described above.

1.5.1 Surgical Left Ventricular Reconstruction

It involves surgical resection and suturing of the left ventricular wall to shape the left ventricle and reduce the left ventricular volume for improving cardiac function. Due to its highly invasive nature and uncertain therapeutic effects, the number of eligible patients for this surgery is limited [10].

1.6 Severe Heart Failure

Heart failure (HF) is not a specific cardiac disease, but rather a condition in which the pumping function of the heart is impaired, impairing blood flow to organs throughout the body. Heart failure is a major cause of death and becomes more serious with the concurrent progression of one or more of the aforementioned cardiac diseases.

1.6.1 Heart Transplantation

Indications for heart transplantation include dilated and hypertrophic cardiomyopathy, ischemic heart disease, and other severe cardiac conditions where the patient's life cannot be saved or prolonged by conventional therapies. After the recipient's heart is removed under artificial heart-lung control, a donor's heart, which meets the matching criteria, is removed and anastomosed to the recipient's blood vessels. Recipients must be treated with immunosuppressive therapy to suppress organ rejection following heart transplantation.

1.6.2 Left Ventricular Assist Device (LVAD) Implantation

LVADs are implanted to assist with significantly reduced cardiac function in patients waiting for heart transplantation [11]. The LVAD assists in pumping of blood from the left ventricle to the aorta. There are two types of LVADs: extracorporeal and implantable.

2 Application of ML Methods in Cardiac Imaging

This section describes the major diagnostic imaging modalities for cardiac diseases and the application of recent ML methods, mainly focusing on deep learning (DL) methods, to the imaging data.

2.1 Echocardiography

Echocardiography (ECHO) is an essential evaluation modality for diagnosing cardiac diseases. Compared to other modalities, such as CT and MRI, ultrasound (US) imaging has the advantage of being small, portable, and real-time. It enables rapid assessment of structure, function, and hemodynamics and provides important information for the initial diagnosis of cardiac diseases. Although B-mode US images include inherent speckle noise, the application of speckle tracking ECHO, a strain imaging technique for the evaluation of cardiac function in several cardiac diseases, has evolved in recent years [12].

ECHO involves transesophageal echocardiography (TEE), intracardiac echocardiography (ICE), and intravascular US (IVUS), in addition to the most common modality, which is transthoracic echocardiography (TTE). Recently, 3D TTE, in addition to 2D TTE, has also been used [13, 14].

2.1.1 Transthoracic and Transesophageal Echocardiography (TTE/TEE)

TTE is the most widely used US imaging modality for assessing structural and functional cardiovascular abnormalities. TTE involves the use of an US probe applied externally to the chest wall. For TEE, an endoscopic US probe is inserted through the mouth into the esophagus. TEE provides clearer images of the upper chambers than TTE but requires conscious sedation of patients.

In a TTE examination, a sonographer measures several parameters related to the structure and function of the chambers, valves, and aorta. ML has the potential to make TTE and TEE examinations more efficient and operator independent. For example, automated-view classification has the potential to help non-experts properly position the US probe and measure US images with sufficient image quality for

Table 1 Summary of machine learning approaches for echocardiography

Type	Year	First author	Purpose	Method
TTE/ TEE	2018	Zhang	EDV/ESV/EF evaluation (comparison with manual)	U-net
	2019	Leclerc		U-net
	2019	Miyoshi		CNN
	2015	Medvedofsky		Philips heart model
	2017	Medvedofsky		
	2018	Barletta	EDV/ESV/EF evaluation (comparison with manual)	
	2018	Levy		
	2019	Wu		
	2015	Gao	View classification	CNN
	2018	Madani		
	2018	Zhang		
	2019	Ostvik		
IVUS	2015	Gao	Detection (lumen and MA border)	Unsupervised clustering
	2017	Su	Detection (lumen and MA border)	Autoencoder
	2018	Sofan	Detection (calcification)	CNN w/ResNet101
	2018	Kim	Segmentation (CA)	U-net
	2018	Yang	Segmentation (lumen, media vessel wall)	U-net
	2019	Lo Vercio	Segmentation (vessel wall)	SVM, RF
	2019	Ko	Segmentation	FCNN w/transfer learning

SVM support vector machine, *RF* random forest, *FCNN* fully convolutional neural network, *CA* coronary artery, *MA* media-adventitia

accurate assessment. In addition, view classification can be used to improve the efficiency of post-examination reviews [15–18].

Left ventricular measurements, particularly the end-diastolic and end-systolic volumes (EDV and ESV, respectively) and ejection fraction (EF), are important parameters for the assessment of cardiac function [19]. Recent studies developed automatic measurements of these parameters based on the automatic segmentation of the left ventricular chamber region in US images and evaluated the accuracy in comparison with criterion measurements based on manual interpretation of TTE or cardiac magnetic resonance (CMR) images (Table 1). In most of these studies, CNN was adopted as the segmentation model. There is also a trial report in which CNN was used for the direct estimation of EF from two US images without image segmentation [20].

2.1.2 Intracardiac Echocardiography (ICE) and Intravascular Ultrasound (IVUS)

For ICE, an ICE catheter with a US probe at its tip is inserted into the patient's vasculature and navigated into the heart chambers. The 2D B-mode image of the ICE catheter enables direct visualization of the myocardial wall, surrounding tissue, and instrument; thus, it can be used for visualization during percutaneous intervention procedures in the chambers, such as trans-septal intervention and catheter ablation of atrial and ventricular tachyarrhythmias. On the other hand, ICE during intervention requires substantial operator expertise. Currently, there are few studies on ML applications to ICE.

For IVUS, an IVUS catheter with a miniaturized US probe at its distal end is inserted into the patient's vasculature. IVUS enables the assessment of the vessel walls, which are difficult to assess using conventional angiography. IVUS is a powerful tool, particularly in PCI, for the quantitative and qualitative evaluation of atherosclerosis and evaluation of implanted coronary stents. ML models for automatic tissue classification (TC) for the assessment of atheromatous plaque and calcification have been developed for IVUS image analysis. In addition to conventional ML approaches based on the combination of feature extraction and classifiers, such as SVM and random forest [21], several recent studies have adopted CNN as the ML model [22–26]. Another major application of ML for IVUS interpretation is the segmentation of anatomical components, especially segmenting the arterial and media-adventitial (MA) walls [15, 27]. There is a publicly available IVUS dataset [28].

2.2 *Cardiac Computed Tomography*

With recent rapid advances in technology such as ECG-gated imaging, dual X-ray sources, and wide multidetector, cardiac CT is currently an important measurement modality for cardiac diseases. There are two major roles: structural and functional assessment of the coronary arteries and assessment of structural heart diseases (Table 2).

2.2.1 Coronary CT Angiography (CTA)

The most popular application of cardiac CT is the assessment of the coronary arteries. With the improvement in CT image quality, it is possible to contrast coronary arteries by CT angiography (CTA) using an iodine contrast agent, instead of conventional invasive coronary angiography (ICA). Coronary CTA is expected to be used for the screening of incident acute coronary syndrome [29], with the assessment of luminal stenosis and atherosclerotic plaques. Moreover, CT fractional flow reserve (FFR-CT), a recent technology that allows non-invasive functional assessment of the coronary arteries, has emerged and been approved by the FDA [30–33]. Instead of conventional invasive FFR measurement using a pressure wire, FFR-CT allows the assessment of the significance of coronary artery lesions in CAD. In addition to coronary CTA assessment, CAC scoring (Agatston CAC score) [34] via non-contrast cardiac CT is also performed to assess the significance of CAD [35].

Table 2 Summary of machine learning approaches for cardiac CT

Target	Year	First author	Purpose	Method
Chamber	2017	Shahzad	Segmentation	3D U-net
	2018	Xu		
	2019	Ye		
CA (non-contrast)	2017	Lessmann	CAC scoring	Two consecutive CNN
	2015	Wolterink		Randomized tree classifier
	2019	Martin		ResNet CNN
	2021	Zeleznik		U-net
CA (CTA)	2019	Wolterink	Centerline extraction	3D dilated CNN
	2016	Merkow	Lumen segmentation	CNN
	2019	Shen		CNN
	2019	Wolterink	CA boundary detection	Graph CNN
	2019	Zreik	Stenosis detection	Multitask recurrent CNN
	2019	Hong		M-net-based CNN
	2016	Itu	FFR-CT	Feature extraction and fully connected NN
	2020	Zreik		Unsupervised ML
	2021	Fossan		Simplified physics based model and fully connected NN

CA coronary artery, *CTA* computed tomography angiography, *CAC* coronary artery calcification

2.2.2 Assessment of Structural Cardiac Diseases

Cardiac CT is useful not only for coronary artery assessment but also for the assessment of other structural cardiac diseases. With the increase in percutaneous interventions, structural assessments using cardiac CT are expanding. For example, assessment of valve anatomy, including regurgitation, is useful in percutaneous valve replacement and valvuloplasty interventions [36–40].

2.2.3 Application of ML Methods

While ML has recently been applied in all aspects of CT imaging, including acquisition, reconstruction, and analysis, ML in cardiac CT has been predominantly used for the analysis of patient-specific risk assessment.

2.3 *Cardiac Magnetic Resonance (CMR)*

Compared to other imaging methods, CMR has the advantage of a better signal-to-noise ratio, higher spatial resolution, and the ability to obtain images in any cardiac plane. CMR also enables flow assessment using phase-contrast velocity mapping. It provides additional information when the assessment of coronary artery and valvular diseases using ECHO, CT, and PET/SPECT is inconclusive [41]. However, CMR has the challenges of long measurement time.

2.3.1 Myocardial Tissue Characterization

An important diagnosis realized by CMR imaging is myocardial tissue characterization using T1 and T2 mapping. Characteristic T1, T2, and T2* magnetization relaxation times enable the differentiation of normal tissue from myocardial interstitial fibrosis and myocardium with iron deposits. Contrast T1 mapping before and after gadolinium contrast use enables the assessment of diffuse interstitial fibrosis [42, 43]. CMR with late gadolinium enhancement (LGE) enables noninvasive visualization of myocardial scars with replacement fibrosis [44], which has been assessed only by invasive biopsies and autopsies.

2.3.2 Application of ML Methods

Although new acquisition sequences have been investigated to speed up CMR [45–47], which is a major challenge in CMR, the image reconstruction process has been a bottleneck. In recent years, several methods have been proposed to speed up CMR by introducing ML and compressed sensing (CS) techniques for acceleration of the image reconstruction process [48, 49]. ML methods have also been studied for CMR analysis to better assess ventricular function [50–52] and myocardial tissue characterization [53–57].

2.4 *Cardiac Nuclear Imaging*

Single-photon emission computed tomography (SPECT) and positron emission tomography (PET) are nuclear medicine imaging modalities used for the assessment of myocardial perfusion and severity of CAD. Although SPECT is a validated and widely available modality, PET is a relatively novel technique. PET provides a higher spatial resolution than SPECT, but the signal-to-noise ratio is limited, and the spatial resolution is not as high as that of other cardiac imaging modalities. For both SPECT and PET imaging, a radiopharmaceutical is injected into the patients. By detecting emitted radiation from the radiopharmaceutical, healthy myocardium can be differentiated from ischemic myocardium. Filtered-back projection (FBP) is the most basic image reconstruction method for these nuclear medicine images.

2.4.1 Application of ML Methods

In SPECT/PET, ML methods are applied in the image reconstruction process to improve the image quality. Recently, end-to-end image reconstruction estimating an image directly from raw measurement data without conventional FBP or iterative reconstruction methods has been studied [58, 59]. Moreover, ML-based correction methods for image degradation caused by attenuation of positron emission [60, 61] and motion of patients [62] have also been studied.

3 Conclusion

Major cardiac diseases and procedures were reviewed. Further, recent representative imaging modalities used for the quantitative diagnosis of these diseases and the application of recent ML methods to each of them were introduced. In the future, further applications of AI technologies are expected, such as the discovery of new risk stratification factors based on measurement results, as seen in radiomics research, and advanced navigation in robotic surgery, to realize less invasive and more effective surgeries.

References

1. Martin DM, Boyle FJ. Drug-eluting stents for coronary artery disease: a review. Med Eng Phys. 2011;33(2):148–63. https://doi.org/10.1016/J.MEDENGPHY.2010.10.009.
2. Bhatt DL. Percutaneous coronary intervention in 2018. JAMA. 2018;319(20):2127–8. https://doi.org/10.1001/JAMA.2018.5281.
3. Bravata DM, Gienger AL, McDonald KM, Sundaram V, Perez MV, Varghese R, Kapoor JR, Ardehali R, Owens DK, Hlatky MA. Systematic review: the comparative effectiveness of percutaneous coronary interventions and coronary artery bypass graft surgery. Ann Intern Med. 2007;147(10):703–16. https://doi.org/10.7326/0003-4819-147-10-200711200-00185.
4. Webb JG, Wood DA. Current status of transcatheter aortic valve replacement. J Am Coll Cardiol. 2012;60(6):483–92. https://doi.org/10.1016/J.JACC.2012.01.071.
5. Chaikof EL, Blankensteijn JD, Harris PL, White GH, Zarins CK, Bernhard VM, Matsumura JS, May J, Veith FJ, Fillinger MF, Rutherford RB, Craig Kent K. Reporting standards for endovascular aortic aneurysm repair. J Vasc Surg. 2002;35(5):1048–60. https://doi.org/10.1067/MVA.2002.123763.
6. Cox JL, Boineau JP, Schuessler RB, Kater KM, Lappas DG. Five-year experience with the maze procedure for atrial fibrillation. Ann Thorac Surg. 1993;56(4):814–24. https://doi.org/10.1016/0003-4975(93)90338-I.

7. Schaff HV, Dearani JA, Daly RC, Orszulak TA, Danielson GK. Cox-maze procedure for atrial fibrillation: Mayo Clinic experience. Semin Thorac Cardiovasc Surg. 2000;12(1):30–7. https://doi.org/10.1016/S1043-0679(00)70014-1.
8. Wazni OM, Dandamudi G, Sood N, Hoyt R, Tyler J, Durrani S, Niebauer M, Makati K, Halperin B, Gauri A, Morales G, Shao M, Cerkvenik J, Kaplon RE, Nissen SE. Cryoballoon ablation as initial therapy for atrial fibrillation. N Engl J Med. 2021;384(4):316–24. https://doi.org/10.1056/NEJMOA2029554/SUPPL_FILE/NEJMOA2029554_DATA-SHARING.PDF.
9. Stabile G, Solimene F, Bertaglia E, La Rocca V, Accogli M, Scaccia A, Marrazzo N, Zoppo F, Turco P, Iuliano A, Shopova G, Ciardiello C, De Simone A. Long-term outcomes of CRT-PM versus CRT-D recipients. Pacing Clin Electrophysiol. 2009;32(Suppl 1):S141–5. https://doi.org/10.1111/J.1540-8159.2008.02271.X.
10. Wakasa S, Matsui Y, Kobayashi J, Cho Y, Yaku H, Matsumiya G, Isomura T, Takanashi S, Usui A, Sakata R, Komiya T, Sawa Y, Saiki Y, Shimizu H, Yamaguchi A, Hamano K, Arai H. Estimating postoperative left ventricular volume: identification of responders to surgical ventricular reconstruction. J Thorac Cardiovasc Surg. 2018;156(6):2088–2096.e3. https://doi.org/10.1016/J.JTCVS.2018.06.090.
11. Miller LW, Rogers JG. Evolution of left ventricular assist device therapy for advanced heart failure: a review. JAMA Cardiol. 2018;3(7):650–8. https://doi.org/10.1001/JAMACARDIO.2018.0522.
12. Inciardi RM, Galderisi M, Nistri S, Santoro C, Cicoira M, Rossi A. Echocardiographic advances in hypertrophic cardiomyopathy: three-dimensional and strain imaging echocardiography. Echocardiography. 2018;35(5):716–26. https://doi.org/10.1111/ECHO.13878.
13. Jenkins C, Tsang W. Three-dimensional echocardiographic acquisition and validity of left ventricular volumes and ejection fraction. Echocardiography. 2020;37(10):1646–53. https://doi.org/10.1111/ECHO.14862.
14. Lang RM, Addetia K, Narang A, Mor-Avi V. 3-dimensional echocardiography: latest developments and future directions. JACC Cardiovasc Imaging. 2018;11(12):1854–78. https://doi.org/10.1016/J.JCMG.2018.06.024.
15. Gao Z, Hau WK, Minhua L, Huang W, Zhang H, Wanqing W, Liu X, Zhang YT. Automated framework for detecting Lumen and Media–Adventitia borders in intravascular ultrasound images. Ultrasound Med Biol. 2015;41(7):2001–21. https://doi.org/10.1016/J.ULTRASMEDBIO.2015.03.022.
16. Madani A, Arnaout R, Mofrad M, Arnaout R. Fast and accurate view classification of echocardiograms using deep learning. NPJ Digit Med. 2018;1(1):1–8. https://doi.org/10.1038/s41746-017-0013-1.
17. Østvik A, Smistad E, Aase SA, Haugen BO, Lovstakken L. Real-time standard view classification in transthoracic echocardiography using convolutional neural networks. Ultrasound Med Biol. 2019;45(2):374–84. https://doi.org/10.1016/J.ULTRASMEDBIO.2018.07.024.
18. Zhang J, Gajjala S, Agrawal P, Tison GH, Hallock LA, Beussink-Nelson L, Lassen MH, Fan E, Aras MA, Jordan CR, Fleischmann KE, Melisko M, Qasim A, Shah SJ, Bajcsy R, Deo RC. Fully automated echocardiogram interpretation in clinical practice: feasibility and diagnostic accuracy. Circulation. 2018;138(16):1623–35. https://doi.org/10.1161/CIRCULATIONAHA.118.034338.
19. Murphy SP, Ibrahim NE, Januzzi JL. Heart failure with reduced ejection fraction: a review. JAMA. 2020;324(5):488–504. https://doi.org/10.1001/JAMA.2020.10262.
20. Asch FM, Poilvert N, Abraham T, Jankowski M, Cleve J, Adams M, Romano N, Hong H, Mor-Avi V, Martin RP, Lang RM. Automated echocardiographic quantification of left ventricular ejection fraction without volume measurements using a machine learning algorithm mimicking a human expert. Circ Cardiovasc Imaging. 2019;12(9):9303. https://doi.org/10.1161/CIRCIMAGING.119.009303.
21. Vercio LL, Del Fresno M, Larrabide I. Lumen-intima and media-adventitia segmentation in IVUS images using supervised classifications of arterial layers and morphologi-

cal structures. Comput Methods Prog Biomed. 2019;177:113–21. https://doi.org/10.1016/J.CMPB.2019.05.021.
22. Ko J, Lee J-G. Lumen and Vessel Wall segmentation on intravascular ultrasound images using fully convolutional network. 2019;11050:120–3. https://doi.org/10.1117/12.2521363.
23. Kim Y, Jeong MH, Kim I, Kim MC, Sim DS, Hong YJ, Kim JH, Ahn Y. Intravascular ultrasound-guided percutaneous coronary intervention with drug-eluting stent for unprotected left Main disease via left snuffbox approach. Korean Circ J. 2018;48(6):532–3. https://doi.org/10.4070/KCJ.2018.0016.
24. Sofian H, Ming JTC, Mohamad S, Noor NM. Calcification detection using deep structured learning in intravascular ultrasound image for coronary artery disease. In: 2nd international conference on BioSignal Analysis, Processing and Systems, vol. 2018. ICBAPS; 2018. p. 47–52. https://doi.org/10.1109/ICBAPS.2018.8527415.
25. Yang J, Faraji M, Basu A. Robust segmentation of arterial walls in intravascular ultrasound images using dual path U-net. Ultrasonics. 2019;96:24–33. https://doi.org/10.1016/J.ULTRAS.2019.03.014.
26. Yang J, Lin T, Faraji M, Basu A. IVUS-Net: an intravascular ultrasound segmentation network, Lecture Notes in Computer Science (Including Subseries Lecture Notes in Artificial Intelligence and Lecture Notes in Bioinformatics), vol. 11010 LNCS; 2018. p. 367–77. https://doi.org/10.1007/978-3-030-04375-9_31/FIGURES/3.
27. Su S, Zhenghui H, Lin Q, Hau WK, Gao Z, Zhang H. An artificial neural network method for lumen and media-adventitia border detection in IVUS. Comput Med Imaging Graph. 2017;57:29–39. https://doi.org/10.1016/J.COMPMEDIMAG.2016.11.003.
28. Balocco S, Gatta C, Ciompi F, Wahle A, Radeva P, Carlier S, Unal G, Sanidas E, Mauri J, Carillo X, Kovarnik T, Wang CW, Chen HC, Exarchos TP, Fotiadis DI, Destrempes F, Cloutier G, Pujol O, Marina Alberti E, Mendizabal-Ruiz G, Rivera M, Aksoy T, Downe RW, Kakadiaris IA. Standardized evaluation methodology and reference database for evaluating IVUS image segmentation. Comput Med Imaging Graph. 2014;38(2):70–90. https://doi.org/10.1016/J.COMPMEDIMAG.2013.07.001.
29. Andreini D, Magnoni M, Conte E, Masson S, Mushtaq S, Berti S, Canestrari M, Casolo G, Gabrielli D, Latini R, Marraccini P, Moccetti T, Modena MG, Pontone G, Gorini M, Maggioni AP, Maseri A. Coronary plaque features on CTA can identify patients at increased risk of cardiovascular events. JACC Cardiovasc Imaging. 2020;13(8):1704–17. https://doi.org/10.1016/J.JCMG.2019.06.019.
30. Al-Mallah MH, Ahmed AM. Controversies in the use of fractional flow reserve form computed tomography (FFRCT) vs. coronary angiography. Curr Cardiovasc Imaging Rep. 2016;9(12):1–7. https://doi.org/10.1007/S12410-016-9396-7/TABLES/1.
31. Chaikriangkrai K, Su Y, eo. Choi, Faisal Nabi, and Su M. i. Chang. Important advances in technology and unique applications to cardiovascular computed tomography. Methodist Debakey Cardiovasc J. 2014;10(3):152. https://doi.org/10.14797/MDCJ-10-3-152.
32. Han D, Lee JH, Rizvi A, Gransar H, Baskaran L, Schulman-Marcus J, Hartaigh B ó, Lin FY, Min JK. Incremental role of resting myocardial computed tomography perfusion for predicting physiologically significant coronary artery disease: a machine learning approach. J Nucl Cardiol. 2018;25(1):223–33. https://doi.org/10.1007/S12350-017-0834-Y/FIGURES/3.
33. Kim JY, Suh YJ, Han K, Kim YJ, Choi BW. Diagnostic value of advanced imaging modalities for the detection and differentiation of prosthetic valve obstruction: a systematic review and meta-analysis. JACC Cardiovasc Imaging. 2019;12(11P1):2182–92. https://doi.org/10.1016/J.JCMG.2018.11.033.
34. Agatston AS, Janowitz WR, Hildner FJ, Zusmer NR, Viamonte M, Detrano R. Quantification of coronary artery calcium using ultrafast computed tomography. J Am Coll Cardiol. 1990;15(4):827–32. https://doi.org/10.1016/0735-1097(90)90282-T.
35. Budoff MJ, Young R, Gregory Burke J, Carr J, Detrano RC, Folsom AR, Kronmal R, Lima JAC, Liu KJ, McClelland RL, Michos E, Post WS, Shea S, Watson KE, Wong ND. Ten-year Association of Coronary Artery Calcium with atherosclerotic cardiovascular disease (ASCVD) events: the multi-ethnic study of atherosclerosis (MESA). Eur Heart J. 2018;39(25):2401–8. https://doi.org/10.1093/EURHEARTJ/EHY217.

36. Feuchtner GM, Dichtl W, Müller S, Jodocy D, Bonatti J, Schachner T, Friedrich G, Alber H, Pachinger O, Friedrich G. 64-MDCT for diagnosis of aortic regurgitation in patients referred to CT coronary angiography. Am J Roentgenol. 2009;192(2):W351–5. https://doi.org/10.2214/AJR.08.2115.
37. Habets J, Symersky P, van Herwerden LA, de Mol BA, Mali WP, Budde RP. A call for routine assessment of left-sided heart valves during cardiac CT. Neth Hear J. 2012;20(12):488–93. https://doi.org/10.1007/s12471-012-0322-9.
38. Ahn Y, Koo HJ, Lee S, Kim DH, Song JM, Kang DH, Song JK, Kim HJ, Kim JB, Jung SH, Choo SJ, Chung CH, Lee JW, Kang JW, Yang DH. Preoperative cardiac computed tomography characteristics associated with recurrent aortic regurgitation after aortic valve re-implantation. Korean J Radiol. 2020;21(2):181–91. https://doi.org/10.3348/kjr.2019.0446.
39. Suchá D, Symersky P, Tanis W, de Mol BA, Budde RP. Multimodality imaging assessment of prosthetic heart valves. Circ Cardiovasc Imaging. 2015;8(9):e003703. https://doi.org/10.1161/CIRCIMAGING.115.003703.
40. Symersky P, Habets J, Budde RP, de Mol BA, Mali WP, van Herwerden LA. Imaging of cardiac valves by computed tomography. Int J Cardiovasc Imaging. 2009;25(5):455–67. https://doi.org/10.1007/s10554-009-9496-0.
41. Zoghbi WA, Adams D, Bonow RO, Enriquez-Sarano M, Foster E, Grayburn PA, Hahn RT, Han Y, Hung J, Lang RM, Little SH, Shah DJ, Shernan S, Thavendiranathan P, Thomas JD, Weissman NJ. Recommendations for noninvasive evaluation of native valvular regurgitation: a report from the American Society of Echocardiography developed in collaboration with the Society for Cardiovascular Magnetic Resonance. J Am Soc Echocardiogr. 2017;30(4):303–71. https://doi.org/10.1016/J.ECHO.2017.01.007.
42. Ghosn MG, Shah DJ. Important advances in technology and unique applications related to cardiac magnetic resonance imaging. Methodist Debakey Cardiovasc J. 2014;10(3):159. https://doi.org/10.14797/MDCJ-10-3-159.
43. Messroghli DR, Moon JC, Ferreira VM, Grosse-Wortmann L, He T, Kellman P, Mascherbauer J, Nezafat R, Salerno M, Schelbert EB, Taylor AJ, Thompson R, Ugander M, Van Heeswijk RB, Matthias G. Friedrich. Clinical recommendations for cardiovascular magnetic resonance mapping of T1, T2, T2* and extracellular volume: a consensus statement by the Society for Cardiovascular Magnetic Resonance (SCMR) endorsed by the European Association for Cardiovascular Imaging (EACVI). J Cardiovasc Magnet Resonance. 2017;19(1):1–24. https://doi.org/10.1186/S12968-017-0389-8.
44. Vöhringer M, Mahrholdt H, Yilmaz A, Sechtem U. Significance of late gadolinium enhancement in cardiovascular magnetic resonance imaging (CMR). Herz Kardiovaskuläre Erkrankungen. 2007;32(2):129–37. https://doi.org/10.1007/S00059-007-2972-5.
45. Jeong D, Schiebler ML, Lai P, Wang K, Vigen KK, François CJ. Single breath hold 3D cardiac cine MRI using kat-ARC: preliminary results at 1.5T. Int J Cardiovasc Imaging. 2015;31(6):851–7. https://doi.org/10.1007/s10554-015-0615-0.
46. Lin ACW, Strugnell W, Riley R, Schmitt M, Cowan B, Young AA. Higher resolution cine imaging with compressed sensing for accelerated clinical left ventricular evaluation. J Magn Reson Imaging. 2017;45(6):1693–9. https://doi.org/10.1002/jmri.25525.
47. Okuda S, Yamada Y, Tanimoto A, Fujita J, Sano M, Fukuda K, Kuribayashi S, Jinzaki M, Nozaki A, Lai P. Three-dimensional cardiac cine imaging using the kat ARC acceleration: initial experience in clinical adult patients at 3T. Magn Reson Imaging. 2015;33(7):911–7. https://doi.org/10.1016/j.mri.2015.04.004.
48. Schlemper J, Yang G, Ferreira P, Scott A, McGill LA, Khalique Z, Gorodezky M, Roehl M, Keegan J, Pennell D, Firmin D, Rueckert D. Stochastic deep compressive sensing for the reconstruction of diffusion tensor cardiac MRI, Lecture notes in Computer Science (Including Subseries Lecture Notes in Artificial Intelligence and Lecture Notes in Bioinformatics), vol. 11070 LNCS; 2018. p. 295–303. https://doi.org/10.1007/978-3-030-00928-1_34/FIGURES/3.
49. Xiang L, Chen Y, Chang W, Zhan Y, Lin W, Wang Q, Shen D. Deep-learning-based multimodal fusion for fast MR reconstruction. IEEE Trans Biomed Eng. 2019;66(7):2105–14. https://doi.org/10.1109/TBME.2018.2883958.

50. Avendi MR, Kheradvar A, Jafarkhani H. A combined deep-learning and deformable-model approach to fully automatic segmentation of the left ventricle in cardiac MRI. Med Image Anal. 2016;30:108–19. https://doi.org/10.1016/J.MEDIA.2016.01.005.
51. Curiale AH, Colavecchia FD, Mato G. Automatic quantification of the LV function and mass: a deep learning approach for cardiovascular MRI. Comput Methods Prog Biomed. 2019;169:37–50. https://doi.org/10.1016/J.CMPB.2018.12.002.
52. Liao F, Chen X, Xiaolin H, Song S. Estimation of the volume of the left ventricle from MRI images using deep neural networks. IEEE Trans Cybern. 2017;49(2):495–504. https://doi.org/10.1109/TCYB.2017.2778799.
53. Baeßler B, Mannil M, Maintz D, Alkadhi H, Manka R. Texture analysis and machine learning of non-contrast T1-weighted MR images in patients with hypertrophic cardiomyopathy—preliminary results. Eur J Radiol. 2018;102:61–7. https://doi.org/10.1016/J.EJRAD.2018.03.013.
54. Li L, Fuping W, Yang G, Lingchao X, Wong T, Mohiaddin R, Firmin D, Keegan J, Zhuang X. Atrial scar quantification via multi-scale CNN in the graph-cuts framework. Med Image Anal. 2020a;60:101595. https://doi.org/10.1016/J.MEDIA.2019.101595.
55. Moccia S, Banali R, Martini C, Muscogiuri G, Pontone G, Pepi M, Caiani EG. Development and testing of a deep learning-based strategy for scar segmentation on CMR-LGE images. MAGMA. 2019;32(2):187–95. https://doi.org/10.1007/S10334-018-0718-4/FIGURES/5.
56. Zabihollahy F, White JA, Ukwatta E. Convolutional neural network-based approach for segmentation of left ventricle myocardial scar from 3D late gadolinium enhancement MR images. Med Phys. 2019;46(4):1740–51. https://doi.org/10.1002/MP.13436.
57. Zhang N, Yang G, Gao Z, Chenchu X, Zhang Y, Shi R, Keegan J, Lei X, Zhang H, Fan Z, Firmin D. Deep learning for diagnosis of chronic myocardial infarction on nonenhanced cardiac cine MRI. Radiology. 2019;291(3):606–7. https://doi.org/10.1148/RADIOL.2019182304/ASSET/IMAGES/LARGE/RADIOL.2019182304.FIG6.JPEG.
58. Häggström I, Ross Schmidtlein C, Campanella G, Fuchs TJ. DeepPET: a deep encoder–decoder network for directly solving the PET image reconstruction inverse problem. Med Image Anal. 2019;54:253–62. https://doi.org/10.1016/J.MEDIA.2019.03.013.
59. Zhu B, Liu JZ, Cauley SF, Rosen BR, Rosen MS. Image reconstruction by domain-transform manifold learning. Nature. 2018;555(7697):487–92. https://doi.org/10.1038/nature25988.
60. Leynes AP, Yang J, Wiesinger F, Kaushik SS, Shanbhag DD, Seo Y, Hope TA, Larson PEZ. Zero-Echo-time and Dixon deep pseudo-CT (ZeDD CT): direct generation of pseudo-CT images for pelvic PET/MRI attenuation correction using deep convolutional neural networks with multiparametric MRI. J Nucl Med. 2018;59(5):852–8. https://doi.org/10.2967/JNUMED.117.198051.
61. Liu F, Jang H, Kijowski R, Zhao G, Bradshaw T, McMillan AB. A deep learning approach For18 F-Fdg pet attenuation correction. EJNMMI Phys. 2018;5(1):1–15. https://doi.org/10.1186/S40658-018-0225-8/TABLES/1.
62. Li T, Zhang M, Qi W, Asma E, Qi J. Motion correction of respiratory-gated PET images using deep learning based image registration framework. Phys Med Biol. 2020b;65(15):155003. https://doi.org/10.1088/1361-6560/AB8688.

AI Surgery in Orthopedics

Yoshinobu Sato, Yoshito Otake, Yoshiyuki Kagiyama, Keisuke Uemura, Masaki Takao, and Nobuhiko Sugano

Abstract The framework of computer-aided design and manufacturing (CAD/CAM) in industrial technology has been naturally applied to orthopedic surgery since the early days of computer-assisted surgery. This chapter describes how AI can bring a paradigm shift of the conventional surgical CAD/CAM framework in orthopedics. AI will optimize and automate the CAD/CAM framework through inference based on comprehensive patient and therapeutic models. These models will be learned from the database of the whole process of orthopedic surgery constructed by the surgical data science (SDS) framework, which will be progressively improved in a closed-loop manner. Toward the comprehensive patient and therapeutic modeling, two aspects of modeling, (1) patient modeling and (2) surgery/therapeutic modeling, are discussed.

Keywords Surgical data science · Surgical CAD/CAM · Automated segmentation · Patient anatomy modeling · Joint function · Surgery/therapeutic modeling · Automated surgical planning · Optimized surgical planning

---

Y. Sato (✉) · Y. Otake
Division of Information Science, Nara Institute of Technology and Science, Nara, Japan
e-mail: yoshi@is.naist.jp; otake@is.naist.jp

Y. Kagiyama
Graduate Faculty of Interdisciplinary Research, University of Yamanashi, Yamanashi, Japan
e-mail: ykagiyama@yamanashi.ac.jp

K. Uemura · N. Sugano
Department of Orthopaedic Medical Engineering, Osaka University Graduate School of Medicine, Osaka, Japan
e-mail: keisuke-uemura@ort.med.osaka-u.ac.jp; sugano@ort.med.osaka-u.ac.jp

M. Takao
Department of Bone and Joint Surgery, Ehime University Graduate School of Medicine, Matsuyama, Ehime, Japan
e-mail: takao.masaki.ti@ehime-u.ac.jp

K. Masamune et al. (eds.), *Artificial Intelligence in Surgery*,
https://doi.org/10.1007/978-981-96-6635-5_10

1 Introduction

Orthopedics mainly deals with processing and assembly of hard tissue (i.e., bone). Unlike soft tissue surgery, its surgical planning and execution are relatively similar to design and manufacturing of industrial materials, and thus the framework of computer-aided design and manufacturing (CAD/CAM) in industrial technology has been naturally applied to orthopedic surgery since the early days of computer-assisted surgery (CAS) [1–4]. Orthopedics has been one of important application areas in surgical robotics, which is regarded as a part of the surgical CAD/CAM framework [1, 4]. While the da Vinci system for soft tissue surgery is currently the most common surgical robot, orthopedic surgical robots have recently become increasingly popular in clinical practice [5, 6]. First question is how AI can bring a paradigm shift of the conventional surgical CAD/CAM framework in orthopedics.

Another notable framework is the concept of "surgery as a closed-loop process" [7, 8], which is a long-term feedback loop of making the best use of accumulated surgical data to improve the models and methods for future surgery. This framework may have not been widely spread, but it can be regarded as a precursor of the recently-emerged "surgical data science (SDS)" framework [9, 10]. While the current most active area of SDS is analysis of intraoperative surgical video data such as endoscopic/laparoscopic/fluoroscopic video data, AI surgery should include optimization of therapeutic selection/planning/execution and pre−/postoperative rehabilitation based on diagnosis and prognosis prediction. Therefore, analysis of pre- and postoperative data and non-video intraoperative data is important as well to understand and model the surgery including preoperative patient conditions and the outcome of surgery. Second question is how AI can contribute to SDS in orthopedics vice versa.

AI will greatly enhance the abovementioned two computer-aided surgery frameworks and unify them to facilitate digital transformation of the whole process of orthopedic surgery, which will include diagnosis such as osteoarthritis (OA) grading, decision about the timing of surgery, pre- and postoperative rehabilitation, and so on, in addition to surgical planning and execution. Regarding the above-raised two questions, the answers could be as follows. AI will optimize and automate the CAD/CAM framework through inference based on comprehensive patient and therapeutic models for the first question. These models will be learned from the database of the whole process of orthopedic surgery constructed by the SDS framework, which will be progressively improved in a closed-loop manner, for the second question. Toward the comprehensive patient and therapeutic modeling, we investigate two aspects of modeling: (1) patient modeling and (2) surgery/therapeutic modeling in total hip arthroplasty (THA) as a typical orthopedic surgery in this chapter.

2 Patient Modeling by AI

The first step of surgical CAD/CAM in orthopedics is reconstruction of the patient-specific musculoskeletal anatomy. AI, for example, U-Net [11], has dramatically improved the performance of automated segmentation from medical images. Automated segmentation of the individual bones is now considered to be ready for practical use in both accuracy and speed for even heavily diseased cases. Segmentation of individual muscles as defined in anatomy books has become possible in much higher accuracy by AI [12] than conventional methods [13] (Fig. 1). Once segmentation is completed, patient-specific tissue properties such as bone mineral density (BMD) [14] and muscle fatty degeneration in muscles [15] are estimated from CT. Further, cartilage and ligament segmentation from MRI and CT is becoming possible.

The CAD/CAM framework is typically coupled with finite element analysis (FEA) and other mechanical analyses [16, 17]. In orthopedic applications, biomechanical analysis of musculoskeletal structures and tissues, e.g., FEA of bone/cartilage tissues and dynamic biomechanical analysis of gait and other motions, is combined. One of the important roles of AI is to drastically facilitate practical use of patient-specific anatomy obtained from medical images in biomechanical analysis, that is, patient-specific biomechanical simulations will be available in clinical routine. More importantly, AI will enable all automatically segmented/annotated patient and surgical data to be increasingly accumulated in the database, including pre-and postoperative patient anatomy from medical images, musculoskeletal function assessment data, and biomechanical simulation data, as well as preoperative planning and intraoperatively acquired data. Further, systematic and automated accumulation of patient follow-up data can be integrated to construct comprehensive patient and surgical database and realize the concept of "surgery as a closed-loop process" [7, 8]. These database accumulation processes will lead to development of AI surgery. Therefore, underlying AIs accelerate the SDS framework, while the SDS framework combined with underlying AIs provides higher-level training data for comprehensive AIs.

One opportunity of applications of automatically accumulated comprehensive database is development of AI for highly capable X-ray image recognition, which is particularly useful for orthopedic surgery and diagnosis. In the computer vision research field, depth maps obtained from depth sensors can be regarded as ground truth training data for AI which predicts depth maps from 2D monocular photo images even though those from the depth sensors may be somewhat noisy [18, 19]. Similarly, original CT data and their automatically segmented data are naturally utilized as ground truth training data for AI of 2D X-ray image analysis. In principle, X-ray images can be viewed as 2D projections of CT. If the patient-wise paired dataset of X-ray images and CT data, which is common in orthopedic patients, is available, automatically segmented/annotated 3D information from CT data can be used as ground truth for training of X-ray image recognition.

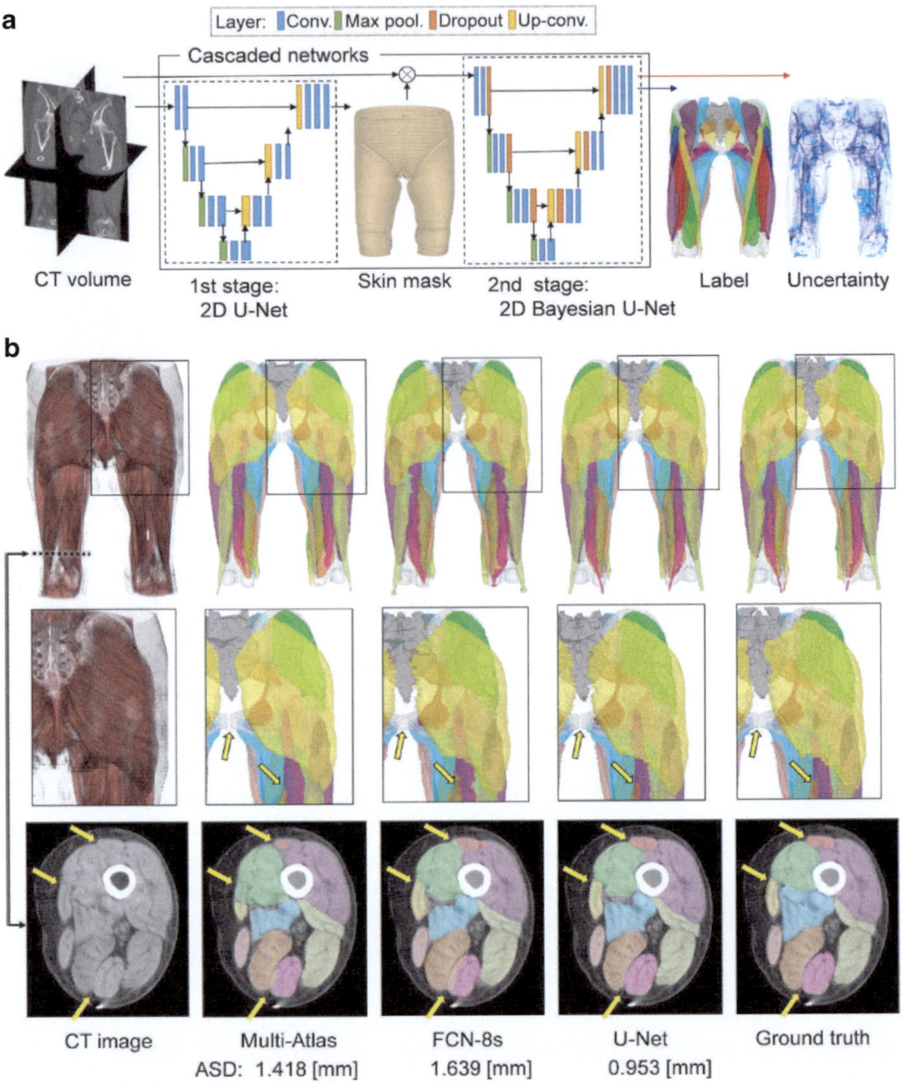

Fig. 1 Musculoskeletal segmentation of the hip and thigh from CT using Bayesian U-Net [12]. (**a**) Schematic diagram of segmentation and uncertainty estimation. The skin surface is first segmented by the deterministic U-Net. Subsequently, the individual muscles are segmented, and the segmentation uncertainty is predicted by Bayesian U-Net. (**b**) Visualization of the predicted labels for a representative patient. The result with U-Net shows distinctly more accurate segmentation near the boundary of the muscles. The region of interest in the slice visualization at the bottom corresponds to the black dotted line in the left-most column. (Copyright © 2020, IEEE)

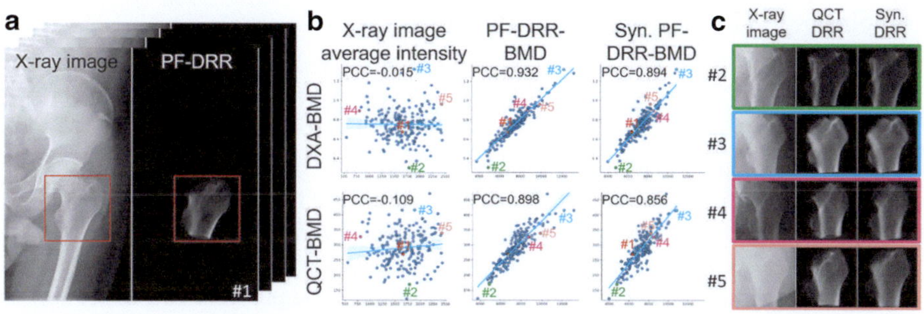

Fig. 2 BMD prediction from a plane X-ray image. Relationships between the intensities of the X-ray image, decomposed digitally reconstructed radiograph (DRR), and BMD values in 200 patient datasets [21]. (**a**) Paired (registered) dataset of X-ray image and decomposed DRR of the proximal femur. (**b**) Scatter plots showing the correlation of the average intensity of X-ray images, predicted BMD from quantitative CT (QCT) DRR, and predicted BMD from the synthesized (decomposed) DRR with DXA-measured BMD and QCT-measured BMD. Pearson correlation coefficient (PCC) was larger than 0.85 between the predicted BMD and the ground-truth BMD of DXA and QCT. (**c**) Proximal femur regions-of-interest (ROIs) of four representative cases. ROIs #2 and #3 have similar X-ray intensity but significantly different BMD, whereas ROIs #4 and #5 have similar BMD but significantly different X-ray intensity. The synthesized DRRs correctly recovered the intensity of QCT DRR, regardless of the intensity of the input X-ray image.

Regarding the bones, accurately registered paired dataset of X-ray image and segmented CT is obtained using automated 2D-3D registration [20]. One illustrative example is the prediction of bone mineral density (BMD) estimates of particular bone regions, which are accurately measured from segmented CT data, from a plane X-ray image [21]. The results show good correlation with DXA (dual-energy X-ray absorptiometry), which is regarded as gold standard of BMD measurement (Fig. 2). Another promising application is 3D shape reconstruction of the bones from X-ray images [22]. Regarding the muscles, muscle mass estimation of individual muscles from a plane X-ray image will be possible from even unpaired dataset of muscle-segmented CT data and X-ray images [23].

Regarding the patient modeling, pathology should be modeled in addition to anatomy. AI for osteoarthritis (OA) detection and severity grading has been intensively studied although these are mostly for total knee arthroplasty (TKA) [24–26]. In addition, AI for prediction on whether the patient undergoes TKA has also been investigated. OA diagnosis is usually based on bones and cartilages. In order to evaluate the joint functions, the evaluation of muscles is important. Muscle atrophy and fatty degeneration associated with hip OA progression were investigated based on manual traces of individual muscles from CT [15]. By using AI-based automated muscle segmentation from CT, muscle atrophy and fatty degeneration will be able to be modeled automatically. Surgery and rehabilitation can be integrated to optimize therapy of OA, and muscle evaluations will play an important role for it.

3 Surgery/Therapeutic Modeling by AI

AI is expected to optimize and automate the CAD/CAM framework. The CAD part in the surgery would correspond to preoperative planning. Automated preoperative planning has been studied for THA surgery. Although one of obstacles against the automation was preoperative patient anatomy modeling from medical images before AI has become commonly used, patient anatomy is now accurately and automatically reconstructed from medical images by AI-based segmentation.

Regarding preoperative planning of THA surgery, the problem can be viewed as prediction of the postoperative patient anatomy and joint functions, X, after THA surgery which involves the selection and placement of the implants as well as design of osteotomy lines, given the preoperative patient data, D, which include anatomy data as well as clinical data, metadata, and so on. One possibility of mathematical modeling for optimal THA planning which predicts the optimal postoperative patient anatomy and joint functions, X_{opt}, will be maximum a posterior (MAP) estimation [27–30]. Assuming that $P(X)$, $P(X|D)$, and $P(D|X)$ are the prior probability of X, the posterior probability of X given D, and the conditional probability (likelihood) of D given X, respectively, prediction of X_{opt} is formulated as

$$X_{opt} = \underset{X}{\operatorname{argmax}}\, P(X|D) = \underset{X}{\operatorname{argmax}} \{P(X)P(D|X)\}$$

according to the Bayesian theorem, $P(X|D) \propto P(X)P(D|X)$.

An intuitive explanation of the above idea is shown in Fig. 3, which is a simplified version of THA planning. In Fig. 3, automated planning of the cup, which is implant placed in the acetabulum of the pelvis (the socket part of the ball-socket

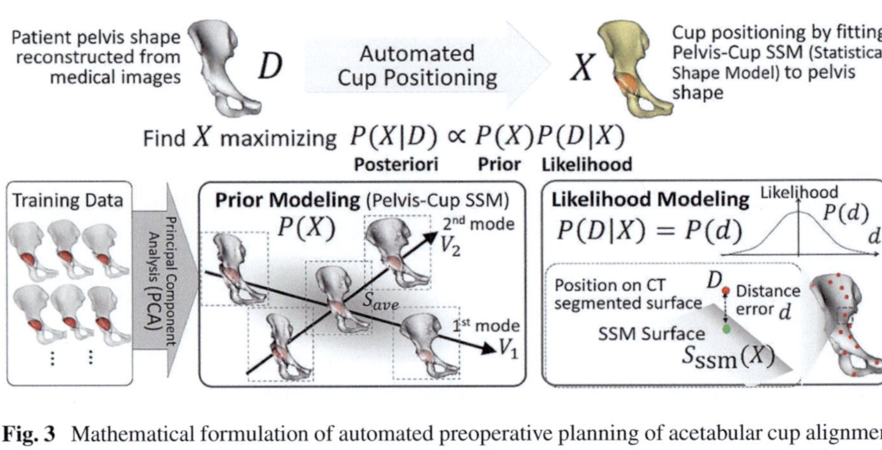

Fig. 3 Mathematical formulation of automated preoperative planning of acetabular cup alignment as Bayesian estimation [27, 29]. Preferable spatial relation between the patient pelvis and cup, X, is encoded in a statistical shape model (SSM), which provides a prior probability distribution $P(X)$. Given patient pelvis shape D, the problem is formulated as finding X maximizing $P(X) \times P(D|X)$. SSM is consider to provide a prior probability distribution, $P(X)$, in Bayes theorem, and $P(X)$ is defined a dimensionality-reduced subspace in the whole shape space. Through analysis of sensory data generation process, a likelihood in Bayes theorem is modeled (e.g., as additive Gaussian noise)

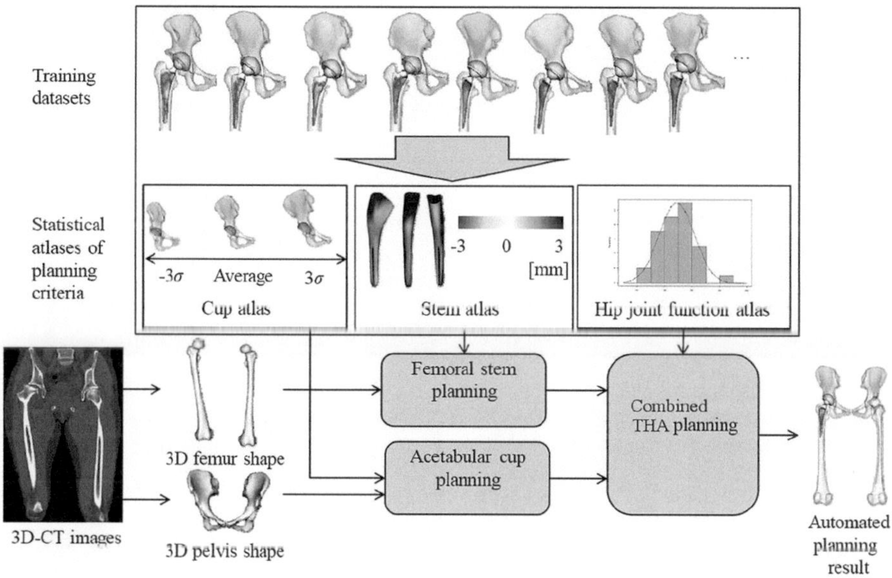

Fig. 4 System overview of automated optimization of preoperative planning for combined pelvic and femoral implants [30]. The SSMs for single-implant planning (acetabular cup and femoral stem) [28, 29] are combined with statistical models of hip joint functions to derive the MAP formulation for automated optimization method of THA planning. (Copyright © 2013, IEEE)

joint), is addressed. Probability distribution $P(X)$ represents the variability of X, that is, the pelvis shape and the placed cup implant on it (with the appropriate size and position) among the different patients, and is modeled by the SDS framework using past surgical data. $P(X|D)$ represents the variability of X, given the measured pelvis shape data, D, which may be perturbated by some noise. The variability of X in $P(X|D)$ will become (much) smaller than that in $P(X)$. X_{opt} which maximizes $P(X|D)$ will be regarded as the most probable X when D is given. The size, position, and orientation of the cup implant with respect to the pelvis are determined from X_{opt}. X can be extended from the combined pelvis and cup to the combined pelvis, femurs, and, all implants needed for THA.

One question is whether the most probable postoperative patient anatomy can be regarded as the optimal plan. Due to regression effects, it is expected that the prediction will not be affected by outlier plans in the training dataset. Therefore, the resulted prediction will provide a typical postoperative anatomy given preoperative patient data, in which implicit clinical knowledge is effectively embedded. Nevertheless, the prediction only provides an anatomically plausible solution from the aspect of implicit clinical knowledge. The probabilistic models of postoperative joint functions, which are constructed from past patient data, can be combined to further optimize the joint functions in the same framework while anatomical plausibility is maintained [30] (Fig. 4). Recent deep learning approaches [31, 32] will effectively enhance this framework to improve the performance in the near future.

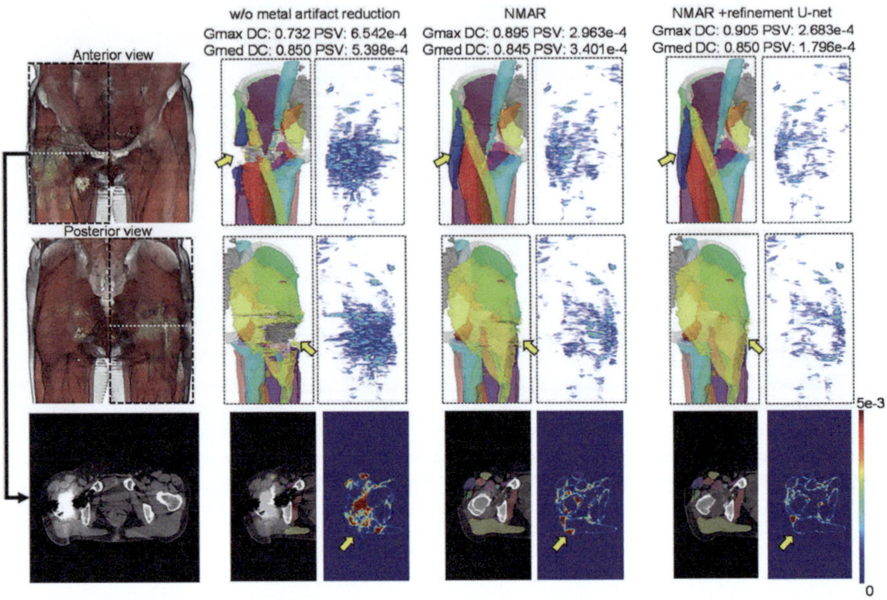

Fig. 5 Real image experiment of metal artifact reduction [33]. 3D renderings and axial cross sections for the real postoperative image of the patient are shown in the left-most column. The segmentation results under three different conditions (without artifact reduction, normalized metal artifact reduction (NMAR) method, and NMAR with refinement U-net) are shown from the second-left to right-most columns. The uncertainty images obtained by Bayesian U-Net segmentation are also shown in the right sides of corresponding segmentation results. The window display of original CT images was [−150,350] HU. Arrows indicate areas where accuracy improvements were observed when the NMAR method [35] and refinement U-Net were used. By combining refinement U-Net, the artifact reduction was improved in comparison with using NMAR only. Note that the uncertainty became smaller as well when the artifact reduction was performed, which shows a possibility that the uncertainty can be used to evaluate the effect of artifact reduction in the real CT images. (Copyright © 2020, Springer Science Business Media, LLC, part of Springer Nature)

There may be two approaches in preparing the training dataset of the postoperative patient anatomy to construct prior $P(X)$ for automated preoperative THA planning. One is to combine the preoperative patient anatomy reconstructed from preoperative CT with preoperative planning data about implant models, sizes, positions, and so on to simulationally reconstruct the postoperative anatomy. The other is to use postoperative CT to reconstruct the postoperative patient anatomy including implants. The former approach may not reflect the actual postoperative anatomy because the actual surgery may be different from the preoperative plans. The latter will reflect the actual postoperative anatomy, but metal artifacts caused by the implants will result in serious degradation in postoperative CT images, which affects the accuracy of automated segmentation. Nevertheless, recently developed metal artifact reduction methods combined with deep learning [33, 34] significantly reduce the unwanted artifacts (Fig. 5). Future work will include modelling of $P(X)$ by a large dataset of postoperative CT data. By using postoperative CT data at multiple time phases, musculoskeletal recovery processes of THA patients can also be modeled [36].

4 Summary and Integration with Robotic Surgery

In this chapter, deep learning and statistical modeling of the musculoskeletal patient anatomy, preoperative planning, and postoperative patient anatomy in orthopedic surgery, especially THA, have been addressed. Fully automated segmentation of pre- and postoperative images is now sufficiently accurate for the automated modeling of pre- and postoperative anatomical structures including muscles, bones, and implants from a large number of the patient image data. Therefore, automated modeling of preoperative planning and postoperative patient anatomy is facilitated.

We mainly addressed optimization and automation of the CAD part of the surgical CAD/CAM framework by the SDS framework, which has been drastically enhanced by AI. We did not address the intraoperative modeling in the CAM part. The Robodoc system for THA and TKA, which is a pre-programmed robot, was one of the earliest surgical robotic systems although the da Vinci system, which is a master-slave type robot, is currently much more popular. Recently, the Mako system for THA and TKA is becoming popular. While the Mako system incorporates both pre-programming and master-slave aspects, it basically guides the surgeons so as to accurately execute the preoperative plan. Therefore, the preoperative planning is particularly important, and its optimality will enhance the value of precise robotic surgery. The surgical CAD/CAM and SDS frameworks will be effectively combined by AI and will lead to better patient care in the future.

References

1. Taylor RH, Mittelstadt BD, Paul HA, Hanson W, Kazanzides P, Zuhars JF, Williamson B, Musits BL, Glassman E, Bargar WL. An image-directed robotic system for precise orthopaedic surgery. IEEE Trans Robot Autom. 1994;10(3):261–75.
2. Taylor RH, Stoiariovici D. Medical robotics in computer-integrated surgery. IEEE Trans Robot Autom. 2003;19(5):922–6.
3. Sugano N, Nishii T, Miki H, Yoshikawa H, Sato Y, Tamura S. Mid-term results of cementless total hip replacement using a ceramic-on-ceramic bearing with and without computer navigation. J Bone Joint Surg Br. 2007;89(4):455–60.
4. Sugano N. Computer-assisted orthopaedic surgery and robotic surgery in total hip arthroplasty. Clin Orthop Surg. 2013;5(1):1–9.
5. Tarwala R, Dorr LD. Robotic assisted total hip arthroplasty using the MAKO platform. Curr Rev Musculoskelet Med. 2011;4(3):151–6.
6. Ando W, Takao M, Hamada H, Uemura K, Sugano N. Comparison of the accuracy of the cup position and orientation in total hip arthroplasty for osteoarthritis secondary to developmental dysplasia of the hip between the Mako robotic arm-assisted system and computed tomography-based navigation. Int Orthop. 2021;45(7):1719–25.
7. Sato Y. Compute aided surgery: current status and future directions. J Inst Electron Inform Commun Eng. 2006;89(2):144–50. (in Japanese)
8. Taylor RH, Kazanzides P, Fischer GS, Simaan N. Medical robotics and computer-integrated interventional medicine. In: Biomedical information technology. Academic; 2020. p. 617–72.
9. Maier-Hein L, Vedula SS, Speidel S, Navab N, Kikinis R, Park A, Eisenmann M, Feussner H, Forestier G, Giannarou S, Hashizume M. Surgical data science for next-generation interventions. Nat Biomed Eng. 2017;1(9):691–6.

10. Maier-Hein L, Eisenmann M, Sarikaya D, März K, Collins T, Malpani A, Fallert J, Feussner H, Giannarou S, Mascagni P, Nakawala H. Surgical data science–from concepts toward clinical translation. Med Image Anal. 2022;76:102306.
11. Ronneberger O, Fischer P, Brox T. U-net: convolutional networks for biomedical image segmentation. In: International conference on medical image computing and computer-assisted intervention. Springer; 2015. p. 234–41.
12. Hiasa Y, Otake Y, Takao M, Ogawa T, Sugano N, Sato Y. Automated muscle segmentation from clinical CT using Bayesian U-net for personalized musculoskeletal modeling. IEEE Trans Med Imaging. 2019;39(4):1030–40.
13. Yokota F, Otake Y, Takao M, Ogawa T, Okada T, Sugano N, Sato Y. Automated muscle segmentation from CT images of the hip and thigh using a hierarchical multi-atlas method. Int J Comput Assist Radiol Surg. 2018;13(7):977–86.
14. Uemura K, Otake Y, Takao M, Makino H, Soufi M, Iwasa M, Sugano N, Sato Y. Development of an open-source measurement system to assess the areal bone mineral density of the proximal femur from clinical CT images. Arch Osteoporos. 2022;17(1):1–1.
15. Ogawa T, Takao M, Otake Y, Yokota F, Hamada H, Sakai T, Sato Y, Sugano N. Validation study of the CT-based cross-sectional evaluation of muscular atrophy and fatty degeneration around the pelvis and the femur. J Orthop Sci. 2020;25(1):139–44.
16. Qian L, Todo M, Matsushita Y, Koyano K. Effects of implant diameter, insertion depth, and loading angle on stress/strain fields in implant/jawbone systems: finite element analysis. Int J Oral Maxillofac Implants. 2009;24(5)
17. Tawara D, Sakamoto J, Murakami H, Kawahara N, Oda J, Tomita K. Mechanical evaluation by patient-specific finite element analyses demonstrates therapeutic effects for osteoporotic vertebrae. J Mech Behav Biomed Mater. 2010;3(1):31–40.
18. Silberman N, Hoiem D, Kohli P, Fergus R. Indoor segmentation and support inference from RGBD images. In: European conference on computer vision. Berlin/Heidelberg: Springer; 2012. p. 746–60.
19. Eigen D, Fergus R. Predicting depth, surface normals and semantic labels with a common multi-scale convolutional architecture. In: Proceedings of the IEEE international conference on computer vision; 2015. p. 2650–8.
20. Otake Y, Armand M, Armiger RS, Kutzer MD, Basafa E, Kazanzides P, Taylor RH. Intraoperative image-based multiview 2D/3D registration for image-guided orthopaedic surgery: incorporation of fiducial-based C-arm tracking and GPU-acceleration. IEEE Trans Med Imaging. 2011;31(4):948–62.
21. Gu Y, Otake Y, Uemura K, Soufi M, Takao M, Sugano N, Sato Y. BMD-GAN: bone mineral density estimation using x-ray image decomposition into projections of bone-segmented quantitative computed tomography using hierarchical learning. In: International conference on medical image computing and computer-assisted intervention. Springer; 2022. p. 644–54.
22. Shiode R, Kabashima M, Hiasa Y, Oka K, Murase T, Sato Y, Otake Y. 2D–3D reconstruction of distal forearm bone from actual X-ray images of the wrist using convolutional neural networks. Sci Rep. 2021;11(1):1–2.
23. Nakanishi N, Otake Y, Hiasa Y, Gu Y, Uemura K, Takao M, Sugano N, Sato Y. Decomposition of musculoskeletal structures from radiography using an improved CycleGAN framework. PREPRINT (Version 1) available at Research Square; 2022. https://doi.org/10.21203/rs.3.rs-2011568/v1.
24. Tiulpin A, Thevenot J, Rahtu E, Lehenkari P, Saarakkala S. Automatic knee osteoarthritis diagnosis from plain radiographs: a deep learning-based approach. Sci Rep. 2018;8(1):1–0.
25. Leung K, Zhang B, Tan J, Shen Y, Geras KJ, Babb JS, Cho K, Chang G, Deniz CM. Prediction of total knee replacement and diagnosis of osteoarthritis by using deep learning on knee radiographs: data from the osteoarthritis initiative. Radiology. 2020;296(3):584.
26. Üreten K, Arslan T, Gültekin KE, Demir AN, Özer HF, Bilgili Y. Detection of hip osteoarthritis by using plain pelvic radiographs with deep learning methods. Skeletal Radiol. 2020;49(9):1369–74.

27. Sato Y. Application of statistical shape modeling for CAOS: a tutorial. Computer Assisted Orthopaedic Surgery for Hip and Knee. 2018:173–82.
28. Otomaru I, Nakamoto M, Kagiyama Y, Takao M, Sugano N, Tomiyama N, Tada Y, Sato Y. Automated preoperative planning of femoral stem in total hip arthroplasty from 3D CT data: atlas-based approach and comparative study. Med Image Anal. 2012;16(2):415–26.
29. Kagiyama Y, Otomaru I, Takao M, Sugano N, Nakamoto M, Yokota F, Tomiyama N, Tada Y, Sato Y. CT-based automated planning of acetabular cup for total hip arthroplasty (THA) based on hybrid use of two statistical atlases. Int J Comput Assist Radiol Surg. 2016;11(12):2253–71.
30. Kagiyama Y, Takao M, Sugano N, Tada Y, Tomiyama N, Sato Y. Optimization of surgical planning of total hip arthroplasty based on computational anatomy. In: 2013 35th annual international conference of the IEEE engineering in medicine and biology society (EMBC). IEEE; 2013. p. 2980–3.
31. Huo J, Huang G, Han D, Wang X, Du Y, Chen Y, Cai D, Zhao C. Value of 3D preoperative planning for primary total hip arthroplasty based on artificial intelligence technology. J Orthop Surg Res. 2021;16(1):1–3.
32. Chen X, Liu X, Wang Y, Ma R, Zhu S, Li S, Li S, Dong X, Li H, Wang G, Wu Y. Development and validation of an artificial intelligence preoperative planning system (AIHIP) for total hip arthroplasty. Front Med. 2022:551.
33. Sakamoto M, Hiasa Y, Otake Y, Takao M, Suzuki Y, Sugano N, Sato Y. Bayesian segmentation of hip and thigh muscles in metal artifact-contaminated CT using convolutional neural network-enhanced normalized metal artifact reduction. J Signal Process Syst. 2020;92(3):335–44.
34. Nakao M, Imanishi K, Ueda N, Imai Y, Kirita T, Matsuda T. Regularized three-dimensional generative adversarial nets for unsupervised metal artifact reduction in head and neck CT images. IEEE Access. 2020;8:109453–65.
35. Meyer E, Raupach R, Lell M, Schmidt B, Kachelrieß M. Normalized metal artifact reduction (NMAR) in computed tomography. Med Phys. 2010;37(10):5482–93.
36. Uemura K, Takao M, Sakai T, Nishii T, Sugano N. Volume increases of the gluteus maximus, gluteus medius, and thigh muscles after hip arthroplasty. J Arthroplast. 2016;31(4):906–12.

Artificial Intelligence in Intraocular Robotic Microsurgery

Iulian I. Iordachita, Nassir Navab, Peter L. Gehlbach, Marin Kobilarov, and M. Ali Nasseri

Abstract Intraocular microsurgery requires surgical skills at the limits of human physiological capability. These minimally invasive procedures require staggering accuracy, precision, and steadiness that typical humans are not able to achieve. Combined with advanced imaging, robotics has become a promising strategy for advancing the field of intraocular microsurgery. Artificial intelligence, especially machine learning, is gradually advancing the practice of surgery with tremendous achievements in imaging, environment perception and understanding, navigation, and robotic assistance. Machine learning applied to intraocular robotic microsurgery is a relatively recent phenomenon that has the potential to revolutionize eye care by combining human strengths with computer and sensor-based technology, in an information-driven environment. Robotic microsurgery, augmented by artificial intelligence, has the potential to enhance a microsurgeon's physical capabilities to superhuman levels, by increasing the precision, safety, efficacy, and efficiency of the surgical tasks and procedures being performed. In this chapter, we analyze present advancements in intraocular robotic microsurgery and the emergence of artificial intelligence applications as an inevitable new strategy for expanding retinal microsurgical techniques into domains that have heretofore been inaccessible frontiers for unassisted human surgeons.

Keywords Artificial intelligence · Machine learning · Intraocular microsurgery · Robotic-assisted microsurgery · Perception · Localizing and mapping · System modelling and control

I. I. Iordachita (✉) · P. L. Gehlbach · M. Kobilarov
Johns Hopkins University, Baltimore, MD, USA
e-mail: iordachita@jhu.edu; pgelbach@jhmi.edu; mkobila1@jhu.edu

N. Navab · M. A. Nasseri
Technical University of Munich, Munich, Germany
e-mail: nassir.navab@tum.de; ali.nasseri@tum.de

K. Masamune et al. (eds.), *Artificial Intelligence in Surgery*,
https://doi.org/10.1007/978-981-96-6635-5_11

1 Introduction

At present there is no longer a question of whether artificial intelligence (AI) will revolutionize the practice of modern surgery. There are now numerous substantial advancements in practice that utilize AI for diagnosis, imaging, tool navigation, surgical instrument utilization, as well as interfacing with robotics [1]. Artificial intelligence and more specifically machine learning are integrated into surgical robotic platforms for environment perception and understanding, real-time decision- making, and to increase precision, safety, and efficiency of the surgical tasks performed. Moreover, advanced machine learning techniques and algorithms (learning from demonstration, reinforcement learning, etc.) can increase the level of robotic autonomy for ever more complicated tasks notably when considering interactions with complex and dynamic surgical environments.

Eye surgery (or ophthalmic surgery) is a type of microsurgery performed on the eye by an ophthalmic surgeon using miniaturized instruments and an operative stereomicroscope, for fine and highly precise tasks, requiring specialized skills and capabilities only acquired through extensive training. Following the current trend in modern surgery, machine learning has become an important tool in advancing eye surgery by extracting data to evaluate, teach, and support the clinician during clinical tasks [2]. Machine learning has been used to increase the accuracy in diagnosis of ophthalmic disease like diabetic retinopathy [3–5], age-related macular degeneration [6, 7], retinopathy of prematurity [8], glaucoma [9], and ocular oncology [10]. Ophthalmic surgical education has benefitted from introducing advanced AI-based and virtual reality technologies into surgical training [11–14], surgical evaluation [15], and now intraoperative guidance [16]. Similarly, cataract surgery, the most performed surgical procedure [2], has proven amendable to machine learning techniques as applied to diagnosis and grading [15], preoperative planning [17, 18], and surgical management [19–21].

Vitreoretinal surgery may be the most technically challenging eye surgery [22] and deals with the surgical treatment of retinal and posterior segment diseases. Following the trend in microsurgery [23], robotic assistance, enhanced by artificial intelligence and combined with advanced imaging, has the potential to fundamentally change and advance the field of intraocular surgery. Still in its early stages, robotic retinal surgery has been cautiously introduced into the operating room and has been successfully evaluated in a limited number of clinical trials [24–26]. Nonetheless, owing to its demonstrated capabilities, robotic intraocular microsurgery, augmented with artificial intelligence, has the potential to assist the surgeon and provide superhuman physical capabilities, enabling unprecedented as well as safer surgical care for patients.

This chapter is organized as follows. Section 2 reviews relevant intraocular surgical procedures, challenges associated with human factors, and the motivation for robotic assistance and artificial intelligence in intraocular retinal microsurgery. Section 3 discusses current approaches utilizing robotic systems and sensorized instruments for intraocular surgery. Sections 4 and 5 review the artificial intelligence techniques employed in intraocular robotic microsurgery for perception, system modeling, and control. Finally, Sect. 6 includes a forward-looking discussion on future directions as well as concluding remarks.

2 Need for Robotic Assistance and Artificial Intelligence in Intraocular Microsurgery

The clinical discipline of ophthalmic surgery consists of delicate extraocular and intraocular microsurgical procedures. Many extraocular procedures occur on the millimeter scale and are routinely performed freehand. Among the exceptions to this are the demanding requirements of refractive and rehabilitative cornea surgery—that may utilize automated robotic lasers, optical coherence tomography (OCT) image guidance, and depth-guided incisions. Intraocular surgery is characterized by further exacting, micrometer-scale requirements. It is performed to strategically alter internal eye anatomy to treat disease and maximize vision. Intraocular procedures require a high-powered stereo operating microscope as well as additional optics, lighting, tissue staining, high precision microsurgical instruments, and highly trained microsurgeons. Even with these requirements met, the globe interior remains a constrained and high-risk workspace. Some portions of the interior eye are poorly visualized and difficult to access. Internal tissues such as the retina are fragile, unforgiving, and with limited ability to regenerate. Importantly, present and emerging surgical procedures may contain essential steps that require dexterity, tremor control, and visualization that may be beyond unassisted human capabilities.

The eye consists of a number of clinically relevant tissues including but not limited to the cornea, lens, trabecular meshwork, and retina [26]. These serve as surgical targets for the major intraocular surgical specialty areas in ophthalmology, namely, cornea, cataract, glaucoma, and vitreoretinal surgery, respectively. Each specialty area presents unique robotic, artificial intelligence, and machine learning opportunities, e.g., precise corneal incisions in corneal refractive and transplant surgery, semi-automation of frequently performed surgical steps in cataract surgery, and enhanced precision in stent and drain placement in glaucoma surgery. It has however been the many challenges of retinal microsurgery that have generated the greatest recent interest from the robotics community.

Retinal microsurgery routinely requires maneuvers directed at single micron scale targets (some of which are optically transparent to the operating surgeon's eye), by surgeons with 50–200 micrometers of physiological hand tremor. Moreover, the retina can be torn/injured with single millinewton forces that are beneath human tactile perception [27]. Once injured the retina and vision may be irreversibly damaged. Recent developments in retinal microsurgery have introduced increasingly advanced, challenging, and presently higher-risk procedures with potential therapeutic benefit. These include but are not limited to subretinal injections, peeling of internal limiting membrane, and endovascular retinal surgery. Of particular interest in retinal surgery is the high level of reliance on preoperative, intraoperative, and postoperative imaging to plan, execute, and evaluate retinal surgery. Fortuitously, retinal surgery is conducted in a high-resolution video-accessible environment. Taken collectively these and other factors make retinal surgery an ideal challenge for artificial intelligence, machine learning, and stepwise advances toward robotic automation.

Algorithms that enable robots to assist surgeons by performing repetitive, ultra-high precision navigational maneuvers, or procedures requiring prolonged endurance are particularly amenable to robotic assistance, as are tasks requiring target recognition. Applications that interpret retinal images and anatomy during the course of surgery (tissue tracking) are well suited to the high-resolution imaging environment that characterizes operative retinal surgery. Machine learning, deep learning, and deep learning recurrent neural networks are presently being applied to preoperative planning and intraoperative tool guidance, while at the same time predictive and seemingly cognitive capabilities are evolving that would be anticipated to be of greatest utility intraoperatively. When fully integrated with the human machine interface decreased intra- and inter-surgeon procedure variability, enhanced precision, enhanced task capabilities, reduced error rates, reduced costs, reduced fatigue, improved ergonomics, and the freeing of a surgeon to focus on the "big-picture" during surgery, all are expected to lead to improved surgical outcomes and patient vision. Such advances in ophthalmic microsurgery would be broadly translational to non-ophthalmic minimally invasive surgical applications.

3 Robotic Systems and Sensorized Instruments for Intraocular Microsurgery

Undoubtedly robotic assistance promises multiple benefits for eye surgery, and there is a strategic role for artificial intelligence to enable access of robotic technology into the ophthalmic operating room. Notable known advantages are the augmentation of capability and safety and eventually efficiency to improve patient outcomes. The integration of various "smart instruments" could further extend robotic functionality, enhance safety, and improve surgical performance. Given current areas of emphasis, force and distance sensing are proposed to be of paramount importance in providing enhanced safety protecting from inadvertent eye movement and to better depth control instrument navigation. This section summarizes state-of-the-art concepts in robotic systems and sensorized instruments for intraocular microsurgery. A comprehensive review is presented in [26].

3.1 Robotic Systems for Intraocular Microsurgery

In the last decades, researchers worldwide have developed numerous robotic systems for intraocular microsurgery. As shown in [24], some of the basic requirements for these robotic systems include (1) requirements that they be lightweight and compliant, to allow safe interactions with patients and clinicians; (2) be easily operated by clinical personnel; (3) be easy to attach to the surgical table or fit into the user's hand; (4) be interfaced with a visualization system having the necessary resolution for microsurgical tasks; (5) be guaranteed safe for instrument manipulation outside and inside the eye via hardware and software constraints; and (6) ensure safety by reacting properly to involuntary patient movements.Currently, there are three main approaches related to robotic system control:

(1) telemanipulation, the systems provide tremor filtering and motion scaling; (2) comanipulation ("co-bots"), the systems support tremor filtering, but lack motion scaling; and (3) handheld devices, which have minimal impact on the workflow. A fourth concept that may become applicable in minimally invasive approaches consists of magnetically controlled microrobots [28, 29]. Some advantages and disadvantages of these approaches are summarized in [24].

Telemanipulation systems: In the telemanipulation approach, the motion controller (leader system) is operated by the surgeon, while the instruments are attached to a separate robotic manipulator (follower system) placed next to the patient. The surgeon-operated system can be positioned either adjacent to the surgical site or at a separate console, and a computer translates the commands from the motion controller to the following manipulator [30–34]. Telemanipulation robots provide tremor filtering and the ability to position an instrument at a predefined position for prolonged periods of time. The main advantages of a telemanipulation robot include variable motion scaling and the possibility to provide (semi) automation of procedures, making this design particularly well suited for a wide range of both static and dynamic tasks. Among the many telemanipulation systems, the PRECEYES Surgical System [33] and the Intraocular Robotic Interventional Surgical System (IRISS) [34] are two relevant examples.

Hand-Over-Hand or Comanipulation Systems In the comanipulation approach, a robotic manipulator and human operator hold and simultaneously control an instrument. The manipulator greatly dampens movements, thereby limiting tremor during a surgical maneuver. Moreover, such systems can maintain a stable position independent of the surgeon's grip, further extending the physiologic reach of a surgeon. Two relevant examples in this category are the Johns Hopkins Steady-Hand Eye Robot [35] and the KU Leuven robot [36]. The stability and possibility to maintain a static position are particularly useful during slow and careful injection of drugs, e.g., during retinal vein cannulation [37–39] and subretinal injections.

Handheld, Smart Surgical Tools In this approach, the smart surgical tools are manually operated by the surgeons, augmenting their surgical capabilities as defined by the specific tool's function [40–42] by, e.g., limiting hand tremor, providing micrometer precision and accuracy, as well as by scaling motion and forces. In this category, a relevant example is Micron [41], a handheld micromanipulator developed at the Robotics Institute, Carnegie Mellon University. Despite their intuitiveness, these tools are often an engineering challenge, with limited abilities to accommodate a wide range of instruments. Their capabilities can be extended by employing complex and intelligent instruments like optical tracking and "snake-like" systems [43, 44]. The requirement that these devices need to be continuously held by the surgeon could be seen as an inherent limitation. However, safe manipulation and unnecessary immobilization of the patient head are inherent benefits for handheld tools.

3.2 Sensorized Instruments for Intraocular Microsurgery

As in other surgical procedures that require physical interaction with patient anatomy through a surgical instrument [45], during intraocular surgery excessive contact forces can result in tissue damage, while insufficient forces prevent task completion [46]. Specific maneuvers and tasks are characterized by safe and often narrow ranges of forces that can also act as quantitative metrics of surgical skill. Furthermore, real-time force data can be used to control robotic platforms or provide feedback to human operators.

Tool-Tip Forces Surgical instruments could come in contact with tissue inside the eye (e.g., tool-tip to retina interaction) or at the eyewall, at the sclerotomy (tool-shaft to sclera interaction). Tool-tip forces are difficult to estimate by hand as the majority are well below human sensory thresholds [27], while scleral forces (typically an order of magnitude larger [47]) obscure them. Consequently, the forces at the instrument tip are able to be measured with sensors embedded in the intraocular segment of the tool, and one possible solution is to employ fiber optic sensors (FOS) [26]. The advantages of using FOS for sub-millimeter sensorized instruments include very small size (diameter 60 to 250μm) [48], high resolution, biocompatibility, sterilizability, electrical immunity, etc. The majority of FOS-based sensorized instruments involve FBG (Fiber Bragg Grating) sensors [49], while some employ the Fabry-Perot Interferometry (FPI) measurement principle [50]. Employing FBGs, prior work has focused on the development of pick tools [51–54], microneedles that could be used for vein cannulation or subretinal injection procedures [55–59], and micro-forceps that could be used for membrane peeling force detection [60–62].

Scleral Interaction Forces Some research [63] investigated the integration of FBG force sensors at the tool-tip and also into the tool shaft, outside the eye, to simultaneously measure forces at the retina, the sclera contact location (tool-tip insertion depth), and the corresponding contact force (scleral force). The information from such multi-function force-sensing tools could be used to augment robotic behavior and create an adaptive remote center-of-motion (RCM) constraint to minimize eye motion and potential damage on the eyewall at the sclerotomy [64–66].

Instruments with OCT for Depth Perception Optical coherence tomography (OCT) with its micrometer-level resolution has been accepted as intraoperative imaging modality for retinal surgery [26]. OCT-based sensorized tools have been developed to visualize retina layers [67–69], to assess the tool-tip distance to anatomy in real time [52], and to conduct subretinal injections at specific depths [70].

More recently, FBG-based force sensing was combined with OCT-based distance-sensing in a cannulation needle [71, 72].

As mentioned above, the smart instruments, employing various sensors, can increase functionality, safety, and performance in robot-assisted intraocular surgery. Furthermore, sensorized instruments augmented with machine learning algorithms to predict and detect the interaction with intraocular microenvironment will be indispensable for assisting the robots to perform surgical steps or eventually the entire procedure, independently [73].

4 Perception in Intraocular Robotic Microsurgery

Generally, surgical robotics can use artificial intelligence techniques for (1) perception, (2) localization and mapping, (3) system modeling and control, and (4) human-robot interaction [1]. Considering the overlap between intraoperative guidance and robot localization and mapping, the most relevant benefits of AI in intraocular robotic microsurgery are perception (presented in this section) and system modeling and control (presented in Sect. 5).

As an AI technique for surgical robotics, perception deals with instrument segmentation and tracking and the interaction between surgical tools and their environment [1]. Instrument tracking in ocular microsurgery depends on the type of visualization: the most relevant ones are stereomicroscopy and optical coherence tomography [26]. Several works have employed machine learning methods to provide fast and robust solutions for instrument tracking overcoming the challenges related to 2D microscopy: illumination changes, cluttered background, deformable shape of the instrument, motion blur, shadows, etc. [2]. Among these, boosting methods [74], random forests [75, 76], and other described methods to update learned models dynamically [77] have been shown to work extremely well for 2D instrument pose localization. However, 2D images from a single microscope are insufficient to estimate an instrument's 6DOF (degrees of freedom) movements during surgery, which is necessary for advanced therapies such as robotic microsurgery and real-time visualization, specifically when the needle is inside the retinal tissue. Traditional navigation solutions such as optical tracking or electromagnetic tracking are not applicable as they usually have an accuracy in the range of 200 to 1400 micrometers, which is worse than the required precision to perform retinal surgery (around $10\mu m$, [26]). To overcome the abovementioned challenges, Probst et al. [78] proposed for the first time to use a stereomicroscope to detect and localize the instrument for applications in robot-assisted retinal surgery. This method, employing convolutional neural networks (CNNs), achieved a precision of 100 micrometers. However, as shown above, intraocular surgery presents unique challenges and has even higher accuracy requirements that limit the stereomicroscope capability method in some scenarios, e.g., subretinal injection. Optical coherence tomography, which was originally used for the diagnosis of ophthalmic diseases because of its excellent

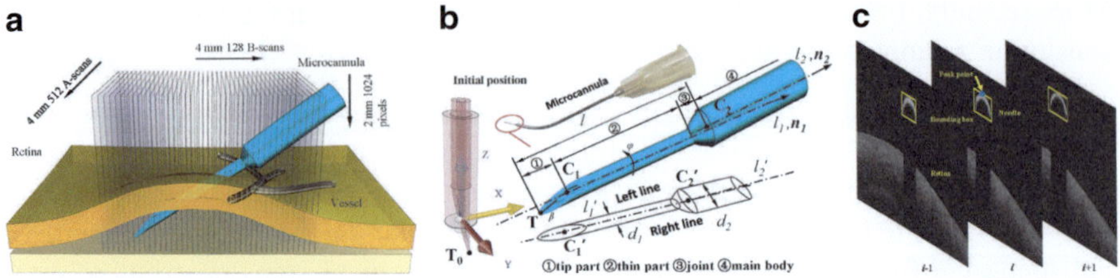

Fig. 1 OCT-based 6DOF needle pose estimation: (**a**) OCT scan setup for subretinal injection. OCT scans a cube with a resolution of 128 × 512 × 1024 pixels in 4 × 4 × 2 mm; (**b**) the structure of the microcannula and its projection; (**c**) the pose and position of the microcannula. (© [2022] IEEE. Reprinted, with permission, from [80])

resolution, has been developed to capture real-time images associated with interactions between the surgical instrument and the retinal tissue. Recently OCT applications have been extended to intraoperative applications. Microscope Integrated OCT (MI-OCT) developed by Carl Zeiss Meditec (Lumera 700 with RESCAN 700 OCT engine), which was first introduced for clinical use in 2014 [79], can share the same optical pathway with the ophthalmic microscope to give real-time cross-sectional information of the target scan area. This is an ideal imaging modality for ophthalmic surgery. MI-OCT imaging modality together with a proper reconstruction framework enables 3D scanning of the target area intraoperatively (Fig. 1a).

Estimating the 6DOF pose of an object from an incomplete point cloud has drawn much attention in computer vision with numerous applications. Kehl et al. [81] introduced a light-weight 3D tracking with 6DOF pose estimation. However, their method cannot be directly applied since the iterative closest point (ICP) with 6DOF parameters relies heavily on the initial guess from the object viewpoint features, e.g., clustered viewpoint feature histogram (CVFH), and the geometrical feature of the needle is cylindrical and has a beveled shape at the needle tip without strong features (Fig. 1b). This can lead to a local optima result and may not be suitable for safety-critical surgical applications.

As a practical alternative, a modified iterative closest point to estimate the 6DOF pose of the needle directly from the OCT volume data was suggested by Zhou et al. [80] (Fig. 1). The premise of this method is that the actual dimensions of the needle are within the range necessary to satisfy the standard for manufacturing medical devices (ISO 9626:2016), typically 6.4 micrometers in diameter and 1 degree in bevel angle. The method consists of two main parts. The first part is a robust needle segmentation method introduced to get the 3D needle point cloud in the OCT volume. Due to the infrared light source of OCT and the geometrical features of the needle, the segmentation result is robust to illumination variation and speck reflection. The second part is a shift-rotate ICP (SR-ICP) to estimate the 6DOF pose of the segmented needle point cloud. Using the geometrical features of the needle, the 6DOF pose is reduced to a 2DOF optimization problem, which can dramatically decrease the chance of getting local optima. Furthermore, different from the typical methods which use object viewpoint features to start the initial guess, Zhou et al.

[82] proposed to align the CAD model tip to the visual needle tip in the OCT volume. This initial guess is very close to the global optimum. To validate these methods, a comparison of the result with brutal grid search (GS) and standard ICP was implemented. Several ex vivo experiments were performed on pig eyes and demonstrated that the AI methods utilizing fundus and intraoperative OCT images are qualified in 6DOF needle pose estimation for retinal surgery applications (Fig. 1c). Notably, the position accuracy can be controlled to within 10 micrometers with 95% confidence, which meets most of the surgical requirements [82].

In addition to tracking the position and orientation of the surgical instruments, automatic analysis of the anatomical target area is of utmost importance to achieve intraoperative OCT (iOCT) supported or even eventual autonomous robotic surgery. This is most applicable to procedures such as subretinal injection that require access to sub-surface areas not visible from conventional microscopic views but benefit from the analysis of iOCT B-scans. Identifying the target area and predicting the point of contact between the robotically controlled instrument and the anatomical structures from a real-time B-scan segmentation can support the appropriate control strategy of the robotic system by continuously monitoring the distance between the tool-tip and the tissue (e.g., Internal Limiting Membrane (ILM) as well as the Retinal Pigment Epithelium (RPE)), therefore reducing the risk of irreversible damage to critical retinal cells. Retinal layer segmentation and analysis have been introduced for diagnostic OCT imaging and extensively investigated by numerous works [83–86] in recent years. However, differences in signal power and speckle noise levels between diagnostic and interventional OCT and the presence of instruments in iOCT imaging generate a translational gap that prevents the direct integration of such algorithms into the surgical context. To overcome this gap, Sommersperger et al. [87] introduced an initial work combining the efforts of instrument identification and retinal layer segmentation to analyze iOCT volumes. A constraint of developing such an intraoperative pipeline for robotic setups (see Fig. 2a) is the efficient volumetric data processing in real time, since advances in spiral scanning [88] and swept-source [89] OCT technology pose the need for efficient processing algorithms that can cope with high acquisition data rates of several GB/s. The proposed pipeline initially reduces the acquired volume to a minimal region of interest (ROI) around the tool-tip to restrict the subsequent analysis to the relevant surgical area (see Fig. 2b). A U-Net-based segmentation network then extracts the retinal layer boundaries of the ILM and RPE along with the instrument surface from the relevant B scans (see Fig. 2c). The joint segmentation of retinal layers and instruments in adjacent B-scans allows the reconstruction of the surgical environment as a set of point clouds. As Fig. 2d illustrates, the generated point clouds finally enable distance estimation between the instrument and the retinal layers, estimation of the cannula insertion direction, the contact point prediction of the robot with the retina surface, and the identification of the injection target area. The overall system showed high potential for (autonomous) robotic subretinal injection by achieving the required distance estimation accuracy with an average error below 10 micrometers, high processing rates of 15Hz, and useful intraoperative visualizations during the insertion procedure.

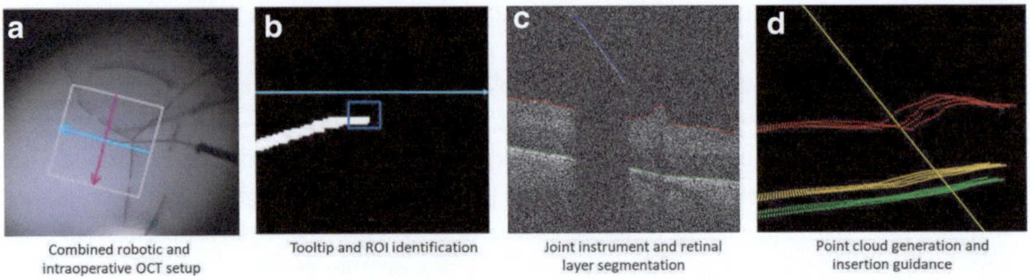

Fig. 2 Setup for iOCT-guided robotic subretinal injection. (**a**) A robotically guided 41 gauge cannula combined with an iOCT device. The blue and magenta arrows, as well as the white bounding box, indicate the volume acquisition area. (**b**) Identification of the ROI around the instrument tip indicated by the blue bounding box. (**c**) Joint segmentation of the ILM (red) and the RPE (green), as well as the surgical instrument (blue). (**d**) The point cloud representation of the retinal layers (red and green) and the injection target area (visualized as the yellow point cloud between ILM and RPE). The tool insertion direction is illustrated using the yellow line. (Adapted with permission from [87]) © The Optical Society

A current limitation to developing algorithms for iOCT-guided robotic intraocular surgery is the restricted availability of dedicated datasets required for learning-based approaches or to test algorithms on datasets with known instrument-tissue configurations. To encourage the development of data-driven algorithms for robotic intraocular surgery, a first work [90] proposed a framework to synthesize iOCT data from a purely virtual environment consisting of retinal layer meshes and virtual instrument models. Given the controllable nature of the virtual setup, the exact configuration of retinal layers and instruments is known and can be modified, which is not possible in the typical model eye or animal experiments. The proposed method to generate the synthetic iOCT data considers this virtual setup. A rendering approach first captures the layer and instrument configuration in a sub-volume of the scene, thereby mimicking the imaging area of an iOCT system.

The extracted positional information of retinal layers and instruments then allows the generation of cross-sectional label maps, including an explicit modeling of iOCT typical imaging artifacts, such as instrument shadowing and mirroring artifacts. A Generative Adversarial Network (GAN) finally converts these label maps to synthetic iOCT B-scans, modeling other physical properties of the image formation process containing iOCT typical speckle noise and signal attenuation. Experiments showed high perceptual similarity between real and synthetic iOCT B-scans and demonstrated the benefit of synthetic data for developing machine learning algorithms to support robotic intraocular surgery.

5 System Modeling and Control for Intraocular Robotic Microsurgery

Safe and efficient intraocular robotic microsurgery requires machine learning techniques for precise and reliable robot localization and mapping and intraoperative guidance as well as to predict and act on any adverse events [2]. The challenge resides in combining the OCT fine detail and depth information, microscopy broad perspective, other sensor (e.g., force) data, and robot precision and steadiness in a consistent framework that will help augment the surgeon's ability to execute any surgical tasks.

5.1 *Video-Based Guidance*

Mapping the robot space onto microscope image space has been widely investigated by many teams for automatic positioning of surgical instruments [26]. Numerous research studies demonstrated the ability to estimate the distance to the retina by employing stereo cameras [78] or reflections of a spotlight [44, 91, 92]. However, only a few of them [44, 91, 93, 94] have achieved automated positioning. For example, Tayama et al. [94], using a teleoperated surgical robot, exploited the dynamics between tool-tip and its casted shadow on the retinal surface to surmise depth. When the surgical tool moved close to the retina, the surgical tip and its shadow in the microscope image converged by a predefined pixel distance, and the robot was signaled to stop thereby ensuring safety. Yang et al. [91] proposed a structured-light approach for retinal surface estimation, employing the handheld robot Micron [41] to provide automatic scanning of a laser probe and creating projected beam patterns on the retina. By analyzing the patterns, geometry was possible to reconstruct the retina surface. The method was validated during automated photocoagulation in realistic eye phantoms. Similarly, Zhou et al. [95] employed a spotlight-based guidance for 3D navigation of a microsurgical instrument in a vessel tracking task with Steady-Hand Eye Robot (SHER) [35]. This technique outperformed manual execution and cooperative control of the SHER in a head-to-head comparison.

More recently, deep networks have been used to output robot controls or waypoint trajectories to solve navigation tasks in retinal surgery. Kim et al. [93, 96] demonstrated a CNN that predicts a distance vector between the surgical tip and the desired target tissue to be reached based on many expert demonstrations of the tool navigation task. The distance vector was then utilized for autonomous navigation of surgical tools and estimation of the retinal geometry by approximating a spherical profile. As an interesting feature of this work, the network could interact with the user via the network input. Specifically, the user was able to specify the desired position to be reached on the retinal surface by directly clicking on the visual feed of the surgery (using a mouse cursor) (Fig. 3a). The advantage of this approach was that the user was only required to specify goals in 2D via a mouse click from top-down view and the network outputted distance vectors in 3D space. The network was shown to be capable of autonomously navigating to various locations across the retinal surface with approximately 100 micrometers in XY accuracy (Fig. 3b–d), which may be sufficient for streamlining surgical tasks such as needle insertion or tissue grasping. Additionally, the learned network was combined with an optimal control framework for safe trajectory generation while satisfying known kinematic constraints, such as the remote-center-of-motion (RCM) constraint and non-penetration constraint of the estimated retinal geometry, which are essential for

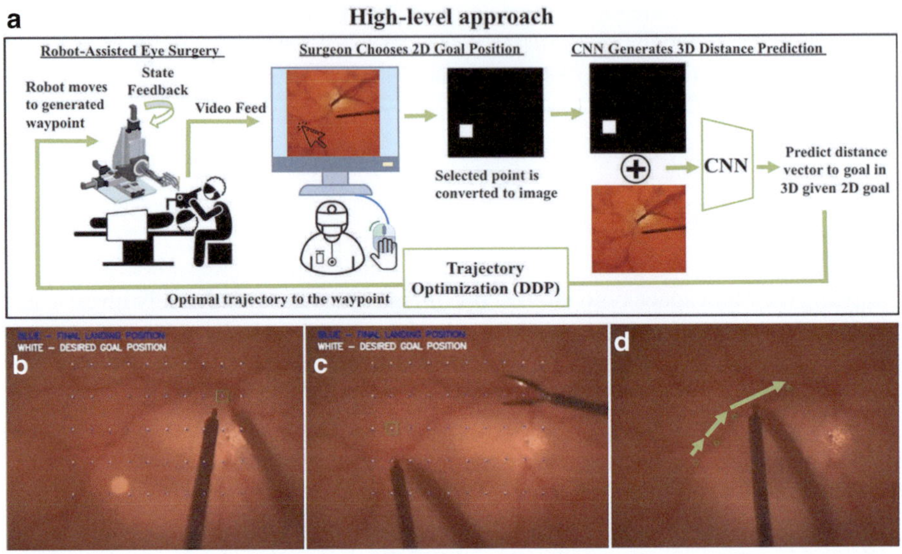

Fig. 3 Surgical tool navigation using a convolutional neural network and optimal control: (**a**) The surgeon selects the desired goal to be reached by directly clicking on the visual feed of the surgery. The network generates a distance vector from the current tool-tip position and the goal location in 3D space. This vector is used for autonomous navigation of surgical tools. (**b**) Benchmark task for assessing the autonomous navigation accuracy; the white squares are the desired positions to be reached, and the blue squares are the final landing position navigated by the network. (**c**) Benchmark task in the presence of unseen distraction such as a forceps to test network robustness. (**d**) The network can be used to reconstruct the eye geometry and perform simple autonomous tasks like vessel following. (Image © Marin Kobilarov)

ensuring safety during surgery. An extension of this work integrated chance-constrained optimal control for autonomous navigation to provide a more natural formulation of safety based on the network's output variance [97].

5.2 *OCT-Based Guidance*

OCT is a non-contact optical imaging modality that provides depth-resolved cross-sectional images in tissues [98]. Comparatively to microscopy, OCT provides higher resolution, although at a higher price. Besides the Microscope Integrated OCT (see Sect. 4), OCT information could be acquired through intraocular surgical instruments [69, 72]. More recently, OCT guidance has been widely employed in robot-assisted intraocular surgery: (1) using iOCT [99–103] and (2) instrument embedded OCT [52, 68, 70, 104]. Comprehensive reviews about OCT- aided systems for vitreoretinal surgery could be found in [26] and [105].

Machine learning techniques could be useful for augmenting the robotic precision and steadiness with OCT fine detail and depth information in intraocular robotic surgery. One recent emerging area of methods for robotic control is deep reinforcement learning (RL) [106, 107], which can solve challenging robotic problems that are otherwise difficult to formulate via supervised learning or classic optimal control strategies mentioned above. One drawback of reinforcement learning is that it takes a substantial amount of time to train and requires real-time interaction with the physical world, which is not feasible in safety-critical applications like surgery. Therefore, RL has shown progress in tasks where simulation training can be easily transferred to the real world or tasks that require low dimensional inputs rather than large dimensional inputs like images to accelerate training time. One interesting application of RL in ophthalmic surgery has been demonstrated in needle insertion in corneal keratoplasty by Keller et al. [108]. However, traditional methods using optimal control with learning-based perception are also effective solutions to this problem as demonstrated by Edwards et al. [109]. Still, since RL methods hold the promise to be a generic method for solving challenging robotic problems, active research is being done to make RL more efficient and transferable to real-world robotic tasks.

5.3 *Force-Base Guidance*

Recently, deep neural networks have emerged as generic black-box models that can be used to tackle a wide array of challenging problems. Several applications in ophthalmic surgery include predicting the surgeon's actions, warning the surgeon of dangerous events, or even automating parts of the surgical task. Various sensor data including force, robot kinematics, and images have been used to build systems for active surgical intervention and automation.

One application of active intervention using force data was demonstrated by He et al. [66], who utilized FBG force sensors to train a recurrent neural network (RNN) to characterize a surgeon's behavior. The novel active interventional control framework (AICF) was shown to enable prediction and prevention of unintentional and potentially risky maneuvers of the surgeon. It should be noted that the system was considered *active* in the sense that it actively interfered with the task, when necessary, in a predictive and intelligent manner, rather than in a passive manner by only damping the motion after the undesired event occurs. Figure 4 top shows the overall scheme of the proposed framework. The framework consisted of an FBG-based force-sensing tool attached to the SHER's end-effector [110], an RNN predictor, and an adaptive admittance controller. To design the RNN, the measurements from the FBG sensors along with velocity of the robot's end-effector and the insertion depth of the tool inside the eyeball were used. The data was fed into an RNN with long short-term memory (LSTM) units to predict undesired instances in terms of forces at the scleral port. When an undesired instance was predicted by the RNN, the adaptive admittance controller then actuated the SHER to partially interrupt the user maneuvers and perform compensatory motions to prevent the excessive range of scleral

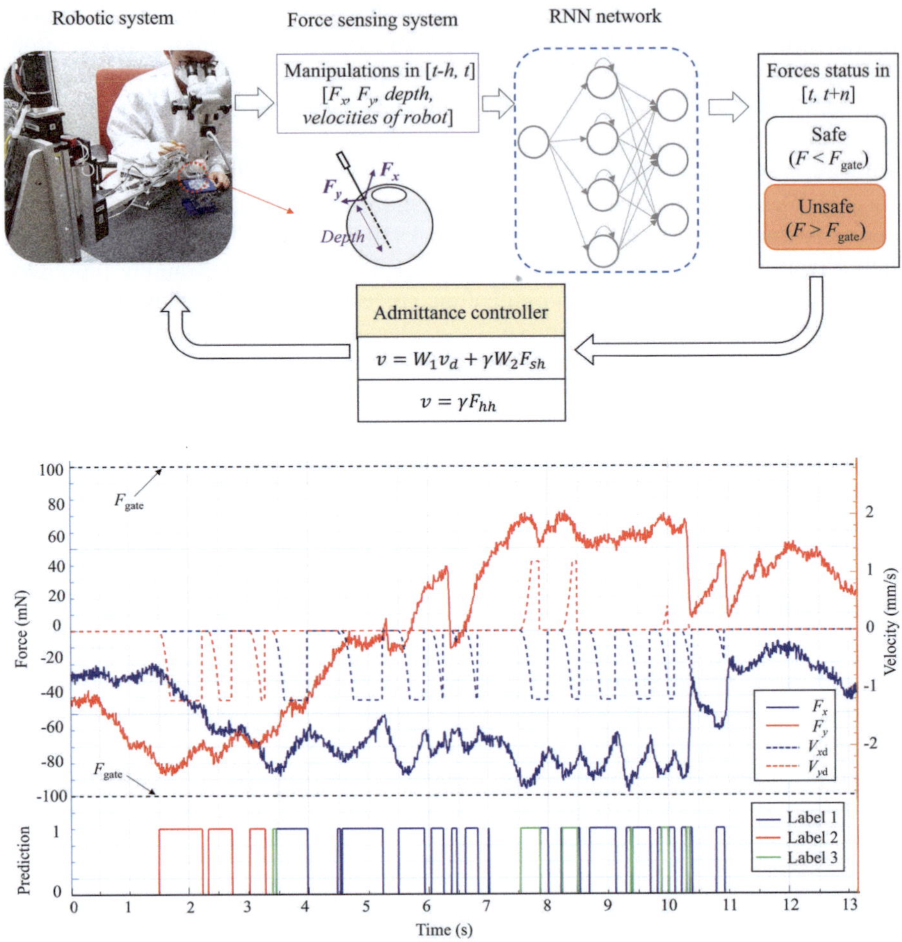

Fig. 4 Active interventional control framework: (Top) overview of the AICF consisting of a force sensing tool, an RNN predictor, an admittance control system, and the SHER research platform [110]. The robotic manipulator is activated to move at a varying speed to decrease the resulting scleral forces. (Bottom) A successful example of AICF intervention on the scleral force. When the label is 0, AICF is inactive; when the label is 1, 2, or 3, AICF is activated, and the desired velocity of the tool at the sclera frame (V_{xd}, V_{yd}) is assigned; as the result, the scleral force (F_x, F_y) is reduced to remain within the safety boundaries (F_{gate}). (Image © Iulian Iordachita)

forces. The force sensing tool was previously developed to measure the scleral force and the insertion depth [63]. In this study, it was assumed that the scleral force characteristics could be captured through a short history of time series of sensor measurements. This assumption was made considering the relatively slow dynamics of human arm motion, especially during microsurgical procedures. An RNN network with LSTM unit [111] was then constructed to make predictions about the scleral force status based on the history.

The scleral force, the insertion depth, and the robot kinematic velocities of past h timesteps were fed into the RNN as the input; the RNN outputs the probabilities of the scleral force status in the t n time steps, labeled as safe and unsafe by comparing it to a safety threshold F_{gate} [112]. The robot admittance control scheme was switched to the interventional mode [64] when the predicted scleral forces were specified as excessive (prediction label = 1, 2, 3). In this mode, the related components of the tool velocity in the sclera frame were assigned a desired value to reduce the scleral force. In a multi-user experiment with a common task during vitreoretinal surgery, called "vessel following" and involving 14 volunteers, the system demonstrated a significant reduction of undesirable force events outperforming two benchmark conditions: one with auditory feedback (AF) [113] and one with real-time feedback (RF) [114]. The intervention effect of AICF on the scleral forces is depicted in Fig. 4 bottom. When an excessive force status is predicted (label = 1, 2, 3), the scleral force is suppressed in the related direction by AICF, thus preventing it from breaching the prescribed safety boundary.

The AICF approach also resulted in statistically significant lower user ratings, where a lower rating indicated a higher rate of assistance provided by the system. The predictive behavior of the AICF also resulted in an ahead-of-time activation of intervention motion, reducing the sudden impact of the safety algorithm as compared to RF. Overall, the results indicated the AICF's effectiveness in increasing the safety level of robot-assisted simulated retinal surgery by reducing the undesired forces applied to the scleral port by the surgical tool.

6 Future Directions and Conclusion

Currently, robotic assistance augmented with artificial intelligence is expeditiously growing and evolving in surgery, and it is doubtless that this process will continue in the future [1]. Following this trend, the highly technical field of robotic ophthalmic surgery has witnessed increasing growth in technological developments and capabilities [2, 25, 115]. To completely realize the potential of robotic assistance in ophthalmic surgery, it is of paramount importance to involve machine learning, to address the known limitations, to discover the still unknown others, and to expand the current achieved benefits. Besides addressing the challenging aspects presented above, future developments may be focused on, but not limited to, safety enhancement, human-robot interaction, and robot autonomy.

Safety is chief among the requirements for robotic assistance in ophthalmic surgery and may be the most challenging one to be properly defined, implemented, and evaluated. For example, safe interaction between tissue and the surgical instrument could be enabled through sensor fusion and machine learning by aggregation of multi-modal data such as camera image [116, 117], iOCT images [100, 101], robot end-effector position [64, 99], and force measurements detected with sensorized tools [63] or vision-based force-sensing [118, 119]. Machine learning techniques can automatically learn accurate mapping between visual-geometric information and applied force [1] and enhance the safety and effectiveness of the robotic-assisted procedures.

As a multidisciplinary field, incorporating knowledge from various disciplines, including artificial intelligence and robotics, human-robot interaction (HRI) can help with developing effective communication between robot and human operator [1]. Owing to the limited number of robotic platforms for eye surgery, the interaction between surgeons and microsurgical robots is a less explored research direction that will very likely require continued efforts for improvement in the future. This development is expected to substantially improve the HRI safety in eye surgery and open the operating room door for intraocular robotic surgery.

Similar to other types of surgery, AI-based automated and even autonomous ophthalmic microsurgery is likely to be implemented [24]. However, owing to the significant challenges involved in surgical robotic autonomy, existing robots have lower degrees of autonomy. In intraocular surgery, there is no example of achieving automation of all surgical steps. As presented above, the relevant research is focused on automation or semi-automation of specific tasks (e.g., [120, 121]). Moving forward, a challenging aspect to be addressed is the need for a robotic system to anticipate, detect, and respond to possible failure modes [122]. Machine learning methods could facilitate this process and will likely require collection and analysis of data from a broad number of surgical procedures to develop the necessary algorithms to correctly, robustly, and reproducibly address the surgical complex decisions [24].

In conclusion, the superhuman challenges associated with intraocular microsurgery could be addressed with robotic assistance. Relevant capabilities enabled by intraocular robotic microsurgery include, but are not limited to, tremor canceling, enhanced dexterity, micrometer-scale distance sensing and positioning precision, haptic feedback, sub-millinewton force sensing, and others. Successfully performed clinical trials on robot-assisted eye interventions have proved the possibility of translating robotic technology into clinical practice. However, medical robotics for eye surgery is still associated with implementation challenges related to learning curves, cost, risks, and complications that make the robotic surgery an ideal target for artificial intelligence. Machine learning techniques (e.g., deep learning with its flavors of neural networks) are presently being applied to preoperative planning, anatomical targets and tool segmentation and recognition, intraoperative tool guidance, and so forth. When fully integrated with the human-machine interface, artificial intelligence and robotics will be able to reduce procedure variability; enhance precision and task capabilities; reduce error rates, costs, and fatigue; and improve ergonomics during surgery, and, at the end, all are expected to lead to improved surgical outcomes and provide advanced and safe surgical care for patients.

Acknowledgments We would like to acknowledge Ji Woong Kim, Michael Sommersperger, and Dr. Changyan He for contributing to this chapter and for their brilliant work in the field.

This work was supported in part by the US National Institutes of Health, under grant numbers R01EB024564 and R01EB025883, by Research to Prevent Blindness, New York, New York, USA, and gifts by the J. Willard and Alice S. Marriott Foundation, the Gale Trust, Mr. Herb Ehlers, Mr. Bill Wilbur, Mr. and Mrs. Rajandre Shaw, Ms. Helen Nassif, Ms. Mary Ellen Keck, Don and Maggie Feiner, and Dick and Gretchen Nielsen.

References

1. Zhou XY, Guo Y, Shen M, Yang GZ. Application of artificial intelligence in surgery. Front Med. 2020;14(4):417–30.
2. Mishra K, Leng T. Artificial intelligence and ophthalmic surgery. Curr Opin Ophthalmol. 2021;32(5):425–30.
3. Takahashi H, Tampo H, Arai Y, Inoue Y, Kawashima H. Applying artificial intelligence to disease staging: deep learning for improved staging of diabetic retinopathy. PLoS One. 2017;12(6):e0179790.
4. Ting DSW, Cheung CYL, Lim G, Tan GSW, Quang ND, Gan A, Hamzah H, Garcia-Franco R, San Yeo IY, Lee SY, et al. Development and validation of a deep learning system for diabetic retinopathy and related eye diseases using retinal images from multiethnic populations with diabetes. JAMA. 2017;318(22):2211–23.
5. Ludwig CA, Perera C, Myung D, Greven MA, Smith SJ, Chang RT, Leng T. Automatic identification of referral-warranted diabetic retinopathy using deep learning on mobile phone images. Transl Vis Sci Technol. 2020;9(2):60.
6. Venhuizen FG, van Ginneken B, van Asten F, van Grinsven MJ, Fauser S, Hoyng CB, Theelen T, Sánchez CI. Automated staging of age-related macular degeneration using optical coherence tomography. Invest Ophthalmol Vis Sci. 2017;58(4):2318–28.
7. Treder M, Lauermann JL, Eter N. Automated detection of exudative age-related macular degeneration in spectral domain optical coherence tomography using deep learning. Graefes Arch Clin Exp Ophthalmol. 2018;256(2):259–65.
8. Bolón-Canedo V, Ataer-Cansizoglu E, Erdogmus D, Kalpathy-Cramer J, Fontenla- Romero O, Alonso-Betanzos A, Chiang MF. Dealing with inter-expert variability in retinopathy of prematurity: a machine learning approach. Comput Methods Prog Biomed. 2015;122(1):1–15.
9. Li Z, He Y, Keel S, Meng W, Chang RT, He M. Efficacy of a deep learning system for detecting glaucomatous optic neuropathy based on color fundus photographs. Ophthalmology. 2018;125(8):1199–206.
10. Damato B, Eleuteri A, Fisher AC, Coupland SE, Taktak AF. Artificial neural networks estimating survival probability after treatment of choroidal melanoma. Ophthalmology. 2008;115(9):1598–607.
11. Bakshi SK, Lin SR, Ting DSW, Chiang MF, Chodosh J. The era of artificial intelligence and virtual reality: transforming surgical education in ophthalmology. Br J Ophthalmol. 2021;105(10):1325–8.
12. Mishra K, Boland MV, Woreta FA. Incorporating a virtual curriculum into ophthalmology education in the coronavirus disease-2019 era. Curr Opin Ophthalmol. 2020;31(5):380–5.
13. Staropoli PC, Gregori NZ, Junk AK, Galor A, Goldhardt R, Goldhagen BE, Shi W, Feuer W. Surgical simulation training reduces intraoperative cataract surgery complications among residents. Simul Healthc. 2018;13(1):11.
14. Castellanos S. Genentech uses virtual reality to train eye surgeons. Wall Street J. 2019;6
15. Kim TS, O'Brien M, Zafar S, Hager GD, Sikder S, Vedula SS. Objective assessment of intraoperative technical skill in capsulorhexis using videos of cataract surgery. Int J Comput Assist Radiol Surg. 2019;14(6):1097–105.
16. Morita S, Tabuchi H, Masumoto H, Yamauchi T, Kamiura N. Real-time extraction of important surgical phases in cataract surgery videos. Sci Rep. 2019;9(1):1–8.
17. Siddiqui AA, Ladas JG, Lee JK. Artificial intelligence in cornea, refractive, and cataract surgery. Curr Opin Ophthalmol. 2020;31(4):253–60.
18. Ladas J, Ladas D, Lin SR, Devgan U, Siddiqui AA, Jun AS. Improvement of multiple generations of intraocular lens calculation formulae with a novel approach using artificial intelligence. Transl Vis Sci Technol. 2021;10(3):7–7.
19. Al Hajj H, Lamard M, Conze PH, Roychowdhury S, Hu X, Maršalkaitė G, Zisimopoulos O, Dedmari MA, Zhao F, Prellberg J, et al. Cataracts: challenge on automatic tool annotation for cataract surgery. Med Image Anal. 2019;52:24–41.

20. Alnafisee N, Zafar S, Vedula SS, Sikder S. Current methods for assessing technical skill in cataract surgery. J Cataract Refract Surg. 2021;47(2):256–64.
21. Sokolova N, Schoeffmann K, Taschwer M, Putzgruber-Adamitsch D, El-Shabrawi Y. Evaluating the generalization performance of instrument classification in cataract surgery videos. In: International conference on multimedia modeling. Springer; 2020. p. 626–36.
22. Channa R, Iordachita I, Handa JT. Robotic eye surgery. Retina (Philadelphia, Pa.). 2017;37(7):1220.
23. Mattos LS, Caldwell DG, Peretti G, Mora F, Guastini L, Cingolani R. Microsurgery robots: addressing the needs of high-precision surgical interventions. Swiss Med Wkly. 2016;146(4344)
24. De Smet MD, Naus GJ, Faridpooya K, Mura M. Robotic-assisted surgery in ophthalmology. Curr Opin Ophthalmol. 2018;29(3):248–53.
25. Roizenblatt M, Edwards TL, Gehlbach PL. Robot-assisted vitreoretinal surgery: current perspectives. Robot Surg Res Rev. 2018;5:1–11.
26. Vander Poorten E, Riviere CN, Abbott JJ, Bergeles C, Nasseri MA, Kang JU, Sznitman R, Faridpooya K, Iordachita I. Robotic retinal surgery. In: Handbook of robotic and image-guided surgery. Elsevier; 2020. p. 627–72.
27. Gupta PK, Jensen PS, de Juan E. Surgical forces and tactile perception during retinal microsurgery. In: International conference on medical image computing and computer- assisted intervention. Springer; 1999. p. 1218–25.
28. Nelson BJ, Kaliakatsos IK, Abbott JJ. Microrobots for minimally invasive medicine. Annu Rev Biomed Eng. 2010;12:55–85.
29. Fusco S, Ullrich F, Pokki J, Chatzipirpiridis G, Özkale B, Sivaraman KM, Ergeneman O, Pane S, Nelson BJ. Microrobots: a new era in ocular drug delivery. Expert Opin Drug Deliv. 2014;11(11):1815–26.
30. Meenink H, Hendrix R, Naus G, Beelen M, Nijmeijer H, Steinbuch M, van Oosterhout E, de Smet M. Robot-assisted vitreoretinal surgery. In: Medical robotics. Elsevier; 2012. p. 185–209.
31. Ueta T, Yamaguchi Y, Shirakawa Y, Nakano T, Ideta R, Noda Y, Morita A, Mochizuki R, Sugita N, Mitsuishi M, et al. Robot-assisted vitreoretinal surgery: development of a prototype and feasibility studies in an animal model. Ophthalmology. 2009;116(8):1538–43.
32. Nasseri MA, Eder M, Nair S, Dean E, Maier M, Zapp D, Lohmann CP, Knoll A. The introduction of a new robot for assistance in ophthalmic surgery. In: 2013 35th annual international conference of the IEEE engineering in medicine and biology society (EMBC). IEEE; 2013. p. 5682–5.
33. de Smet MD, Meenink TC, Janssens T, Vanheukelom V, Naus GJ, Beelen MJ, Meers C, Jonckx B, Stassen JM. Robotic assisted cannulation of occluded retinal veins. PLoS One. 2016;11(9):e0162037.
34. Wilson JT, Gerber MJ, Prince SW, Chen CW, Schwartz SD, Hubschman JP, Tsao TC. Intraocular robotic interventional surgical system (IRISS): mechanical design, evaluation, and master–slave manipulation. Int J Med Robot Comput Assist Surg. 2018;14(1):e1842.
35. Üneri A, Balicki MA, Handa J, Gehlbach P, Taylor RH, Iordachita I. New steady- hand eye robot with micro-force sensing for vitreoretinal surgery. In: 2010 3rd IEEE RAS & EMBS international conference on biomedical robotics and biomechatronics. IEEE; 2010. p. 814–9.
36. Gijbels A, Wouters N, Stalmans P, Van Brussel H, Reynaerts D, Vander Poorten E. Design and realisation of a novel robotic manipulator for retinal surgery. In: 2013 IEEE/RSJ international conference on intelligent robots and systems. IEEE; 2013. p. 3598–603.
37. de Smet MD, Stassen JM, Meenink TC, Janssens T, Vanheukelom V, Naus GJ, Beelen MJ, Jonckx B. Release of experimental retinal vein occlusions by direct intraluminal injection of ocriplasmin. Br J Ophthalmol. 2016;100(12):1742–6.
38. Gijbels A, Vander Poorten EB, Gorissen B, Devreker A, Stalmans P, Reynaerts D. Experimental validation of a robotic comanipulation and telemanipulation system for

retinal surgery. In: 5th IEEE RAS/EMBS international conference on biomedical robotics and biomechatronics. IEEE; 2014. p. 144–50.
39. Willekens K, Gijbels A, Schoevaerdts L, Esteveny L, Janssens T, Jonckx B, Feyen JH, Meers C, Reynaerts D, Vander Poorten E, et al. Robot-assisted retinal vein cannulation in an in vivo porcine retinal vein occlusion model. Acta Ophthalmol. 2017;95(3):270–5.
40. MacLachlan RA, Becker BC, Tabarés JC, Podnar GW, Lobes LA, Riviere CN. Micron: an actively stabilized handheld tool for microsurgery. IEEE Trans Robot. 2011;28(1):195–212.
41. Yang S, MacLachlan RA, Riviere CN. Manipulator design and operation of a six-degree-of-freedom handheld tremor-canceling microsurgical instrument. IEEE/ASME Trans Mechatron. 2014;20(2):761–72.
42. Kuru I, Gonenc B, Balicki M, Handa J, Gehlbach P, Taylor RH, Iordachita I. Force sensing micro-forceps for robot assisted retinal surgery. In: 2012 annual international conference of the IEEE engineering in medicine and biology society. IEEE; 2012. p. 1401–4.
43. He X, Van Geirt V, Gehlbach P, Taylor R, Iordachita I. Iris: integrated robotic intraocular snake. In: 2015 IEEE international conference on robotics and automation (ICRA). IEEE; 2015. p. 1764–9.
44. Yang S, MacLachlan RA, Martel JN, Lobes LA, Riviere CN. Comparative evaluation of handheld robot-aided intraocular laser surgery. IEEE Trans Robot. 2016;32(1):246–51.
45. Taylor RH, Menciassi A, Fichtinger G, Fiorini P, Dario P. Medical robotics and computer-integrated surgery. Springer Handbook of Robotics; 2016. p. 1657–84.
46. Golahmadi AK, Khan DZ, Mylonas GP, Marcus HJ. Tool-tissue forces in surgery: a systematic review. Ann Med Surg. 2021:102268.
47. Jagtap AD, Riviere CN. Applied force during vitreoretinal microsurgery with handheld instruments. In: 26th annual international conference of the IEEE engineering in medicine and biology society, vol. 1. IEEE; 2004. p. 2771–3.
48. Tosi D, Poeggel S, Iordachita I, Schena E. Fiber optic sensors for biomedical applications. In: Opto-mechanical fiber optic sensors. Elsevier; 2018. p. 301–33.
49. Presti DL, Massaroni C, Leitão CSJ, Domingues MDF, Sypabekova M, Barrera D, Floris I, Massari L, Oddo CM, Sales S, et al. Fiber Bragg gratings for medical applications and future challenges: a review. IEEE Access. 2020;8:156863–88.
50. Liu X, Iordachita II, He X, Taylor RH, Kang JU. Miniature fiber-optic force sensor based on low-coherence Fabry-Pérot interferometry for vitreoretinal microsurgery. Biomed Opt Exp. 2012;3(5):1062–76.
51. Iordachita I, Sun Z, Balicki M, Kang JU, Phee SJ, Handa J, Gehlbach P, Taylor R. A submillimetric, 0.25 mn resolution fully integrated fiber-optic force-sensing tool for retinal microsurgery. Int J Comput Assist Radiol Surg. 2009;4(4):383–90.
52. Balicki M, Han JH, Iordachita I, Gehlbach P, Handa J, Taylor R, Kang J. Single fiber optical coherence tomography microsurgical instruments for computer and robot-assisted retinal surgery. In: International conference on medical image computing and computer- assisted intervention. Springer; 2009. p. 108–15.
53. Sunshine S, Balicki M, He X, Olds K, Kang JU, Gehlbach P, Taylor R, Iordachita I, Handa JT. A force-sensing microsurgical instrument that detects forces below human tactile sensation. Retina (Philadelphia, Pa.). 2013;33(1)
54. He X, Handa J, Gehlbach P, Taylor R, Iordachita I. A submillimetric 3-dof force sensing instrument with integrated fiber Bragg grating for retinal microsurgery. IEEE Trans Biomed Eng. 2013;61(2):522–34.
55. Gijbels A, Vander Poorten EB, Stalmans P, Reynaerts D. Development and experimental validation of a force sensing needle for robotically assisted retinal vein cannulations. In: 2015 IEEE international conference on robotics and automation (ICRA). IEEE; 2015. p. 2270–6.
56. Gijbels A, Willekens K, Esteveny L, Stalmans P, Reynaerts D, Vander Poorten EB. Towards a clinically applicable robotic assistance system for retinal vein cannulation. In: 2016 6th IEEE international conference on biomedical robotics and biomechatronics (BioRob). IEEE; 2016. p. 284–91.

57. Gonenc B, Tran N, Riviere CN, Gehlbach P, Taylor RH, Iordachita I. Force-based puncture detection and active position holding for assisted retinal vein cannulation. In: 2015 IEEE international conference on multisensor fusion and integration for intelligent systems (MFI). IEEE; 2015. p. 322–7.
58. Gonenc B, Tran N, Gehlbach P, Taylor RH, Iordachita I. Robot-assisted retinal vein cannulation with force-based puncture detection: Micron vs. the steady-hand eye robot. In: 2016 38th annual international conference of the IEEE engineering in medicine and biology society (EMBC). IEEE; 2016. p. 5107–11.
59. Gonenc B, Patel N, Iordachita I. Evaluation of a force-sensing handheld robot for assisted retinal vein cannulation. In: 2018 40th annual international conference of the IEEE engineering in medicine and biology society (EMBC). IEEE; 2018. p. 1–5.
60. Gonenc B, Chae J, Gehlbach P, Taylor RH, Iordachita I. Towards robot-assisted retinal vein cannulation: a motorized force-sensing microneedle integrated with a handheld micromanipulator. Sensors. 2017;17(10):2195.
61. He X, Balicki MA, Kang JU, Gehlbach PL, Handa JT, Taylor RH, Iordachita II. Force sensing micro-forceps with integrated fiber Bragg grating for vitreoretinal surgery. In: Optical fibers and sensors for medical diagnostics and treatment applications XII, vol. 8218. International Society for Optics and Photonics; 2012. p. 82180W.
62. Gonenc B, Gehlbach P, Handa J, Taylor RH, Iordachita I. Motorized force-sensing micro-forceps with tremor cancelling and controlled micro-vibrations for easier membrane peeling. In: 5th IEEE RAS/EMBS international conference on biomedical robotics and biomechatronics. IEEE; 2014. p. 244–51.
63. He X, Balicki M, Gehlbach P, Handa J, Taylor R, Iordachita I. A multi-function force sensing instrument for variable admittance robot control in retinal microsurgery. In: 2014 IEEE International Conference on Robotics and Automation (ICRA). IEEE; 2014. p. 1411–8.
64. Ebrahimi A, Patel N, He C, Gehlbach P, Kobilarov M, Iordachita I. Adaptive control of sclera force and insertion depth for safe robot-assisted retinal surgery. In: 2019 international conference on robotics and automation (ICRA). IEEE; 2019. p. 9073–9.
65. He C, Roizenblatt M, Patel N, Ebrahimi A, Yang Y, Gehlbach PL, et al. Towards bimanual robot-assisted retinal surgery: tool-to-sclera force evaluation. In: IEEE sensors. IEEE; 2018. p. 1–4.
66. He C, Ebrahimi A, Yang E, Urias M, Yang Y, Gehlbach P, Iordachita I. Towards bimanual vein cannulation: preliminary study of a bimanual robotic system with a dual force constraint controller. In: 2020 IEEE international conference on robotics and automation (ICRA). IEEE; 2020. p. 4441–7.
67. Liu X, Li X, Kim DH, Ilev I, Kang JU. Fiber-optic Fourier-domain common-path OCT. Chin Opt Lett. 2008;6(12):899–901.
68. Yang S, Balicki M, MacLachlan RA, Liu X, Kang JU, Taylor RH, Riviere CN. Optical coherence tomography scanning with a handheld vitreoretinal micromanipulator. In: 2012 annual international conference of the IEEE engineering in medicine and biology society. IEEE; 2012. p. 948–51.
69. Song C, Park DY, Gehlbach PL, Park SJ, Kang JU. Fiber-optic OCT sensor guided "SMART" micro-forceps for microsurgery. Biomed Opt Express. 2013;4(7):1045–50.
70. Kang JU, Cheon GW. Demonstration of subretinal injection using common-path swept source OCT guided microinjector. Appl Sci. 2018;8(8):1287.
71. Smits J, Ourak M, Gijbels A, Esteveny L, Borghesan G, Schoevaerdts L, Willekens K, Stalmans P, Lankenau E, Schulz-Hildebrandt H, et al. Development and experimental validation of a combined FBG force and OCT distance sensing needle for robot-assisted retinal vein cannulation. In: 2018 IEEE international conference on robotics and automation (ICRA). IEEE; 2018. p. 129–34.
72. Ourak M, Smits J, Esteveny L, Borghesan G, Gijbels A, Schoevaerdts L, Douven Y, Scholtes J, Lankenau E, Eixmann T, et al. Combined OCT distance and FBG force sensing cannula-

tion needle for retinal vein cannulation: in vivo animal validation. Int J Comput Assist Radiol Surg. 2019;14(2):301–9.

73. Zhu I, Mieler WF. Robotic retinal surgery. In: Macular surgery. Springer; 2020. p. 565–74.
74. Sznitman R, Richa R, Taylor RH, Jedynak B, Hager GD. Unified detection and tracking of instruments during retinal microsurgery. IEEE Trans Pattern Anal Mach Intell. 2012;35(5):1263–73.
75. Alsheakhali M, Eslami A, Roodaki H, Navab N. Crf-based model for instrument detection and pose estimation in retinal microsurgery. Comput Math Methods Med. 2016;2016
76. Laina I, Rieke N, Rupprecht C, Vizcaíno JP, Eslami A, Tombari F, Navab N. Concurrent segmentation and localization for tracking of surgical instruments. In: International conference on medical image computing and computer-assisted intervention. Springer; 2017. p. 664–72.
77. Rieke N, Tan DJ, Tombari F, Vizcaíno JP, San Filippo CAd, Eslami A, Navab N. Real-time online adaption for robust instrument tracking and pose estimation. In: International conference on medical image computing and computer-assisted intervention. Springer; 2016. p. 422–30.
78. Probst T, Maninis KK, Chhatkuli A, Ourak M, Vander Poorten E, Van Gool L. Automatic tool landmark detection for stereo vision in robot-assisted retinal surgery. IEEE Robot Automat Lett. 2017;3(1):612–9.
79. Ehlers JP, Kaiser PK, Srivastava SK. Intraoperative optical coherence tomography using the rescan 700: preliminary results from the discover study. Br J Ophthalmol. 2014;98(10):1329–32.
80. Zhou M, Huang K, Eslami A, Roodaki H, Zapp D, Maier M, Lohmann CP, Knoll A, Nasseri MA. Precision needle tip localization using optical coherence tomography images for subretinal injection. In: 2018 IEEE international conference on robotics and automation (ICRA). IEEE; 2018. p. 4033–40.
81. Kehl W, Tombari F, Ilic S, Navab N. Real-time 3d model tracking in color and depth on a single CPU core. In: Proceedings of the IEEE Conference on Computer Vision and Pattern Recognition; 2017. p. 745–53.
82. Zhou M, Hao X, Eslami A, Huang K, Cai C, Lohmann CP, Navab N, Knoll A, Nasseri MA. 6dof needle pose estimation for robot-assisted vitreoretinal surgery. IEEE Access. 2019;7:63113–22.
83. Roy AG, Conjeti S, Karri SPK, Sheet D, Katouzian A, Wachinger C, Navab N. Relaynet: retinal layer and fluid segmentation of macular optical coherence tomography using fully convolutional networks. Biomed Opt Express. 2017;8(8):3627–42.
84. Borkovkina S, Camino A, Janpongsri W, Sarunic MV, Jian Y. Real-time retinal layer segmentation of OCT volumes with GPU accelerated inferencing using a compressed, low- latency neural network. Biomed Opt Express. 2020;11(7):3968–84.
85. Tran A, Weiss J, Albarqouni S, Faghi Roohi S, Navab N. Retinal layer segmentation reformulated as OCT language processing. In: International conference on medical image computing and computer-assisted intervention. Springer; 2020. p. 694–703.
86. Maier H, Faghihroohi S, Navab N. A line to align: deep dynamic time warping for retinal OCT segmentation. In: International conference on medical image computing and computer-assisted intervention. Springer; 2021. p. 709–19.
87. Sommersperger M, Weiss J, Nasseri MA, Gehlbach P, Iordachita I, Navab N. Real- time tool to layer distance estimation for robotic subretinal injection using intraoperative 4d OCT. Biomed Opt Express. 2021;12(2):1085–104.
88. Carrasco-Zevallos OM, Viehland C, Keller B, McNabb RP, Kuo AN, Izatt JA. Constant linear velocity spiral scanning for near video rate 4d OCT ophthalmic and surgical imaging with isotropic transverse sampling. Biomed Opt Express. 2018;9(10):5052–70.
89. Carrasco-Zevallos O, Keller B, Viehland C, Hahn P, Kuo AN, DeSouza PJ, Toth CA, Izatt JA. Real-time 4d visualization of surgical maneuvers with 100khz swept-source microscope integrated optical coherence tomography (mioct) in model eyes. Invest Ophthalmol Vis Sci. 2014;55(13):1633.

90. Sommersperger M, Martin-Gomez A, Mach K, Gehlbach PL, Nasseri MA, Iordachita I, Navab N. Surgical scene generation and adversarial networks for physics-based iOCT synthesis. Biomed Opt Express. 2022;13(4):2414–30.
91. Yang S, Martel JN, Lobes LA Jr, Riviere CN. Techniques for robot-aided intraocular surgery using monocular vision. Int J Robot Res. 2018;37(8):931–52.
92. Zhou M, Wu J, Ebrahimi A, Patel N, He C, Gehlbach P, Taylor RH, Knoll A, Nasseri MA, Iordachita I. Spotlight-based 3D instrument guidance for retinal surgery. In: 2020 international symposium on medical robotics (ISMR). IEEE; 2020. p. 69–75.
93. Kim JW, Zhang P, Gehlbach P, Iordachita I, Kobilarov M. Towards autonomous eye surgery by combining deep imitation learning with optimal control. arXiv preprint arXiv. 2020;2011.07778
94. Tayama T, Kurose Y, Marinho MM, Koyama Y, Harada K, Omata S, Arai F, Sugimoto K, Araki F, Totsuka K, et al. Autonomous positioning of eye surgical robot using the tool shadow and Kalman filtering. In: 2018 40th annual international conference of the IEEE engineering in medicine and biology society (EMBC). IEEE; 2018. p. 1723–6.
95. Zhou M, Wu J, Ebrahimi A, Patel N, Liu Y, Navab N, Gehlbach P, Knoll A, Nasseri MA, Iordachita I. Spotlight-based 3D instrument guidance for autonomous task in robot-assisted retinal surgery. IEEE Robot Automat Lett. 2021;6(4):7750–7.
96. Kim JW, He C, Urias M, Gehlbach P, Hager GD, Iordachita I, Kobilarov M. Autonomously navigating a surgical tool inside the eye by learning from demonstration. In: 2020 IEEE international conference on robotics and automation (ICRA). IEEE; 2020. p. 7351–7.
97. Zhang P, Kim JW, Kobilarov M. Towards safer retinal surgery through chance constraint optimization and real-time geometry estimation. In: 2021 60th IEEE conference on decision and control (CDC). IEEE; 2021. p. 5175–80.
98. Huang D, Swanson EA, Lin CP, Schuman JS, Stinson WG, Chang W, Hee MR, Flotte T, Gregory K, Puliafito CA, et al. Optical coherence tomography. Science. 1991;254(5035):1178–81.
99. Yu H, Shen JH, Joos KM, Simaan N. Design, calibration and preliminary testing of a robotic telemanipulator for OCT guided retinal surgery. In: 2013 IEEE international conference on robotics and automation. IEEE; 2013. p. 225–31.
100. Weiss J, Rieke N, Nasseri MA, Maier M, Eslami A, Navab N. Fast 5DOF needle tracking in iOCT. Int J Comput Assist Radiol Surg. 2018;13(6):787–96.
101. Zhou M, Hamad M, Weiss J, Eslami A, Huang K, Maier M, Lohmann CP, Navab N, Knoll A, Nasseri MA. Towards robotic eye surgery: marker-free, online hand-eye calibration using optical coherence tomography images. IEEE Robot Automat Lett. 2018;3(4):3944–51.
102. Yu H, Shen JH, Shah RJ, Simaan N, Joos KM. Evaluation of microsurgical tasks with OCT-guided and/or robot-assisted ophthalmic forceps. Biomed Opt Express. 2015;6(2):457–72.
103. Draelos M, Tang G, Keller B, Kuo A, Hauser K, Izatt JA. Optical coherence tomography guided robotic needle insertion for deep anterior lamellar keratoplasty. IEEE Trans Biomed Eng. 2019;67(7):2073–83.
104. Gerber MJ, Hubschman JP, Tsao TC. Automated retinal vein cannulation on silicone phantoms using optical coherence tomography-guided robotic manipulations. IEEE/ASME Trans Mechatron. 2020;
105. Ahronovich EZ, Simaan N, Joos KM. A review of robotic and OCT-aided systems for vitreoretinal surgery. Adv Ther. 2021;38(5):2114–29.
106. Vecerik M, Hester T, Scholz J, Wang F, Pietquin O, Piot B, Heess N, Rothörl T, Lampe T, Riedmiller M. Leveraging demonstrations for deep reinforcement learning on robotics problems with sparse rewards. arXiv preprint arXiv. 2017;1707.08817
107. Sun W, Bagnell JA, Boots B. Truncated horizon policy search: Combining reinforcement learning & imitation learning. arXiv preprint arXiv. 2018;1805:11240.
108. Keller B, Draelos M, Zhou K, Qian R, Kuo AN, Konidaris G, Hauser K, Izatt JA. Optical coherence tomography-guided robotic ophthalmic microsurgery via reinforcement learning from demonstration. IEEE Trans Robot. 2020;36(4):1207–18.

109. Edwards W, Tang G, Tian Y, Draelos M, Izatt J, Kuo A, Hauser K. Data-driven modelling and control for robot needle insertion in deep anterior lamellar keratoplasty. IEEE Robot Automat Lett. 2022;
110. He X, Roppenecker D, Gierlach D, Balicki M, Olds K, Gehlbach P, Handa J, Taylor R, Iordachita I. Toward clinically applicable steady-hand eye robot for vitreoretinal surgery. In: ASME International Mechanical Engineering Congress and Exposition, vol. 45189. American Society of Mechanical Engineers; 2012. p. 145–53.
111. Hochreiter S, Schmidhuber J. Long short-term memory. Neural Comput. 1997;9(8):1735–80.
112. He C, Ebrahimi A, Roizenblatt M, Patel N, Yang Y, Gehlbach PL, Iordachita I. User behavior evaluation in robot-assisted retinal surgery. In: 2018 27th IEEE international symposium on robot and human interactive communication (RO-MAN). IEEE; 2018. p. 174–9.
113. Cutler N, Balicki M, Finkelstein M, Wang J, Gehlbach P, McGready J, Iordachita I, Taylor R, Handa JT. Auditory force feedback substitution improves surgical precision during simulated ophthalmic surgery. Invest Ophthalmol Vis Sci. 2013;54(2):1316–24.
114. Ebrahimi A, He C, Roizenblatt M, Patel N, Sefati S, Gehlbach P, Iordachita I. Real- time sclera force feedback for enabling safe robot-assisted vitreoretinal surgery. In: 2018 40th annual international conference of the IEEE engineering in medicine and biology society (EMBC). IEEE; 2018. p. 3650–5.
115. Urias MG, Patel N, He C, Ebrahimi A, Kim JW, Iordachita I, Gehlbach PL. Artificial intelligence, robotics and eye surgery: are we overfitted? Int J Retin Vitr. 2019;5(1):1–4.
116. Sarikaya D, Corso JJ, Guru KA. Detection and localization of robotic tools in robot- assisted surgery videos using deep neural networks for region proposal and detection. IEEE Trans Med Imaging. 2017;36(7):1542–9.
117. Volkov M, Hashimoto DA, Rosman G, Meireles OR, Rus D. Machine learning and coresets for automated real-time video segmentation of laparoscopic and robot-assisted surgery. In: 2017 IEEE international conference on robotics and automation (ICRA). IEEE; 2017. p. 754–9.
118. Aviles AI, Alsaleh SM, Hahn JK, Casals A. Towards retrieving force feedback in robotic-assisted surgery: a supervised neuro-recurrent-vision approach. IEEE Trans Haptics. 2016;10(3):431–43.
119. Marban A, Srinivasan V, Samek W, Fernández J, Casals A. A recurrent convolutional neural network approach for sensorless force estimation in robotic surgery. Biomed Signal Process Contr. 2019;50:134–50.
120. Xia J, Bergunder SJ, Lin D, Yan Y, Lin S, Nasseri MA, Zhou M, Lin H, Huang K. Microscope-guided autonomous clear corneal incision. In: 2020 IEEE international conference on robotics and automation (ICRA). IEEE; 2020. p. 3867–73.
121. Becker BC, MacLachlan RA, Lobes LA Jr, Riviere CN. Semiautomated intraocular laser surgery using handheld instruments. Lasers Surg Med. 2010;42(3):264–73.
122. Yang GZ, Bellingham J, Dupont PE, Fischer P, Floridi L, Full R, Jacobstein N, Kumar V, McNutt M, Merrifield R, et al. The grand challenges of science robotics. Sci Robot. 2018;3(14):eaar7650.

Clinical Case: Laparoscopic Surgery

Nobuyoshi Takeshita and Masaaki Ito

Abstract Artificial intelligence (AI) has been gradually introduced into the fields of radiological and endoscopic diagnosis as supports for clinical practices. In the field of laparoscopic surgery, AI-based image recognition technology is also promising for the development of surgical navigation, skill assessment, and OR (operating room) management. Some of the active research and developments in this area using deep learning approach include the identification of surgical phases, surgical instruments, and anatomical structures. The major tasks of AI can be divided into image classification (the task of assigning a whole image to a specific class), object detection (the identification of the location of lesions, organs, or other objects with a circle or a box region of interest), and semantic segmentation (the recognition of the precise pixel-wise borders of objects). To develop these AI-based systems, a large number of still images from surgical videos are required as the training set, a dataset of annotations for each still image. Therefore, the construction of the high-quality surgery video database which contributes to the development is desired. We need to establish this infrastructure to boost the developments of AI-based surgical systems with global collaborations.

Keywords Laparoscopic surgery · Image recognition · Deep learning · Surgical phase recognition · Surgical video database

1 Introduction

In recent years, the number of laparoscopic surgeries being performed has increased at a rapid pace, and their safety and efficacy have been studied in a recent report [1]. In contrast, laparoscopic surgery requires a high level of skill, and it is known that

N. Takeshita (✉) · M. Ito
NEXT Medical Device Innovation Center, Surgical Device Innovation Office,
National Cancer Center Hospital East, Kashiwa, Japan
e-mail: ntakeshi@east.ncc.go.jp

K. Masamune et al. (eds.), *Artificial Intelligence in Surgery*,
https://doi.org/10.1007/978-981-96-6635-5_12

there are disparities in outcomes between facilities and surgeons. Taking colorectal cancer as an example, it has been reported that treatment outcomes, such as anorectal preservation and local control rates, are superior in facilities that conduct a higher number of surgeries per year [2]. In addition, recurrence-free survival is superior in these facilities when surgeries are performed by trained colorectal surgery teams compared with when they are performed by general surgery teams [3]. Thus, the quality of surgery is greatly influenced by the skill of the surgeon, which affects not only short-term outcomes such as perioperative complication rates but also long-term outcomes such as survival rates.

The equalization of laparoscopic surgery and the shortage of surgeons are urgent issues in surgical practice, and in conjunction with the COVID-19 pandemic and shortage of medical resources, solutions that improve surgical efficiency and save human resources, such as surgical robots and other surgical support devices and systems, are needed in clinical practice. In the field of surgery, there is an increasing need for such methods. Visualization of surgical techniques, which until now has been performed in the form of tacit knowledge based on surgeons' skills and judgment stemming from their experience and knowledge, is extremely important as an approach to solving the above issues, both from the perspective of surgical education and the development of new surgical support systems. Since a large number of surgical videos have been accumulated due to the spread of laparoscopic surgery, attempts to quantify and digitize surgery based on this vast amount of data have been initiated. These data can be utilized as a training dataset to create an algorithm for machine learning, one of the subdomains of artificial intelligence (AI). The development of a surgical support system by utilizing these data has been initiated, and high expectations are placed on these systems to support intraoperative decision-making and automation of surgery.

2 Image Recognition Using Deep Learning Models for Laparoscopic Surgery

In laparoscopic surgery, surgical videos are widely used for educational and research purposes. Laparoscopic surgery provides a great deal of information to the surgical team due to its magnification effect and improved image quality, but it is difficult for team members to interpret all of this information equally in real time. In contrast, this visual information is considered to be the most essential information generated during the surgical procedure compared to other information such as tactile information. The image recognition approach is a very reasonable method to help the surgical team interpret visual information.

Deep learning is a type of machine learning method that is based on neural networks, and the most important feature of deep learning is that it automatically extracts the features that should be focused on for analysis during the learning process. Some of the active research and developments in the area of laparoscopic surgery using image recognition and deep learning include the identification of surgical phases, surgical instruments, and anatomical structures. The major tasks of AI can be divided into the following: image classification (the task of assigning a whole image to a specific class), object detection (the identification of the location of lesions, organs, or other objects with a circle or a box region of interest), and semantic segmentation (the recognition of the precise pixel-wise borders of objects). These AI models are constructed by preparing a large number of still images from surgical videos and a dataset of annotations for each still image and then using them to train the machine learning algorithm.

2.1 *Identification of Surgical Phase in Laparoscopic Surgery*

Understanding and recognizing the process and context of surgery is the first step in learning surgery for medical students and others. In the development of image recognition in laparoscopic surgery, surgical action recognition has been used in various ways, but the most widely used method is surgical phase recognition (Fig. 1). Automatic surgical phase recognition can be useful for surgical training of surgeons and indexing of documented procedures, as well as for intraoperative information sharing, efficient operation room management, providing alerts on upcoming adverse events, and in efforts to automate surgery [4]. If the surgeon himself can recognize which surgical process is taking a long time, he can know where to focus training, and if he can look back on the surgery efficiently, the burden on the surgeon will be reduced. If it is possible to share in real time the information regarding which process is currently being performed in surgery, the operating room management leader can consider preparations for the next surgery, staffing, timing of replacement, and so on. If we know in real time that a particular surgical process is taking a long time, we can quickly detect the possibility that something unexpected is happening, and we can consider the need for intervention or prepare for adverse events. These ideas are similar to those used in many industrial process engineering applications.

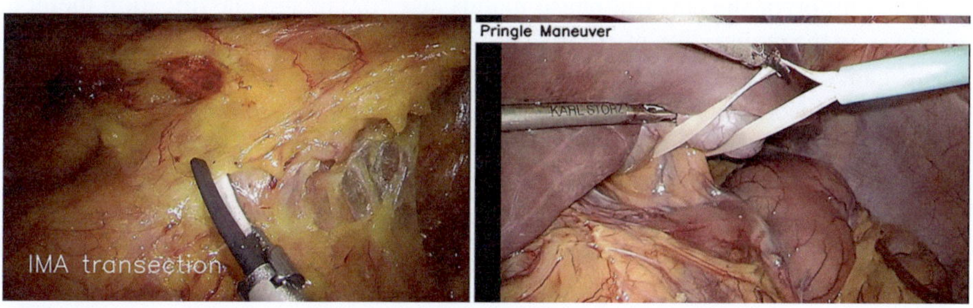

Fig. 1 Surgical phase recognition using image classification in laparoscopic sigmoid/liver resection

The development of surgical phase recognition has been studied most actively with respect to laparoscopic cholecystectomy. Laparoscopic cholecystectomy is the oldest and most commonly performed laparoscopic procedure. The operative field is relatively fixed, which makes it a good first step in the training of beginning surgeons, as well as in image recognition and other engineering techniques. However, even in laparoscopic cholecystectomy, the surgical phase itself is defined in a wide range of ways [4], and there are still many issues to be solved before a general-purpose system can be developed. Naturally, a greater number of processes that are to be classified lead to an increase in the difficulty of the task of image classification and a concomitant decrease in the accuracy of the method. The accuracy will similarly decrease when it comes to atypical surgical fields and procedures. Other types of surgeries that utilize surgical phase recognition include laparoscopic sleeve gastrectomy [5], laparoscopic colectomy [6, 7], robot-assisted prostatectomy [8], peroral endoscopic myotomy [9], etc., with accuracy rates ranging from about 92% for the most accurate to about 69% for the least accurate. This variation is thought to be largely due to the presence or absence of standardization of the surgical processes and techniques. In addition, as discussed below, the accuracy will also be highly dependent on the number of cases in the surgical video database to be utilized as the training set.

2.2 *Identification of Surgical Tools in Laparoscopic Surgery*

Recognizing the use and movement of surgical tools is valuable for the analysis of surgeon's performance, surgical training, and even market analysis. If the movement of forceps during surgery can be evaluated objectively and quantitatively, it will help in the analyses of the surgical economy, efficiency of the performance, the characteristics of forceps movement, and its correlation with adverse events. In the field of robot-assisted surgery, in addition to sensor information attached to forceps, the status and movement of the forceps on the image are also very important complementary information.

Recognition of the surgical phase mainly uses the image classification method, whereas, in the recognition of surgical tools, location and tracking the tips of instruments can also be useful information (Fig. 2). Therefore, in addition to image classification, object detection methods are often used. In image classification of surgical tools, the recognition of the tools is reported to have an accuracy of 85–92% [10, 11], whereas detection of the location of the tools is reported to have an accuracy of 38–86% [12–14]. Attempts to improve the accuracy of surgical phase recognition by using these tools together have also been reported [15]. Furthermore, attempts using semantic segmentation methods have been initiated [16]. However, since the recognition of surgical instruments by semantic segmentation requires the creation of AI models by annotating the outlines of the instruments, it is a time-intensive task, and it is difficult to address the variations in surgical instruments. There is a requirement for efficient annotation and learning methods [17, 18].

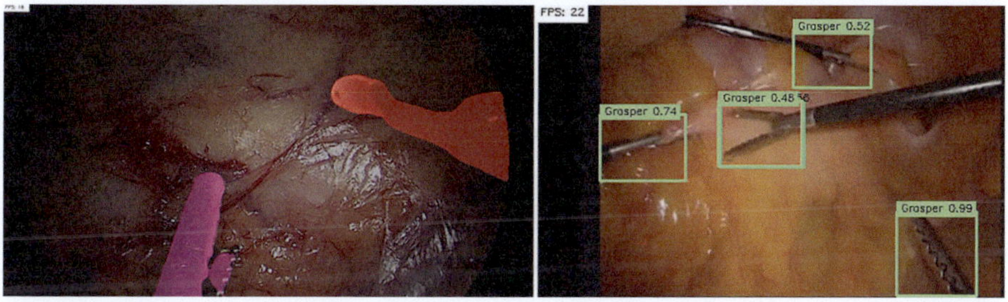

Fig. 2 Surgical tool recognition using semantic segmentation and object detection in laparoscopic sigmoid resection

Although inorganic objects in the surgical field are relatively easy to recognize visually compared to other anatomical structures, the wide variety of surgical tools that need to be recognized by the algorithm also reduces the accuracy for each tool. Moreover, unlike surgical phases and anatomical structures, usage of surgical tools is subject to change continuously in the real world as time goes by, and it is difficult to adapt them to a system that can be continually utilized in clinical practice without constantly updating the AI models. For the development of continuously updating tool detection AI models, other approaches that do not require manual annotation must be developed.

2.3 *Identification of Anatomical Structures in Laparoscopic Surgery*

During surgery, there are many anatomical structures that need to be marked or road-signed to perform the surgery efficiently and avoid intraoperative organ injury. It is known that intraoperative organ injury is mainly caused by misidentification or lack of confirmation of anatomical structures. It has been found that the risk of intraoperative injury is higher in surgeries performed by less experienced surgeons. In contrast, it is also known that intraoperative injuries occur with a certain frequency even when surgeries are performed by surgeons with the experience of a large number of cases. This indicates that it is difficult to maintain concentration and continue to perform anatomical structure recognition with high accuracy during long surgeries. In the intra-abdominal region, where anatomical structures are intermingled, intraoperative organ injuries that require prolonged hospitalization and additional procedures, large vessel injuries that are sometimes fatal, and nerve injuries that reduce the quality of life occur with a certain frequency. Therefore, image recognition for helping with the surgeon's identification of anatomical structures is valuable for surgical safety. Development of models that highlight key areas of anatomy and safe or unsafe areas of dissection and assist and alert the surgeon using object detection or semantic segmentation is also being attempted (Fig. 3) [19, 20].

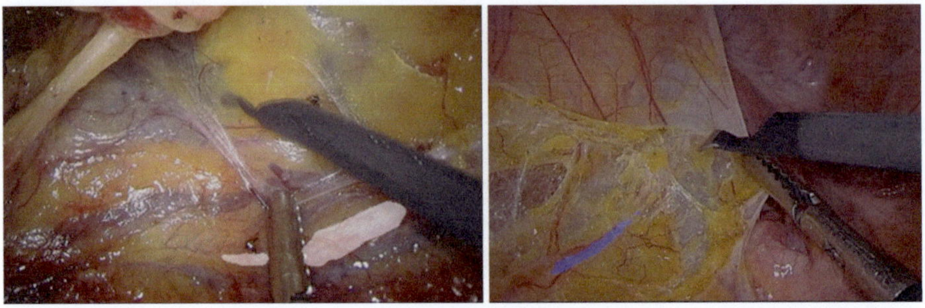

Fig. 3 Ureter and nerve recognition using semantic segmentation in laparoscopic sigmoid resection

In cholecystectomy, the development of image navigation for anatomical structures and the recognition of critical view of safety and quality evaluation of it are topics that are being actively pursued [21, 22], and it is hoped that this will lead to avoidance of bile duct injuries during surgery.

For the development of an AI navigation system using image recognition of anatomical structures, we have to consider the regulatory processes and ethical issues associated with the use of such medical devices. In the case of clinical implementation of these initiatives, the concept directly affects surgical safety and the surgeon's decision. Therefore, there is a strong need for high-quality manual annotation for training data, appropriate management of clinical data, and highly accurate AI performance. Also, to be widely used in the clinical field, it must be versatile in terms of recognition accuracy. As for the manual annotation to create training data, trained surgeons need to guarantee the quality of the dataset, and inter-annotator agreement based on well-maintained standard operating procedures is necessary. In the area of endoscopic and radiological diagnostics, AI-powered systems have been developed and are beginning to be introduced to the market to provide physicians with AI support. It will not be long before surgeons may operate while using Google Maps-like navigation of anatomical structures. This will also be a great first step toward the automation of surgery.

3 Construction of Surgical Video Database

Without exception, the development of image recognition as described so far must begin with the construction of surgical video databases. The construction of such databases must be surgeon-driven and will require an enormous amount of effort and management of ethical issues. The databases of laparoscopic surgery videos reported to date include laparoscopic cholecystectomy [15, 23, 24], laparoscopic colectomy [16, 25], laparoscopic sleeve gastrectomy [26], laparoscopic gastric bypass [27], laparoscopic hysterectomy [28], other general surgery [29],

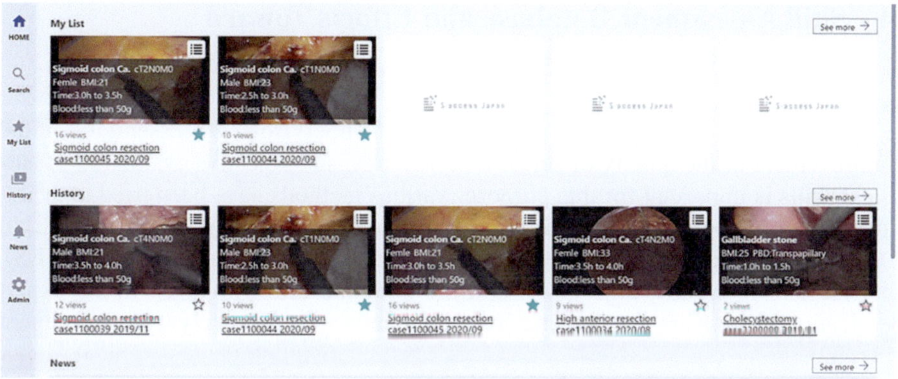

Fig. 4 Surgical video database constructed in our project, "S-access JAPAN"

gynecological area [11, 30], etc. The number of data included can range from a few cases to several hundred cases. In considering a database useful for AI development, the variation within the data is as important as the amount of data. Data for AI model training can easily lead to overfitting, which reduces the generality and external accuracy of the model. In order to utilize the database for research and development, it is also important to determine whether it is necessary to obtain consent from the patient. The treatment of personal information and the attribution of rights to surgical videos are very important topics to be discussed, although there are regional differences.

We have built databases of laparoscopic surgery videos from 2017, named LapSig300, which contains surgical videos of laparoscopic sigmoid resection, phase classifications, and other data from 19 centers and 300 cases [16]. A series of surgical workflows were classified into nine phases and three actions, and the areas of five tools were assigned by annotations. More than 82 million frames were annotated for a phase and action classification task, and 4000 frames were annotated for a tool segmentation task. Furthermore, we started the "S-access JAPAN project" in 2019 as an industrially available database based on patient consent. A total of 3000 surgical video data were collected from all over Japan for laparoscopic cholecystectomy, laparoscopic colectomy, laparoscopic/robot-assisted low anterior resection, laparoscopic liver resection, laparoscopic/robot-assisted gastrectomy, laparoscopic pancreatectomy, robot-assisted prostatectomy, etc. (Fig. 4). This database included the annotation of surgical phases, and background clinical information on the patient and surgeon was compiled. Moves are underway to extend these databases to gynecology and esophageal surgery. In addition, in collaboration with international collaborators, we have started to set up a framework for the construction of databases in Asia, Europe, and the United States for the validation of AI models developed using data from outside of Japan. In order to develop AI support systems for laparoscopic surgery that can be used globally, it is essential to build a surgical video database based on data collected from many countries worldwide.

4 Skill Assessment Database and Efforts Toward Automatic Evaluation

Education of young surgeons and training of supervisors are essential for the improvement of the quality of surgical procedures, and objective evaluation of surgical skills is important for this purpose. Various methods have been tried to evaluate surgical skills, such as the Objective Structured Assessment of Technical Skill (OSATS) and the Global Operative Assessment of Laparoscopic Skills (GOALS), but most of them lack objectivity, and the time and effort involved in the expert evaluation process are problematic, even though they are relatively widely accepted [31, 32].

In an approach to objectively quantify the surgeon's performance, the use of AI makes a lot of sense. Moreover, such an AI-driven approach can also be used to efficiently implement the performance measurement system. Image recognition of surgical tools, surgical phases and actions, and other objects that can be the subject of surgical performance evaluation, as described above, has the potential to automatically quantify surgeon performance in a full surgical video. By quantifying every action and total procedure during surgery, we can compare them objectively and at the same time evaluate the growth of surgical techniques after training. Another approach is the three-dimensional convolutional neural network approach that can be used to evaluate surgical skills from videos [33]. This approach can be fully automatic and easy to use for various types of surgery, and no special annotations or kinetics data extraction are required. In any case, to streamline and automate skill evaluation, in addition to the image recognition approaches described so far, it is necessary to define what constitutes good surgical skills and then create a database of the results of skill evaluation by experts in the form of surgical videos and data sets.

We are exploring an objective and quantitative method for evaluation of surgical skill in laparoscopic surgery using AI-based image recognition, utilizing data from the Japan Society for Endoscopic Surgery (JSES) initiative of surgical skill accreditation review [34]. The data from the technical evaluation results will be used to develop an AI automated surgical skill evaluation system. First, some kinds of surgical phase recognition models, surgical tool recognition models, and other object and action recognition models have been developed through machine learning so far. As described above, we will be able to quantify surgeons' performance completely in every surgical video by using these models. By linking these quantified results to the expert's scoring results for every case, parameters and correlations to assess surgical skills and performance in videos will be determined. Finally, a prototype of the AI automated skill evaluation system will be constructed. We think it can be used in various applications in education and training in the field of laparoscopic surgery. Firstly, we need to validate this new system through a prospective comparison study in a JSES surgical skill accreditation review in the future. Then, this AI automated skill evaluation system will be useful for the first screening tool and evaluation support in JSES surgical skill accreditation review by reducing the burden on evaluators. Also, this system can provide feedback to surgeons based on the objective assessment results by clarifying the points that lack surgical skills and require training. It will lead to efficient and effective training for young surgeons.

5 Future of AI in Laparoscopic Surgery

AI development efforts in laparoscopic surgery have only just begun. The main approach is image recognition, which is a concept to improve efficiency and safety of surgery and operating room management through visual information support, such as surgical phase recognition, surgical instrument recognition, and anatomical structure recognition. In the approach of image recognition for navigation using laparoscopic surgical view, it can provide real-time superficial information but cannot address invisible information such as deeply located or hidden anatomical structures which can be more valuable for surgeons to perform operations safely and securely. By using preoperative imaging methods such as computed tomography and magnetic resonance imaging, we can obtain the non-superficial information of target anatomy. However, deformation and displacement of organs due to dissection and pneumoperitoneum cannot be ignored in laparoscopic surgery; thus, preoperative images are sometimes not useful enough to provide precise anatomical information during operation. To address this issue, we need to work on complementing the advantages of both preoperative and laparoscopic imaging or incorporating new technologies to give real-time information on anatomical structures located deep in the body.

In terms of steps taken toward the automation of surgery, efforts are underway to facilitate surgeon's decision-making and automate surgical skill evaluation for the first step in visual approach. The automation of surgery itself requires collaboration with surgical robot systems, and this will be possible by using robots as sensors and loggers to accumulate information other than images, which can then be utilized in the development of further AI models. As we make further progress in the process of automation of surgery, we will encounter more challenges. There are many technical and ethical hurdles in moving from the phase of assisting the surgeon in making decisions to the phase of proactively performing surgical procedures by surgical robots.

Although the day when we will be operated by automated surgical robots does not seem to be near and we cannot easily imagine that day yet, it could result from an extension of the step-by-step development of these surgical innovations.

References

1. John AS, Caturegli I, Kubicki NS, et al. The rise of minimally invasive surgery: 16 year analysis of the progressive replacement of open surgery with laparoscopy. JSLS. 2020;24(4):e2020.00076.
2. Wibe A, Eriksen MT, Syse A, et al. Effect of hospital caseload on long-term outcome after standardization of rectal cancer surgery at a national level. Br J Surg. 2005;92(2):217–24.
3. Renzulli P, Lowy A, Maibach R, et al. The influence of the surgeon's and the hospital's caseload on survival and local recurrence after colorectal cancer surgery. Surgery. 2006;139(3):296–304.
4. Garrow CR, Kowalewski KF, Li L, et al. Machine learning for surgical phase recognition: a systematic review. Ann Surg. 2021;273(4):684–93.
5. Hashimoto DA, Rosman G, Volkov M, et al. Artificial intelligence for intraoperative video analysis: machine learning's role in surgical education. J Am Coll Surg. 2017;225:S171.
6. Kitaguchi D, Takeshita N, Matsuzaki, et al. Real-time automatic surgical phase recognition in laparoscopic sigmoidectomy using the convolutional neural network-based deep learning approach. Surg Endosc. 2020;34(11):4924–31.
7. Jalal NA, Alshirbaji TA, Möller K. Predicting surgical phases using CNN-NARX neural network. Biomed Tech. 2019;64:S188.
8. Zia A, Guo L, Zhou L, et al. Novel evaluation of surgical activity recognition models using task-based efficiency metrics. Int J Comput Assist Radiol Surg. 2019;14(12):2155–63.
9. Ward TM, Hashimoto DA, Ban Y, et al. Automated operative phase identification in peroral endoscopic myotomy. Surg Endosc. 2021;35(7):4008–15.
10. Kletz S, Schoeffmann K, Husslein H. Learning the representation of instrument images in laparoscopy videos. Healthc Technol Lett. 2019;6:197–203.
11. Leibetseder A, Petscharnig S, Primus MJ, et al. Lapgyn4: a dataset for 4 automatic content analysis problems in the domain of laparoscopic gynecology. In: Proceedings of the 9th ACM multimedia systems conference; 2018. p. 357–62.
12. Nwoye CI, Mutter D, Marescaux J, Padoy N. Weakly supervised convolutional LSTM approach for tool tracking in laparoscopic videos. Int J Comput Assist Radiol Surg. 2019;14:1059–67.
13. Zhang B, Wang S, Dong L, Chen P. Surgical tools detection based on modulated anchoring network in laparoscopic videos. IEEE Access. 2020;8:23748–58.
14. Madad Zadeh S, Francois T, Calvet L, et al. SurgAI: deep learning for computerized laparoscopic image understanding in gynaecology. Surg Endosc. 2020;34:5377–83.
15. Twinanda AP, Shehata S, Mutter D, Marescaux J, Mathelin MD, Padoy N. EndoNet: a deep architecture for recognition tasks on laparoscopic videos. IEEE Trans Med Imaging. 2017;36:86–97.
16. Kitaguchi D, Takeshita N, Matsuzaki H, et al. Automated laparoscopic colorectal surgery workflow recognition using artificial intelligence: experimental research. Int J Surg. 2020;79:88–94.
17. Nwoye CI, Mutter D, Marescaux J, Padoy N. Weakly supervised convolutional LSTM approach for tool tracking in laparoscopic videos. Int J Comput Assist Radiol Surg. 2019;14(6):1059–67.
18. Ross T, Zimmerer D, Vemuri A, et al. Exploiting the potential of unlabeled endoscopic video data with self-supervised learning. Int J Comput Assist Radiol Surg. 2018;13(6):925–33.
19. Kitaguchi D, Takeshita N, Matsuzaki H, et al. Computer-assisted real-time automatic prostate segmentation during TaTME: a single-center feasibility study. Surg Endosc. 2021;35(6):2493–9.
20. Madani A, Namazi B, Altieri MS, et al. Artificial intelligence for intraoperative guidance: using semantic segmentation to identify surgical anatomy during laparoscopic cholecystectomy. Ann Surg. 2020;13 https://doi.org/10.1097/SLA.0000000000004594.
21. Mascagni P, Vardazaryan A, Alapatt D, et al. Artificial intelligence for surgical safety: automatic assessment of the critical view of safety in laparoscopic cholecystectomy using deep learning. Ann Surg. 2020; https://doi.org/10.1097/SLA.0000000000004351.

22. Tokuyasu T, Iwashita Y, Matsunobu Y, et al. Development of an artificial intelligence system using deep learning to indicate anatomical landmarks during laparoscopic cholecystectomy. Surg Endosc. 2021;35(4):1651–8.
23. Stauder R, Okur A, Peter L, et al. Random forests for phase detection in surgical workflow analysis. In: International conference on information processing in computer-assisted interventions. Springer; 2014. p. 148–57.
24. Stauder R, Ostler D, Kranzfelder M, Koller S, Feußner H, Navab N. The TUM LapChole dataset for the M2CAI 2016 workflow challenge. arXiv preprint arXiv. 2016;161009278
25. Maier-Hein L, Wagner M, Ross T, et al. Heidelberg colorectal data set for surgical data science in the sensor operating room. arXiv preprint arXiv. 2020:200503501.
26. Hashimoto DA, Rosman G, Witkowski ER, et al. Computer vision analysis of intraoperative video: automated recognition of operative steps in laparoscopic sleeve gastrectomy. Ann Surg. 2019;270:414–21.
27. Twinanda AP, Yengera G, Mutter D, Marescaux J, Padoy N. RSDNet: learning to predict remaining surgery duration from laparoscopic videos without manual annotations. IEEE Trans Med Imaging. 2019;38:1069–78.
28. Madad Zadeh S, Francois T, Calvet L, Chauvet P, Canis M, Bartoli A, Bourdel N. SurgAI: deep learning for computerized laparoscopic image understanding in gynaecology. Surg Endosc. 2020;34:5377–83.
29. Bodenstedt S, Wagner M, Mündermann L, et al. Prediction of laparoscopic procedure duration using unlabeled, multimodal sensor data. Int J Comput Assist Radiol Surg. 2019;14:1089–95.
30. Petscharnig S, Schoffmann K. Learning laparoscopic video shot classification for gynecological surgery. Multimed Tools Appl. 2018;77:8061–79.
31. Martin JA, Regehr G, Reznick R, et al. Objective structured assessment of technical skill (OSATS) for surgical residents. Br J Surg. 1997;84(2):273–8.
32. Vassiliou MC, Feldman LS, Andrew CG, et al. A global assessment tool for evaluation of intraoperative laparoscopic skills. Am J Surg. 2005;190(1):107–13.
33. Kitaguchi D, Takeshita N, Matsuzaki H, et al. Development and validation of a 3-dimensional convolutional neural network for automatic surgical skill assessment based on spatiotemporal video analysis. JAMA Netw Open. 2021;4(8):e2120786.
34. Tatsuo Yamakawa T, et al. Endoscopic surgical skill qualification system (ESSQS) of the Japanese Society of Endoscopic Surgery (JSES). BH Surg. 2013;3:6–8.

Clinical Case: Maxillofacial Surgery

Qingchuan Ma

Abstract Surgeons are under an increasing workload due to the fast-growing patient population of oral and maxillofacial surgery (OMS). Previously proposed methods have a limited benefit to surgeons' manual work because of the significant individual diversity in OMS patients. Artificial intelligence (AI) offers a promising tool to mimic surgeons' decision-making mechanisms to reduce the workload. In this chapter, our recent achievements in OMS by using a machine learning-based approach to assist surgical planning were introduced. We collected both preoperative and 1-year-later postoperative CT images of 56 patients to train a 12-layer cascaded deep neural network structure with two successive models. A virtual surgery planning approach was also presented to illustrate how the model-predicted results were further used to assist the surgeon's planning work during Lefort I treatment. Current limitations and future trends of AI in OMS were also briefly discussed. AI demonstrates its feasibility in assisting the human surgeon and shows great potential for reducing the workload. Preparation of annotated medical data, high computing power hardware, efficient feature-extracting network, and ethical issues will be key challenges for a wide application of AI in OMS.

Keywords Artificial intelligence · Surgical planning · Oral and maxillofacial surgery · 3D cephalometry

1 Introduction

Oral and maxillofacial surgery (OMS) is a discipline that involved the diagnosis and treatment of anatomical defects in the mouth, jaw, face, neck, skull, and surrounding structures [1]. During OMS, surgeons need to perform a series of intricate operations in a very limited workspace while not causing fatal damage to the important

Q. Ma (✉)
School of Engineering Medicine, Beihang University, Beijing, China
e-mail: maqingchuan@buaa.edu.cn

K. Masamune et al. (eds.), *Artificial Intelligence in Surgery*,
https://doi.org/10.1007/978-981-96-6635-5_13

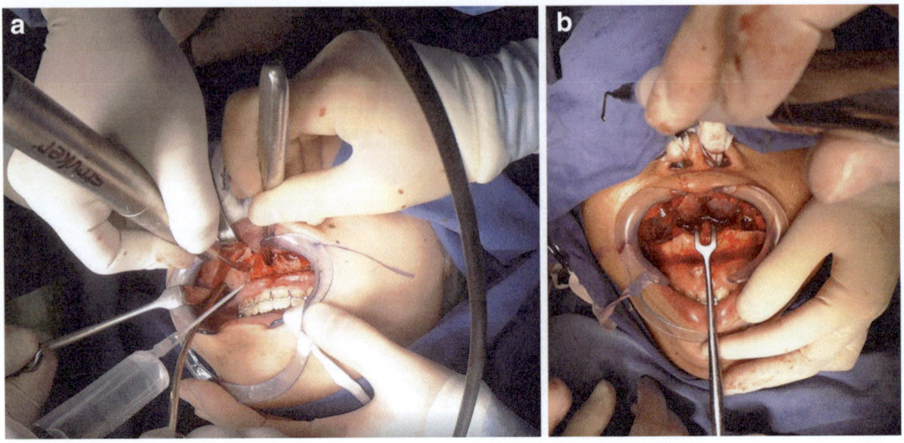

Fig. 1 Actual operation images during (**a**) and after (**b**) maxilla separations

nerves and blood vessels, as shown in Fig. 1. The surgeon's view may be blocked by the soft tissues and cannot observe the surgical site using the naked eyes [2]. Typical OMS may last 8 h or even longer with the help of many surgical instruments and close cooperation between surgeon and assistant. The long-time and intense surgical procedure is a critical challenge of physical endurance even for highly experienced surgeons. In addition, the surgeon needs to make a detailed surgical plan before surgery and recall it during surgery, which becomes an additional mental workload to the surgeon [3].

Some computer-assisted surgery (CAS) or robot-assisted surgery (RAS) has been applied to assist surgeons and relieve their workload during OMS [4]. However, these technologies heavily rely on surgeons' own experience and still need human direct involvement in critical surgical steps. With the huge success of artificial intelligence (AI) in image classification and computer vision (CV), there are increasing interests among medical researchers to apply AI in OMS for developing intelligent surgical tools [5] or integrate AI with existing CAS/RAS technologies for improving the intelligence of surgical equipment [6]. In general definition, AI-based surgery is a research topic trying to reproduce surgeons' professional intelligence in the medical field. As the specific application of AI, machine learning, especially deep learning, focuses on training intelligent models using medical data for relieving the workload of medical staff and augments their capability [7]. As for OMS, preoperatively planning is currently the most active research topic that AI (machine learning) has a promising potential to replace the old planning approaches [8].

In conventional OMS, surgical planning is an inevitable procedure in OMS for simulating the skeletal changes before actual surgery to ensure safety and develop detailed operation programs [9]. In clinical practice, surgeons usually use 3D-printed models or surgical templates based on the computerized tomography (CT) image of the patient to measure and observe potential skeletal changes in advance [10]. However, such type of method is time-consuming and only allows limited trials. Therefore, various approaches have been proposed to assist so-called virtual surgery, which enables the surgeon to conduct as many simulations as they want without the need for a surgical model or template [11]. In the current workflow of virtual surgical planning, surgeons usually conducted a cephalometric analysis for indicating the key biomechanical information of the patient's head [12]. Thus, one technological category called landmark-based or landmark-oriented planning method was further developed, which selected specifically landmarks to indicate critical skeleton features and used their locations to reflect the changes of the surgical regions [13, 14].

Recently, the application of AI in medical imaging has substantially increased and achieved remarkable success in various fields [15]. However, OMS still is an experience-centered surgical category and is not fully benefited from the recent research progress in AI [16]. In this chapter, we introduced our group's research case that used a machine learning-based approach for assisting surgical planning in OMS, which adopted a cascaded network structure to automatically predict optimal postoperative skeletal changes indicated by specifically selected anatomical landmarks. A custom virtual surgery planning (VSP) module was also developed to interpret the model-predicted result and make double-check. The proposed approach aims to learn and subsequently imitate the decision-making mechanism of surgeons during surgical planning, showing great potential for exploiting the valuable experience of some top-level surgeons and making a balance between AI and human intelligence.

We also discussed the challenges of AI in OMS application and predicted future trends from a wider perspective. The discussion not only focuses on the technological limitations of AI applications but also involved non-technological issues. The predictions of future trends are not limited to the preoperative planning that is the main topic of our research case; we also try to discuss the AI's potential for covering the entire surgical circle of OMS from preoperative, intraoperative, to postoperative phase. We hope this chapter could give readers a specific application of AI in OMS while also providing a brief big picture to show the current challenges and future trends.

2 Research Case: AI-Based Assisted Model for OMS Surgical Planning

2.1 Data Pre-processing

Both preoperative and postoperative CT images from a database of patients undertaking OMS from 2008 to 2017 at the University of Tokyo Hospital were evaluated in this study. The patients were screened by a professional surgeon according to inclusion criteria. First, only the CT images with the whole skull scanned were included, where the CT slices should cover at least a range from the nasion point to the menton point. Second, the CT data should have at least 330 slices. Third, both preoperative and postoperative CT images of a patient should meet the inclusion criteria. Fourth, the postoperative data should be 1 year later after the surgery. CT

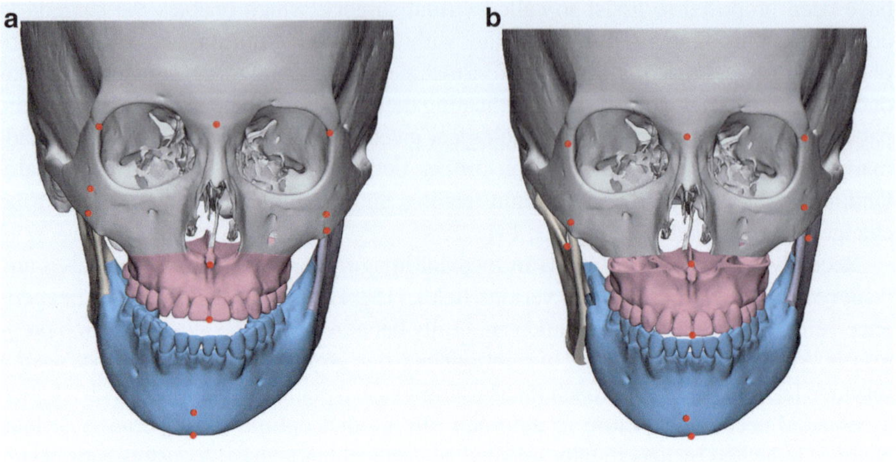

Fig. 2 Landmarks' location and corresponding skeletal changes before (**a**) and after (**b**) AI-based model prediction

images of 56 patients were qualified and selected finally; we allocated 50 of them to the training group and 6 of them to the testing group.

All medical images were generated using a Canon CT with a pixel size of 0.35 mm/pixel and slice thickness of 0.5 mm/pixel. The original DICOM data of the patient were imported into MIMICS to create a bone mask while deleting the irrelevant medical information. Subsequently, all mask slices in axial coordinate were exported as BMP pictures to be used as training materials. Afterward, the 3D model of the bone mask was created in MIMICS using a high-resolution mode. Finally, manual landmarking was conducted on the created 3D head model for preparing the ground-truth landmarks.

In this study, we empirically selected 11 landmarks to indicate the key characteristics of the head of the patient, as shown in Fig. 2. The three landmarks at the skull region functioned as references, and the rest of the landmarks might be subject to location changes after OMS. Manual landmarking was conducted by one of the authors. Each patient's landmark data was saved as an 11 × 3 matrix, where the first column represented the image sequence and the second and third columns were landmarks' horizontal and vertical locations in the image.

2.2 *Specific Processing for Preoperative and Postoperative Data*

The exported slice images of each preoperative CT volume were standardized to 330 slices and saved to a [330, 512, 512, 1] tensor. We adopted principal component analysis (PCA) to correlate the inter-landmark relationship and subsequently transfer them to a lower-dimensional space. To correlate both pre- and postoperative landmarks into the same coordinate, we adopted the iterative closest point (ICP) algorithm to calculate the transfer matrix between two datasets using three landmarks at the skull part to register the rest of the landmarks. After the PCA and ICP adjustments, the processed preoperative and postoperative landmarks were used as training data for the first model and second model, respectively.

2.3 Network Architecture

The proposed deep neural network structure has two successive models. The first one is the landmarking model that extracts landmarks from 2D patches of 3D volume. The second model is the regression model that uses the results of the first model and predicts postoperative skeletal changes. Feeding the entire 3D medical data directly into the landmarking model network may result in high computational cost and memory requirements. Therefore, we adopted a patch-based method using 2.5D representations of 3D volume data [17]. For a certain point in the 3D volume, three 2D patches were extracted centering on the point to represent input image data sent to the network, which consisted of 3n patches with each patch having the same patch size. Consequently, the 2D patches were remapped as three-channel image data and fed into the CNN model. Another principle in the landmarking model is to jointly conduct the classification and regression tasks for predicting the displacement and direction of the movement of the point toward the annotated landmark. These two tasks shared the same backbone network as shown in Fig. 3a. The backbone network of the first model consisted of three convolution blocks, and each block had a standard Conv-BatchNorm-ReLU operation. All convolution layers had the same kernel size as 3x3 with stride = 1. A max-pooling layer followed every block to reduce the spatial dimension of the feature maps by half.

The first model had two subnets following the backbone network for joint classification and regression tasks. They shared a similar structure, including three fully connected (FC) layers. ReLU activation and dropout layer were added to each FC layer, except the last one. The loss function of the first model consisted of two separate losses from two subnets. The loss of the regression subnet L_{1r} was calculated as the mean square error (MSE). The loss for classification subnet L_{1c} is the standard cross-entropy loss. A scale factor α was applied to weigh two losses, and we empirically set α as 0.5. The extracted landmarks from the first model were subsequently fed into the second model with a three-layer multi-layer perceptron (MLP) for the prediction of corresponding postoperative landmarks. The first and second FC layers had 32 and 64 neurons, respectively, and were followed by ReLU activation. The final output FC layer had 33 neurons, corresponding to the 11 landmarks of the postoperative phase. The loss function of the second model was also MSE.

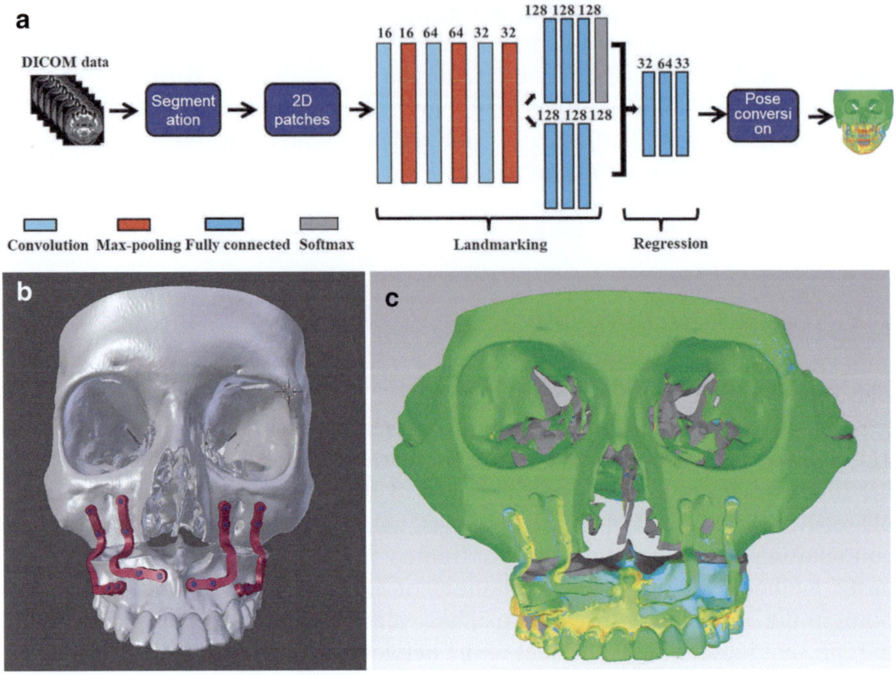

Fig. 3 Detailed network structure (**a**), virtual surgery planning results (**b**), and comparisons between model predicted and actual results (**c**)

2.4 *Virtual Surgery Planning*

The model-predicted result was interpreted and double-checked using a custom virtual surgery planning (VSP) module implemented in a commercial software 3-Matics (Version 13, Materialise NV), which can automatically generate the digital fixing plate and navigation models based on the topological feature of the patient's skull. The patient's head bone was first grouped into five parts: skull, maxilla, mandible body, right ramus, and left ramus. The maxilla and skull were merged in 3-Matics after duplicating the new ones. Then the planned relocating gap between them was fixed for drawing guiding curves. Afterward, the custom fixing plates were created in sequence based on the guiding curve. The width and thickness of the plate were set as 3 and 2 mm, respectively, and the outer and inner diameter of the screw holes were set as 4 and 3 mm, respectively. The drilling holes were created by clicking preferred drilling locations and then creating the fixing plate based on surface topography. Finally, the digital fixing plates can be exported for 3D printing the actual fixing plates, and drilling holes can be used for creating navigation models for guiding the surgical movement of surgeons. The final results after custom VSP are shown in Fig. 3b,c.

3 Experiments and Discussions of Research Case

We conducted an experiment to evaluate the performance of the proposed AI model and corresponding VSP modules when compared with the human surgeon. The result showed that the overall average accuracy of the AI model in the landmark level is 5.4 ± 0.6 mm. The total time from extracting the landmark to finishing the surgical planning is 42.9 ± 0.1 seconds for each volume. The VSP results were compared with the actual results after a robotic surgical experiment based on 3D printed models by using the software Geomagic Control X (3D Systems Corp., Rock Hill, South Carolina, USA). It was indicated that the average RMS error of the whole models and the fixing plates are 0.87 ± 0.16 mm and 1.00 ± 0.05 mm, respectively.

The comparison between the model-predict results and the real human surgeon's surgical outcomes demonstrates the feasibility of the proposed methodology. The real medical CT volumes used in this study provided valuable research resources to develop an approach that can be potentially used in actual healthcare facilities. By contrast, some studies used medical data of healthy subjects [18] or excluded images with severe skeletal deformities [19], which may pose severe challenges during real-world application. The present study includes patients with various anatomical conditions, ranging from mild to severe. Therefore, the obtained experimental results are closely similar to the clinical results.

The use of the custom VSP approach enables the surgeon to generate custom fixing plates based on the topography characteristics of patients. Some surgical steps can be avoided such as using surgical splint and wire to fix the maxilla to the mandible, bending the titanium plates during surgery for maintaining planned displacement, and using the glabellar reference screw for the fixed skeletal marker. The cooperation between artificial intelligence and human intelligence allows the surgeon to conduct a double-check and make some manual adjustments if the AI-produced results are slightly different from the real medical practice, thus significantly simplifying the current workflow while still giving the surgeon the highest priority for controlling the surgical outcomes. Such kind of working philosophy could also solve the problem of ethical issue that concerns surgical safety by directly relying on AI for the human vital operation [20]. The custom manufacture of fixing plate could yield personalized treatment for making the plates closely contact the bone in most connecting areas rather than only around the plate's holes. This characteristic could potentially solve the rebounding problem of titanium plates after surgery and reduce the possibility of a second surgery for re-fixing the plates.

4 Key Challenges of AI in Maxillofacial Surgery

4.1 Lack of Annotated Training Materials

The larger number of annotated databases is the key contributor to the current success of AI (machine learning). For example, the well-known ImageNet has more than 14 million labeled images, which becomes valuable research resources for testing the latest network architecture in ILSVRC (ImageNet Large Scale Visual Recognition Challenge) [21]. However, there is still a lack of publicly available databases with a larger number of annotated medical data in OMS. Three factors may attribute to these limitations. The first one is the difficulty to obtain abundant medical data. Unlike the common 2D images that can be easily obtained by using a common camera or collected from the internet, OMS images require professional surgeons to use expensive medical equipment like CT scanners to collect. The second one is the difficulty to annotate the medical images. Annotation of the medical image was still limited to the professionals with medical backgrounds by using medical image software, which is more time-consuming and requires more image preprocessing. By contrast, common 2D images can be easily annotated even by common people without professional knowledge. The third difficulty is the ethical issue during data analysis and sharing. OMS image contains patients' facial and anatomic information, which is under strict regulations of ethical issues [22]. Consequently, researchers need to anonymize personal information and only use the data within the medical facility, which forbade the researchers to combine their small datasets with other research institutes and publicly share the annotated data. Without enough training data, the performance of the AI model will be limited. Unfortunately, this problem currently cannot be solved by merely using the technological method; regulation changes such as giving limited permission of data sharing for research purposes could be a possible way.

4.2 High Computing Power Hardware

The widespread use of the high-performance computing platform is another key factor of AI success, especially the use of NVidia GPU and its corresponding CUDA toolkit [23]. However, for the same amount of data, the requirement of computing power and memory is larger in 3D medical images than in common 2D images. To solve this problem, some researchers adopted the compromise methods such as using the 2D representation of 3D data [18]; nevertheless, the requirement of computing power is still much higher than the pure 2D images. A multi-GPU array is a possible way to solve this problem. But the cost will also significantly increase, easily beyond the researcher's affordability. More investment in hardware is still a highly desirable way to train more clinical-applicable AI models in the future.

4.3 *Efficient Feature-Extracting Network*

Common 2D pictures only need 2D CNN to extract the key features. By contrast, OMS images are mostly CT images; some compromising approaches have to be adopted such as using the image preprocessing method by discarding the redundant information or resizing the image into smaller ones. Nevertheless, the network design and hyperparameter tuning are still much more difficult for 3D images. To efficiently extract the useful image features, the network needs to be designed deep and large; more Conv layers and optimization layers (Dropout, BN) with more neurons will be needed. For 2D images, there are some successful network templates such as U-net [24], V net [25], Resnet50 [26], VGG19 [27], and YOLO [28], which allow researchers to use these backbone network structures and connect them with additional layers, only need to fine-tune the last several layers for their specific research purpose. By contrast, there still lack mature backbone networks that researchers can migrate for extracting the features of 3D medical images. Consequently, researchers have to spend much time designing and tuning the networks by themselves. The development of widely accepted pre-trained backbone networks for 3D medical images could be a major contribution to the research community.

4.4 *Regulations and Ethical Issues*

As aforementioned, OMS medical data includes highly sensitive patients' anatomical and personal information; the regulations and requirement of ethical issues can protect the patients' information from any unauthorized use and regulate research conduct [20]. However, on the one hand, the performance of the medical-used AI model is directly affected by the database size. On the other hand, current strict regulations limited the database expansion and only allow the limited person to have limited access to the data [29]. Regulations are necessary for proper medical data use, whereas too strict regulations will have a negative impact on the wider application of AI in OMS. Compared with the fast-evolving AI research, current regulations and ethical issues still lack updates for helping the researchers fully use medical data while still protecting the patients' personal information. Some technological methods may be adopted such as anonymizing and encrypting the medical data; then these data can be used for a more widespread use such as database sharing and limited public use. Nevertheless, given the difference between AI and common biomedical research, a highly specialized regulation and ethical issue guidance could be a more practical way to solve the discrepancy between data utilization and data protection.

Given the above, if we compare AI to a car, the database like the gas, the hardware like the engine, the network like the shape, the ethical issue like the traffic rule, as shown in Fig. 4a. Only when we fueled enough gas, equipped with a powerful

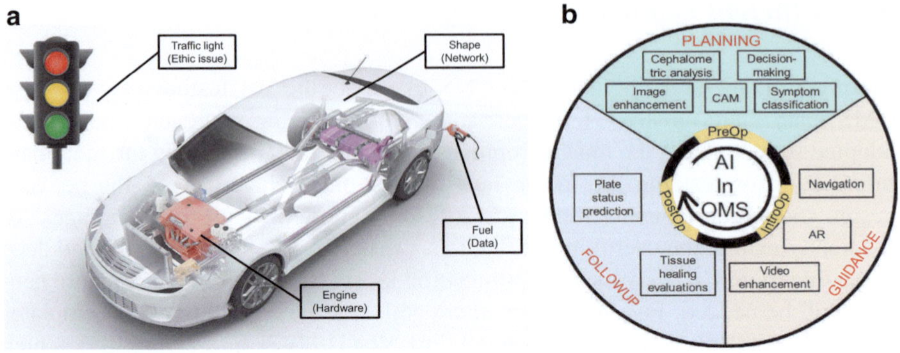

Fig. 4 The similarity between AI's application in medical filed and the four factors influencing a car's performance (**a**), current application and future trends of AI in the full life circle of OMS (**b**)

engine, designed the car with an air dynamic shape, and enacted the driver-friendly traffic rule, then we can make the car run longer and faster.

5 Future Trends of AI in Maxillofacial Surgery

A full life circle of OMS includes the preoperative, intraoperative, and postoperative phases throughout the treatment. AI researchers are currently trying to make contributions in all three operational phases. Nevertheless, the research activity and research amount are interestingly different in different phases. Hereafter, a brief discussion was given to analyze current research achievements and predict future trends.

5.1 *Preoperative Planning*

Currently, the preoperative phase is the most active research section in the AI-based OMS [30]. There are three possible reasons for this phenomenon. First, all patients need to do CT scans before surgery, and surgeon can easily access these medical data. Second, there are numerous conventional researches in this phase available in the literature, which provides theoretical support for researchers when they try to use AI-based methods to solve previously proposed problems. Third, the AI models trained in this phase are mostly offline models, and researchers have enough time to conduct model inferring before surgery. The models also have no requirement of real-time performance and have less dependence on high computing power. Therefore, there are a remarkable amount of AI-based research which can be found in this surgical phase to replace or assist surgeon's work, such as AI-based cephalometric analysis to extract anatomical landmarks from medical images [17], AI-based decision-making to mimic surgeon's thinking mechanism [15], AI-based image enhancement to delete noise from raw images [31], AI-based computer-assisted manufacture (CAM) to make fixing plate and surgical splints [32], and AI-based symptom classification to detect the types of disease from medical images [33].

5.2 Intraoperative Guidance

By comparison, the AI-based research for surgical guidance in the intraoperative phase has a higher requirement of real-time performance and model accuracy, because the models need to give on-site and on-time responses during the surgery. Some researches in this area directly transferred from non-medical used applications and made some adaptions for specific use. For example, YOLO is a very successful backbone network structure originally developed for vehicle navigation. Some researchers have successfully migrated YOLO to medical navigation for tracking the target tissue [28]. AI-based AR/VR is also a hot topic in OMS given that the intricate working condition hampered surgeon's observation by soft tissue and other organs [34]. Besides, AI-based surgical video enhancement can give the surgeon clearer video streams compared with originally blurred ones [35]. However, AI-based models aiming for real clinic applications are still challenging in the intraoperative phase due to the limited annotation data, high computing power, and high requirement of real-time performance.

5.3 Postoperative Follow-Up

Postoperative AI-based researches are very limited in OMS. This is mainly because some affecting factors of postoperative healing and evolving mechanisms caused by implant and surgical interventions are still unclear [36]. There is also less basic medical research to support AI-based follow-up research despite its high research value. In clinic, it is common that the post-6-month or post-1-year outcomes of patients differed from the surgeon's original expectation; some patients even need to do re-treatment because of poor healing or loose fixation plates [37]. What are the causes of such kind phenomenon and how to counteract are still unclear. An AI-based predicting model is a promising tool that can potentially solve this problem by building a multi-input network considering the influences of the skeleton, soft tissue, fixing plate, dental occlusion, and gender using pre-, post-6-month, and post-1-year medical images. Unfortunately, there still has no adequate research regarding this topic.

6 Conclusions

This chapter introduced the basic characteristics of OMS and the promising potential of AI in this surgical type. A research case regarding AI-assisted surgical planning approach was introduced, which consists of two successive models and a virtual surgical planning module. The current challenges of AI in the OMS and the future trends were also discussed for clarifying the limitations and possible applications of AI in OMS. From our previous research and observation of the current research community, we believe that AI in OMS is still in a child phase, but it is currently growing fast and will become a powerful adult to support the human surgeon in the future if some technological and medical barriers can be removed properly. A promising working concept is to use AI to finish most tedious and high-duty work while still allowing the human surgeon to interfere and supervise the AI for a more responsible surgical result. Thus human's higher intelligence and machine's artificial intelligence can be both fully utilized.

References

1. Mitchell DA. An introduction to oral and maxillofacial surgery. CRC Press; 2014.
2. Fonseca RJ. Oral and maxillofacial surgery-E-book: 3-volume set. Elsevier Health Sciences; 2017.
3. Chen X, Xu L, Sun Y, Politis C. A review of computer-aided oral and maxillofacial surgery: planning, simulation and navigation. Expert Rev Med Devices. 2016:1.
4. Kong X, Duan X, Wang Y. An integrated system for planning, navigation and robotic assistance for mandible reconstruction surgery. Intell Serv Robot. 2016;9(2):113–21.
5. Yu KH, Beam AL, Kohane IS. Artificial intelligence in healthcare. Nat Biomed Eng. 2018;2(10):719–31.
6. Hashimoto DA, Ward TM, Meireles OR. The role of artificial intelligence in surgery. Adv Surg. 2020;54
7. Etienne H, Hamdi S, Roux ML, Camuset J, Khalifehocquemiller T, Giol M, et al. Artificial intelligence in thoracic surgery: past, present, perspective and limits. 2020.
8. Litjens G, Kooi T, Bejnordi BE, Setio A, Sánchez C. A survey on deep learning in medical image analysis. Med Image Anal. 2017;42(9):60–88.
9. Reyneke JP. Essentials of orthognathic surgery. Chicago: Quintessence; 2003.
10. Mani V. Surgical correction of facial deformities. JP Medical Ltd; 2010.
11. Kau CH, Richmond S. Three-dimensional imaging for orthodontics and maxillofacial surgery. Wiley; 2011.
12. Swennen GR, Schutyser FA, Hausamen J-E. Three-dimensional cephalometry: a color atlas and manual. Springer; 2005.
13. Lin H-H, Chuang Y-F, Weng J-L, Lo L-J. Comparative validity and reproducibility study of various landmark-oriented reference planes in 3-dimensional computed tomographic analysis for patients receiving orthognathic surgery. PLoS One. 2015;10(2):e0117604.
14. Meehan M, Teschner M, Girod S. Three-dimensional simulation and prediction of craniofacial surgery. Orthod Craniofac Res. 2003;6:102–7.
15. Loftus TJ, Vlaar APJ, Hung AJ, Bihorac A, Dennis BM, Juillard C, Hashimoto DA, Kaafarani HMA, Tighe PJ, Kuo PC, Miyashita S, Wexner SD, Behrns KE. Executive summary of the

artificial intelligence in surgery series. Surgery. 2021;171(5):1435–9. https://doi.org/10.1016/j.surg.2021.10.047.
16. Costa F, Robiony M, Toro C, Sembronio S, Polini F, Politi M. Condylar positioning devices for orthognathic surgery: a literature review. Oral Surg Oral Med Oral Pathol Oral Radiol Endod. 2008;106(2):179–90.
17. Ma Q, Kobayashi E, Fan B, Nakagawa K, Sakuma I, Masamune K, et al. Automatic 3D landmarking model using patch-based deep neural networks for CT image of oral and maxillofacial surgery. Int J Med Robot Comput Assist Surg. 2020;16(3):e2093.
18. Lee SM, Kim HP, Jeon K, Lee S-H, Seo JK. Automatic 3D cephalometric annotation system using shadowed 2D image-based machine learning. Phys Med Biol. 2019;64(5):055002.
19. Brunso J, Franco M, Constantinescu T, Barbier L, Santamaría JA, Alvarez J. Custom-machined miniplates and bone-supported guides for orthognathic surgery: a new surgical procedure. J Oral Maxillofac Surg. 2016;74(5):1061.e1–1061.e12.
20. Shane O'S, Nathalie N, Colin A, et al. Legal, regulatory, and ethical frameworks for development of standards in artificial intelligence (AI) and autonomous robotic surgery. Int J Med Robot Comput Assist Surg. 2019.
21. Jia D, Wei D, Socher R, Li LJ, Kai L, Li FF. ImageNet: a large-scale hierarchical image database. 2009. p. 248–255.
22. Yang GZ, Cambias J, Cleary K, Daimler E, Drake J, Dupont PE, et al. Medical robotics—regulatory, ethical, and legal considerations for increasing levels of autonomy. Sci Robot. 2017;2(4):eaam8638.
23. Li W, Jin G, Cui X, See S. IEEE. An evaluation of unified memory technology on NVIDIA GPUs. In: 2015 15th IEEE ACM international symposium on cluster cloud and grid computing (CCGrid 2015). Shenzhen, P R China; 2015. p. 1092–8.
24. Siddique N, Paheding S, Elkin CP, Devabhaktuni V. U-net and its variants for medical image segmentation: a review of theory and applications. IEEE Access. 2021;9:82031–57.
25. Milletari F, Navab N, Ahmadi S-A, Ieee. V-net: fully convolutional neural networks for volumetric medical image segmentation. In: 4th IEEE international conference on 3D vision (3DV). Stanford: Stanford University; 2016. p. 565–71.
26. Wen L, Li X, Gao L. A transfer convolutional neural network for fault diagnosis based on ResNet-50. Neural Comput Applic. 2020;32(10):6111–24.
27. Carvalho T, de Rezende ERS, Alves MTP, Balieiro FKC, Sovat RB. Exposing computer generated images by eye's region classification via transfer learning of VGG19 CNN. In: 16th IEEE International Conference on Machine Learning and Applications (ICMLA). Cancun, Mexico; 2017. p. 866–70.
28. Al-masni MA, Al-antari MA, Park J-M, Gi G, Kim T-Y, Rivera P, et al. Simultaneous detection and classification of breast masses in digital mammograms via a deep learning YOLO-based CAD system. Comput Methods Prog Biomed. 2018;157:85–94.
29. Lee LM, Gostin LO. Ethical collection, storage, and use of public health data a proposal for a national privacy protection. JAMA. 2009;302(1):82–4. https://doi.org/10.1001/jama.2009.958.
30. Zhou X-Y, Guo Y, Shen M, Yang G-Z. Application of artificial intelligence in surgery. Front Med. 2020;14(4):417–30.
31. Sun Y, Liu X, Cong P, Li L, Zhao Z. Digital radiography image denoising using a generative adversarial network. J Xray Sci Technol. 2018;26(4):523–34.
32. Pascal E, Majoufre C, Bondaz M, Courtemanche A, Berger M, Bouletreau P. Current status of surgical planning and transfer methods in orthognathic surgery. J Stomatol Oral Maxillofac Surg. 2018;119(3):245–8.
33. Chilamkurthy S, Ghosh R, Tanamala S, Biviji M, Campeau NG, Venugopal VK, et al. Deep learning algorithms for detection of critical findings in head CT scans: a retrospective study. Lancet. 2018;392(10162):2388–96. https://doi.org/10.1016/s0140-6736(18)31645-3.

34. Wang J, Suenaga H, Hoshi K, Yang L, Kobayashi E, Sakuma I, et al. Augmented reality navigation with automatic marker-free image registration using 3-D image overlay for dental surgery. IEEE Trans Biomed Eng. 2014;61(4):1295–304.
35. Ghamsarian N, Taschwer M, Schoeffmann K, Ieee. Deblurring cataract surgery videos using a multi-scale deconvolutional neural network. In: IEEE 17th international symposium on biomedical imaging (ISBI). Iowa; 2020. p. 872–6.
36. Ho CL, McAdory L. Postoperative imaging of complications following cranial implants. J Belgian Soc Radiol. 2019;103(1)
37. Amjad S, Kalim Ansari MD, Ahmad SS, Rahman T. Comparative study of outcomes between locking plates and three-dimensional plates in mandibular fractures. Natl J Maxillofac Surg. 2020;11(2):263–9.

Future Trends: AI × Robot

Renáta Levendovics, Tamás Levendovics, and Tamás Haidegger

Abstract Robotic surgery has become part of the clinical practice and an extensively studied research domain. Extending the traditional concept of image guidance, capsule, continuum, and microrobots and the dominating robot-assisted minimally invasive surgery (RAMIS) systems support the work of the surgeons. The global-scale adoption in the data age brings new challenges to researchers, engineers, ethics professionals, and legal regulatory experts. Even today, commercialized systems are almost exclusively based on human-in-the-loop control or deterministic algorithmic solutions (such as registration techniques for image-guided technologies), and adaptive decision-making expert systems are lagging. Artificial Intelligence (AI) is one of the most studied research areas; learning from big data shows very promising results in the critical parts of surgery, such as vision, decision support, reasoning, diagnostics, and situation awareness. AI can reduce the complexity of intra-operative workflow, provide predictions on patient outcomes, and enhance efficiency in postoperative reporting. AI-based solutions can create a completely new sub-field, dubbed autonomous robotic surgery, where the systems can provide autonomy supported by proper decision-making and problem-solving capabilities. In this chapter, the most significant, already advanced (research prototypes and commercialized) surgical robotic systems (RAMIS, image-guided, cooperative, continuum, micro, and capsule robots) are introduced, along with the domain's legal and ethical considerations. The most thoroughly studied research

---

R. Levendovics · T. Levendovics (✉)
University Research and Innovation Center (EKIK), Obuda University, Budapest, Hungary

John von Neumann Faculty of Informatics, Obuda University, Budapest, Hungary

Austrian Center for Medical Innovation and Technology (ACMIT), Wiener Neustadt, Austria
e-mail: renata.levendovics@irob.uni-obuda.hu; tamas.levendovics@irob.uni-obuda.hu

T. Haidegger
University Research and Innovation Center (EKIK), Obuda University, Budapest, Hungary

Austrian Center for Medical Innovation and Technology (ACMIT), Wiener Neustadt, Austria
e-mail: haidegger@irob.uni-obuda.hu; https://irob.uni-obuda.hu/en/main/

K. Masamune et al. (eds.), *Artificial Intelligence in Surgery*,
https://doi.org/10.1007/978-981-96-6635-5_14

topics are introduced based on the current global trends, highlighting the AI-based approaches having the highest possible impact on the clinical practice. Additionally, future trends and challenges to tackle in AI-driven robotic surgery are presented.

Keywords Surgical robotics · Artificial intelligence · Automation of surgery Computer-integrated surgery · Robot-assisted minimally invasive surgery

1 Introduction

The history of surgical robotics started in the early 1960s—the US National Aeronautics and Space Administration (NASA) and the US Department of Defense Defense Advanced Research Projects Agency (DARPA) laid the foundations of telerobotic surgical systems [1]. Originally, their aim was to provide medical assistance for astronauts or wounded soldiers during their remote missions. For this, teleoperated robots would have been used, operated from the Earth or from the more safety background. At the end of the Cold War, the technology was released for commercial purposes, the attention from telesurgery in space shifted to shorter-distance telesurgery solutions, and soon, the first surgical robot prototypes received their Food and Drug Administration (FDA) clearances and entered the market [2].

The basic concept of computer-integrated surgery (CIS) can be fitted to the computer-aided design/computer-aided manufacturing (CAD/CAM) paradigm known from the manufacturing industry, which involves the data–model–plan–execution–evaluation circle, where surgical robotics takes the most important role in the execution step [3, 4] (Fig. 1). The evolution of advanced information sources mainly images (such as endoscopic, computed tomography, magnetic resonance imaging, etc.) and the development of robotic devices led to the concept of

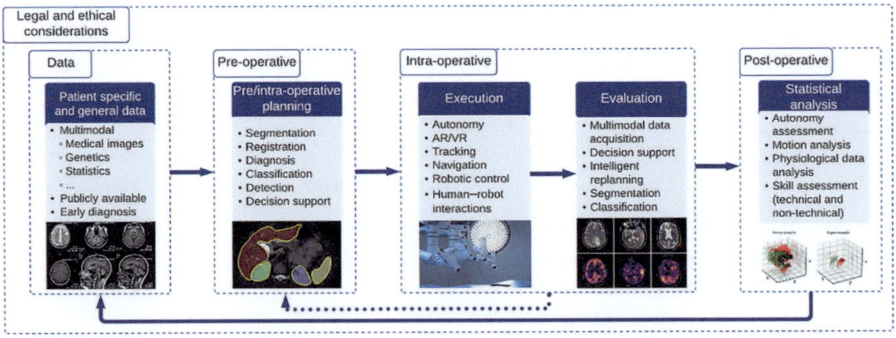

Fig. 1 AI-based surgical CAD/CAM model, based on the original model by Taylor et al. [3]. AI can support computer-integrated surgery in every phase in the future (see Chapters "Development of AI Analysis Platform—Smart Cyber Operating Theater (SCOT)—For Medical Information in Neurosurgery", "Deployment of Smart Cyber Operating Theater-Based Digital Operating Room to a Mobile Operating Theater", "Surgical Processing Models", and "Semantic Data Modeling")

robot-assisted or robot-executed surgeries. However, against the everyday terminology, surgical robotics does not necessarily mean high-level automation: there are devices, which only perform low-level, assistance-based automation, such as the market leading da Vinci surgical system (Intuitive Surgical Inc., Sunnyvale, CA). Advanced image-guided surgical systems, such as CyberKnife (Accuray Inc., Sunnyvale, CA), can perform high-level autonomy (see Sect. 2) [5].

In most of the cases, the pre-operative and intra-operative surgical planning in CIS is based on the human operator; however, with autonomous image segmentation, registration, classification, and diagnosis techniques, the accuracy can be increased, and the workload of the surgeon can be decreased [6] (Fig. 1). In the case of implementation, autonomy, augmented reality (AR)/virtual reality (VR), tracking, navigation, and robotic control can be added values in the future [7, 8]. For the future CIS concept, the intra-operative evaluation might include decision support, intelligent re-planning, data acquisition, and image processing steps. The post-operative analysis can be extended with autonomy assessment, motion analysis, and autonomous surgical skill assessment. *AI is the ability of a digital computer or computer-controlled robot to perform tasks commonly associated with intelligent beings. The term is frequently applied to the project of developing systems endowed with the intellectual processes characteristic of humans, such as the ability to reason, discover meaning, generalize, or learn from past experience* [9] (see Chapter "Introduction/Definition of "AI Surgery""). With advanced AI approaches, higher accuracy can be achieved in surgical robotics, which can improve patient safety [10] (see Chapter "Development of AI Analysis Platform—Smart Cyber Operating Theater (SCOT)—For Medical Information in Neurosurgery"). In this chapter, commercialized and research projects are introduced in the field of surgical robotics, highlighting the AI-based components, the legal and ethical considerations, and the future directions of research [11–14].

2 Autonomy in Surgical Robotics: The Present and the Future

Autonomy is considered as a fundamental component of robots, yet it is one of the hardest terms to define, assess, and regulate [5]. The autonomy in surgical robotics was defined by expert surgeons and engineers, which follows a six-level scale, similar to autonomy levels in the case of self-driving cars (Fig. 2). Levels of autonomy (LoAs) of surgical robots are the following:

LoA 0: No autonomy
LoA 1: Robot assistance
LoA 2: Task-level autonomy
LoA 3: Supervised autonomy
LoA 4: High-level autonomy
LoA 5: Full autonomy

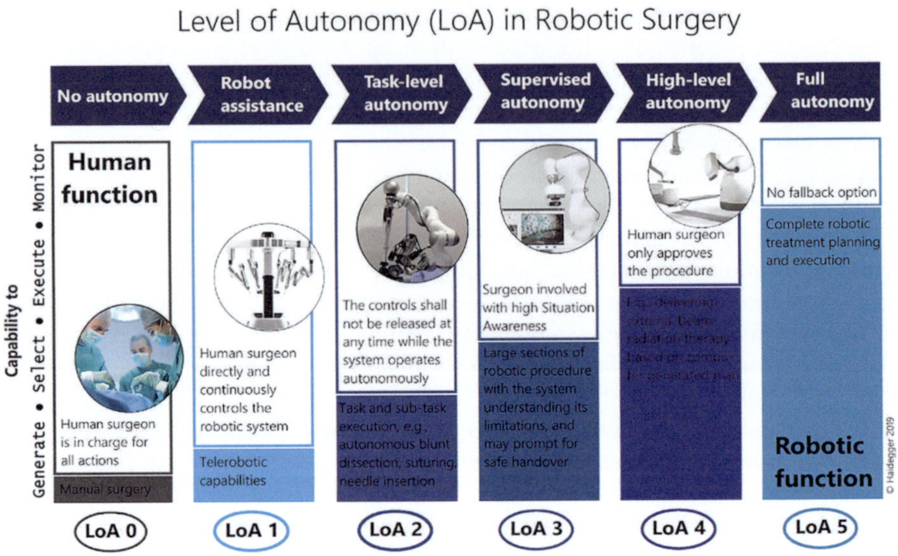

Fig. 2 Levels of autonomy (LoAs) in robotic surgery [5]. The six-stage classification follows the ISO/IEC standardization framework, determining LoA based on the human versus robotic functions of the system

In the case of LoA 0, during the intervention no active robotic equipment is used; thus it may be considered identical to a nonrobotic case. LoA 1 means that the surgical robot performs only specific, low-level functions. Teleoperation, tremor filtering, and abrupt motion filtering belong to LoA 1, such as the market dominating da Vinci surgical system (Sect. 3.1). LoA 2 is where the robotic system performs tasks and subtasks autonomously, such as endoscope handling, needle insertion, suturing, etc. AutoLap autonomous endoscope-handling robot (developed by the Medical Surgery Technologies Ltd.) represents LoA 2 with visual servoing for MIS operations. LoA 3 denotes the level of supervised autonomy, where the system can autonomously complete a large section of a surgical procedure and make low-level cognitive decisions. Situation awareness (*the perception of the elements in the environment within a volume of time and space, the comprehension of their meaning, and the projection of their status in the near future* [15]) is a key factor at this level since human oversight is necessary. For LoA 3, TSolution-One (formerly ROBODOC, THINK Surgical Inc., Fremont, CA) total knee arthroplasty image-guided surgical system is a good example, which is introduced in Sect. 3.2. LoA 4 means the high-level autonomy, where the robotic system executes complete procedures based on a pre-operative surgical plan, approved by a human operator, while the human has only the possibility to abort the procedure. The key difference between LoA 3 and LoA 4 is that at LoA 4, the robotic system must be able to finish the procedure even if the human operator fails to respond appropriately to a handover request even if the system understands that the conditions changed, allowing only suboptimal performance [5]. The typical commercially available example for LoA 4 is the CyberKnife stereotactic radiosurgery system. CyberKnife uses a linear accelerator to deliver high-energy X-rays or photons used in radiation therapy. CyberKnife moves around the patient to deliver the right amount of radiation and to minimize the radiation exposure of healthy tissues. CyberKnife is an image-guided robotic system, where the treatment plan, the execution, and patient motion compensation are autonomously performed. In the case of LoA 5, there is no need for human supervision; cognitive abilities of the robotic system allow for adapting to every situation and environment. Till now, there is no commercially available robotic system which reached LoA 5 level [5, 16–18]. Autonomy can be an added value in the future of robotic surgery, and AI can be a basis of it. AI-based surgical planning can involve data-based, autonomous outlining the surgery with intelligent computer vision, data science, and AI-based robotic motion planning techniques. AI can also play a role in the subtask automation, such as in RAMIS. In that case, AI can be a part of reasoning, decision support, endoscopic image processing, and situation awareness.

3 Robotics Approaches in CIS: Control Types

3.1 Human-in-the-Loop Surgical Robots

For soft tissue manipulation, the most typical approach is the human-in-the-loop control, i.e., teleoperation, which leaves the surgeon in the control loop. Teleoperation is mainly used in robot-assisted minimally invasive surgery (RAMIS). Undoubtedly, the most successful surgical robotic system is the da Vinci surgical system (dVSS) with over 9000 clinical devices used in hospitals (Fig. 3). DVSS is a teleoperational RAMIS system; the human operator is always in the control loop, which means robot assistance (LoA 1) in autonomy without any cognitive functions or decision-making from the robot [19]. However, dVSS can help with tremor filtering, precision, ergonomics, and 3D vision. Since dVSS patient-side arms do only what the surgeon does at the surgeon-side console, surgeon's actions can be recorded with image and kinematic data, which can lead to AI-driven surgical skill assessment, automation, and advanced decision-making support. There are other commercially available and ready-to-launch RAMIS platforms, such as the Senhance Surgical Robotic System, the Bitrack, the Versius, the Mantra, etc., (Fig. 3), but until now, these systems' commercial/clinical impact has remained at low level [20].

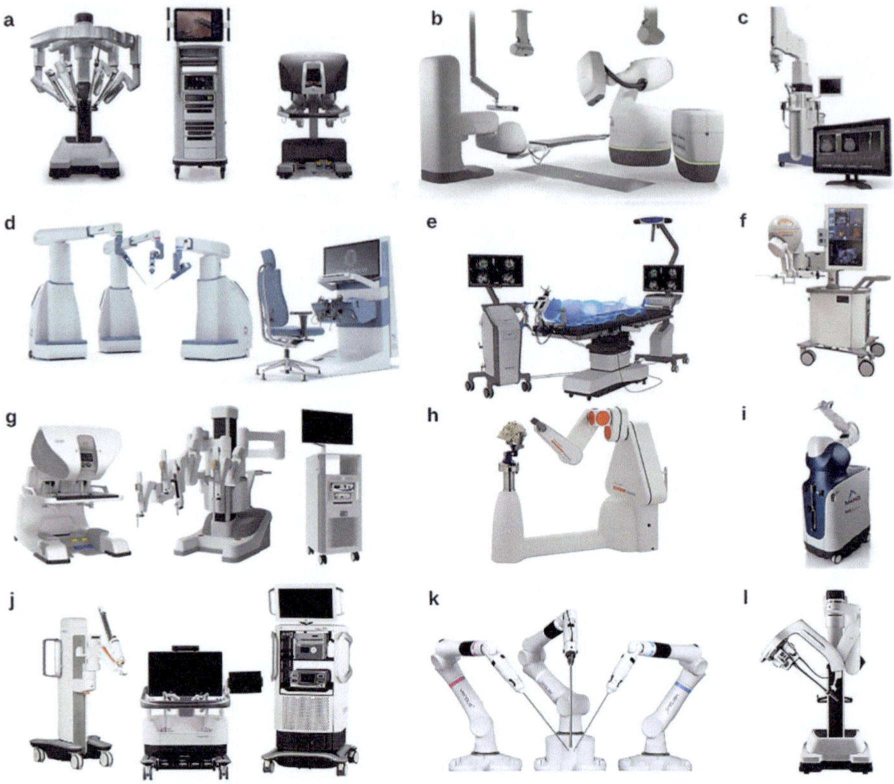

Fig. 3 Commercialized, ready-to-launch, and advanced research prototype robotic surgical systems along the three main control approaches (teleoperational, cooperative, image-guided)(**a**) Da Vinci Xi, (**b**) CyberKnife, (**c**) TSolution-One, (**d**) Senhance Surgical Robotic System, (**e**) iSYS/Micromate/Stealth autoguide robot, (**f**) Eigen ARTEMIS, (**g**) Revo-i, (**h**) Neuromate, (**i**) Mako, (**j**) Hugo RAS system, (**k**) Versius, (**1**) da Vinci SP

3.2 Image-Guided Surgical Robots

CIS is based on a priori information, and the most important input information is usually the set of medical images of the patient. The improvement of medical imaging provided the basis of the image-guided techniques, which resulted more accurate organ targeting, more safety, and better patient outcome [21]. Image-guided robotic systems are guided by pre-operative and/or intra-operative images (most commonly, computed tomography (CT), magnetic resonance imaging (MRI), fluoroscopy, ultrasound, or RGB). For image-guided interventions, real-time, intra-operative tracking (defining the pose) of the surgical tools is crucial. It requires tracking techniques, such as optical (with passive or active markers), electromagnetic, or other modalities [22]. For image guidance, the coordinate systems employed by the controller (patient, navigation system, tool, etc.) have to be registered to the physical surroundings. Since the pose of the patients and tools can be calculated, thus with proper robotic devices and surgical plan, image-guided procedures can be automated on a task or subtask level, and the human operator can supervise the intervention in the meantime. TSolution-One is a good example for the image-guided surgical device that is commercially available since 2008 for total knee and hip replacement. It relies on a pre-operative CT scan and adequate surgical plan to implement bone drilling with a very high accuracy [5, 23] (Fig. 3). Furthermore, LoA 4 CyberKnife is an image-guided surgical robotic system as well (Sect. 2).

3.3 *Cooperatively Controlled Surgical Robots*

Cooperative robotic systems implement a specific teleoperation control paradigm (so-called shared control or hands-on surgery), where the surgeon and patientside devices are identical [2]. The surgeon always has physical contact with the surgical system, but the robotic device can support the surgeon with special features and effectors. In the case of cooperative control, the human operator remains in the control loop. This can help with compensation of hand tremor, which can increase the precision and decrease the workload on the surgeon [24]. Furthermore, additional functions can be implemented in cooperative control mode, such as virtual fixtures (spatial boundaries), which can help avoid restricted areas based on defined pre-operative and intra-operative safety zones. Cooperative systems can support micro-surgical cases and the orthopedic surgery. A commercially available cooperative robotic system is the MAKO Rio (Stryker Inc., Kalamazoo, MI), which combines image guidance and cooperative approaches for total and partial knee replacements (Fig. 3). In the case of cooperatively controlled surgical robots, data-based features, such as autonomously restricted areas (virtual fixtures) and autonomous subtask co-execution, can mean added safety with heavily relying on AI in the future.

4 Increasing Accuracy, Decreasing Invasiveness: Capsule Robots, Microrobots, Continuum Robots

The discussed commercially available robotic approaches (teleoperation, image-guided robots, and cooperative systems) typically require large spaces in the operating room and use rigid tools with functional articulated devices [21–23]. Minimally invasive procedures are available for many surgical interventions; however, there are organ targets that cannot be easily reached by these rigid, large-scale robotic devices. For MIS, minimizing the size or the rigidity of the tools/systems/devices is necessary. To achieve this, capsule robotics, microrobotics, and continuum robotics have been developed. On the other hand, surgical robots are now parts of the clinical practice, advanced devices are on the market, and just a few from the mentioned devices are commercially available.

4.1 Capsule Robots

Capsule robotics, which originally aims at inspecting the gastrointestinal tract in a minimally invasive manner without wires, holds a great prospect in diagnostics and treatment methods. It is a well-known technique to collect endoscopic images with a small, swallow-able device by a wide-angle camera, but usually these devices are passive (their movement is based on the peristaltic of the gastrointestinal tract) and do not implement adaptive or cognitive functions; however, there is a need to see more anatomy and be less invasive [25]. The actuation of these devices can be difficult due to the size of a capsule robot (typically 24 mm x 11 mm). In the literature, two main approaches for capsule robots can be found: onboard and magnetic actuation. Onboard actuation employs very small locomotion mechanisms (legs, wheels, crawling systems), and it can be very challenging to develop these in miniature sizes, mainly because of their power supplies. In the case of magnetic actuation, the swallow-able devices can be actuated by an externally generated magnetic field (permanent magnets or electromagnets). This approach can decrease the size and complexity of the device; however, it requires complex control approaches due to the nonlinear properties of the magnetic field, which can be a target in AI applications. In this case, it is critical to know the pose of the device to plan the magnetic force and torque. Commercially available example for active capsule robots is the NaviCam (AnX Robotica, Plano, TX), which received FDA approval in 2020. NaviCam is a magnetically actuated capsule endoscopy system for visualizing the desired anatomy of the gastrointestinal tract. According to Dupont et al., the future of capsule robotics may involve intelligent magnetic control, multimodal imaging, and wireless power transfer [25]. AI solutions can be parts of capsule robots' cognitive functions, intelligent motion, and adaptivity for diagnostics and treatment in a miniature scale soon [26].

4.2 Microrobots and Nanorobots

Microrobotics employs microscopic-scale automated solutions for diagnostics and treatment. Capsule robotics requires very small size solutions, but even those can be too large for the minimally invasive treatment of the circulatory system, the urinary tract, the eye, or the neural system [27–29]. Micro-scale technology solutions are still challenging due to the specific physical effects, such as fluid viscosity and surface effects. The movement of these miniature devices can be achieved by piezoelectric motors or external magnets with a swimming-like motion in fluids, but battery technology is not applicable in this scale [30]. Targeted therapy, material removal (ablation and biopsy), controllable structures, and telemetry can be the future of microrobots according to Nelson et al. [27]. Adaptivity, cognitive functions, and decision-making in the case of microrobots can be implemented in the future, especially in case the microrobot takes active part in the surgery [31]. Nanorobots are planned to target individual cells, and *many proposed nanorobots are more like pharmaceuticals than machines, utilizing concepts from synthetic biology and requiring large numbers of them to complete a task*; however, they are still in theoretical phase [27].

4.3 Continuum Robots

Redundant robots have more degrees of freedom (DoF) than necessary to execute a kinematic task. Continuum robots achieve extreme redundancy with infinite number of DoF, which means their kinematic structure can change its shape along its length, so it can adapt to different, complex environments where conventional robotic systems cannot, which could be a great benefit in medical approaches [32]. Continuum robots can be employed in the following interventions:

- **Neurosurgery**: intracerebral drug delivery, intracerebral hemorrhage evacuation.
- **Otolaryngology**: functional endoscopic, sinus surgery, transnasal skull base surgery, throat surgery.
- **Cardiac surgery**: percutaneous intracardiac surgery, robotic catheters for electrophysiology, robotic catheters for cardiac surgery.
- **Vascular surgery**: treatment of angioplasties, aneurysms, embolization.
- **Abdominal interventions**: percutaneous interventions.
- **Urology**: transurethral surgery, handheld robot for transurethral prostate surgery.

Examples for continuum robotic systems include the ones for bronchoscopy as Monarch (Auris Health Inc., Redwood City, CA, USA) and Ion (Intuitive Surgical Inc.) platforms [33]. According to the literature, there are six main technical challenges of continuum robots: instrumentation, visualization, OR integration, human-machine interaction, shape, and force sensing [25].

5 Legal and Regulatory Considerations of Surgical Robots

The diversity of surgical robots makes the standardization of the domain extremely difficult [5]. Industrial robots are defined by ISO 8373:2015 as *programmed actuated mechanism with a degree of autonomy, moving within its environment, to perform intended tasks*, and a service robot was defined as *a robot that performs useful tasks for humans or equipment excluding industrial automation applications*. Since the da Vinci surgical system employs only teleoperation control, it does not belong to the above defined systems. This nomenclature issue has been addressed with a more recent definition of robots: *A robot is a complex mechatronic system enabled with electronics, sensors, actuators, and software, executing tasks with a certain degree of autonomy. It may be pre-programmed, teleoperated or carrying out computations to make decisions* [34]. Nevertheless, authorities consider and regulate all medical devices according to the medical device standards. The IEC 60601-1 Medical electrical equipment standard and the 93/42/EEC Medical Devices Directive are applicable to all surgical robotic systems with a "medical intended use." In recent decades in the European medical legislation, the Regulation (EU) 2017/745, Medical Device Regulation (MDR), which came into force in May 2021, forms the change. The new regulation increased the safety-related expectations and the requisite documentation for certifying medical devices, disproportionately affecting medical robots [4]. ISO/IEC defined the following domains for medical robots: rehabilitation robots, neuro-rehabilitation robots, assistive/daycare robots, nursing/rounding robots, invasive/surgical robots (endoscopy, biopsy), and diagnostic robots. However, the boundaries of these domains are still not definite. In 2018, a new standardization working group was launched, IEEE P2730 Standard for Classification, Terminologies, and Definitions of Medical Robots, with the scope to "specify the categories, naming, and definition of medical robots". The more recent IEEE 7007 Ontological Standard for Ethically Driven Robotics and Automation Systems is dealing with ethical considerations for robotic systems, which can support AI-based products as well. The development of robotic technologies can have an important role in efforts to achieve the United Nations' (UN) Sustainable Development Goals (SDGs) as well [35, 36].

6 AI × Surgical Robotics

6.1 Rationale

In medical technologies, clinical outcome is the most important consideration [29, 37]. Special attention is needed when the technological approach is not practical and hard to use and results in great stress or workload of the patient and/or to the doctor. The general goal of robotic surgery and especially of the new, intelligent approaches in the medical research is to make surgery safer and to achieve better clinical outcome with accuracy, repeatability, intelligent decisions, etc. Surgery – in case it is performed by a human operator – gives great fatigue to the surgeon; it can be stressful, and the human-related limitations (stability, dexterity, etc.) may cause problems during the interventions [38]. The main promise is that AI-based technologies will exceed these human-related limitations, making appropriate decisions with stability, dexterity, accuracy, and repeatability, without dealing with stress, situation awareness, or fatigue. For this, a huge amount of data is necessary, which can be provided along the principles of Surgical Data Science (SDS).

6.2 AI × Surgical Robotics State of the Art

AI-based technological approaches form the biggest trend now; however, in commercial surgical robots, these features have not appeared widely yet. A good example is the market dominating RAMIS systems that leave the surgeon in the control loop or the IGS systems that rely on a surgical plan created by a human operator. On the other hand, in research phase, there are projects and publications reported daily dealing with AI-based surgical support. In this section, we introduce the most important research domains in AI-based robotic surgical solutions, involving surgical automation, skill training and assessment, gesture/workflow segmentation, and surgical tool segmentation. Since RAMIS dominates in the surgical robotics market, and other robotic AI approaches mainly focus on image processing [39–44], in this section, RAMIS AI-based solutions are presented. In Table 1, the publications on RAMIS AI-based solutions are summarized based on novelty and/or citation metrics, categorized by the utilized AI approach (supervised learning, unsupervised learning, learning by demonstration, and reinforcement learning).

6.3 RAMIS Databases and Data Collection Approaches

The well-known key to AI is data – without the proper amount of data, AI in surgery will not be applicable. Furthermore, data is needed for validation as well. Image databases, RAMIS kinematic databases, and skill and gesture datasets are widely used in the research domain to train and test AI algorithms. For RAMIS data collection and research in general, the da Vinci Research Kit (DVRK) was introduced by the Johns Hopkins University and partners with the support of the Intuitive Surgical Inc. DVRK involves open-source hardware and software elements and provides complete read and write access to the da Vinci device's arms, video stream, etc. The DVRK community is a relatively small but growing group, including 40 research

Table 1 AI examples in RAMIS research, based on novelty and/or citation metrics

	Target task	Ref.
Unsupervised learning	Tool segmentation Skill assessment Gesture segmentation	[45–48]
Supervised learning	Tool segmentation Skill assessment Gesture segmentation Automation	[49–57]
Semi-supervised learning	Force estimation	[58]
Learning by demonstration	Automation	[59–61]
Reinforcement learning	Automation Skill training Gesture recognition	[60, 62–65]

groups [66]. The annual MICCAI conference of the Medical Image Computing and Computer Assisted Intervention (MICCAI) Society presents every year a robotic surgical tool segmentation challenge (Endoscopic Vision Challenge Robotic Instruments, “EndoVis,” https://endovis.grand-challenge.org/), providing a dataset with labeled surgical tools ground truth. The MICCAI EndoVis dataset consists of ten sequences of abdominal porcine procedures recorded by da Vinci Xi systems. The stereo image data with the ground truth labels include seven different robotic surgical instruments: the Large Needle Driver, the Prograsp Forceps, the Monopolar Curved Scissors, the Cadiere Forceps, the Bipolar Forceps, the Vessel Sealer, and additionally a drop-in ultrasound probe [67]. Synthetic MICCAI dataset (created by the University College London, https://www.ucl.ac.uk/interventional-surgical-sciences/) was recorded with the DVRK. In Synthetic MICCAI, da Vinci’s EndoWrist Large Needle Drivers were used to perform a surgical movement. Synthetic MICCAI contains the same surgical movements with ex vivo and green screen background as well. Tool segmentation ground truth was generated with the green screen elimination. Synthetic MICCAI contains 15 scenarios with different tool movements; each scenario contains 300 video frames [68]. JIGSAWS (JHU-ISI Gesture and Skill Assessment Working Set https://cirl.lcsr.jhu.edu/research/hmm/datasets/jigsaws_release/) was created through a collaboration between the Johns Hopkins University and Intuitive Surgical, Inc. It is a complex RAMIS skill assessment dataset, widely used for testing endoscopic image-based and kinematic data-based surgical skill assessment methods [69]. JIGSAWS was captured using the dVSS, with eight surgeons, having different skill levels (expert, intermediate, and novice) while performing well-known surgical training tasks (knot-tying, needle passing, and suturing). JIGSAWS contains not only the kinematic and stereo video data but the skill level of the surgeons and the gesture annotations as well. While JIGSAWS’s video data is available, it is not annotated with the instrument segmentation ground truth. These databases with reduced complexity and ground truth labels fit AI solutions and needs.

6.4 Subtask Automation in RAMIS

Since RAMIS operates with soft tissues, automation in this domain can be extremely difficult due to the constantly changing surroundings. This time, on the market there is no autonomy over LoA 1 in RAMIS, but subtask automation is widely researched [5]. For RAMIS automation, workflow and movement hierarchical decomposition were introduced [17]. In order to understand the key motions and ontologies in RAMIS in a machine-readable format, the main levels of surgical workflow were defined as the following:

1. **Operation**: the complete invasive part of the intervention (such as laparoscopic cholecystectomy).
2. **Task**: well-defined surgical activity with a high-level goal (exposing the Calot’s triangle.

3. **Subtask**: activity segments to achieve landmarks of tasks (e.g., blunt dissection).
4. **Surgeme**: atomic unit of a surgical activity (e.g., approach the tissue, perform dissecting motion).
5. **Motion primitive**: machine-readable motion patterns (e.g., open the dissector).

RAMIS automation research is mainly focusing on surgical subtask automation, which belongs to partial/conditional automation, where the automation of surgemes and motion primitives are necessary. However, the workflow of RAMIS contains subtask elements, where choosing the proper subtask can be extremely difficult since it can be critical in the patient outcome. These subtasks can be monotonous and time-consuming; thus, their automation could decrease the workload of the surgeon as well.

A typical example for this is the first RAMIS subtask automation research, automating multilateral debridement and shape cutting by the UC Berkeley AUTOLAB and the Center for Automation and Learning for Medical Robotics (CALMR) [70]. In this subtask automation research, a learning by observation approach was employed: human motion patterns were recorded and segmented, and then those patterns were used to generate robot trajectories during autonomous implementation. While a surgical phantom was used with traditional image processing algorithms, the project was mainly focused on robot motion generation. In another work of the research group, autonomous multilateral tumor resection based on palpation was also done in a phantom environment [71]. For this subtask's automation, a state machine was compiled. In another work of the group, the needle size, trajectory, and control parameter usage were optimized using sequential convex programming for automating suturing. Blunt dissection was automated by the IROB Center, Obuda University, based on stereo image processing and motion primitives on specific silicone phantom [72]. This research was validated on ex vivo environments as well. Soft tissue retraction [73] and peg transfer automation were also done by our research group [18].

The first 10 years of surgical subtask automation research focused mainly on traditional, deterministic approaches (except learning by observation-based studies) and lower-level automation. However, recent works showed promising results in AI usage for RAMIS subtask automation, even in higher-level task automation. A peg transfer solution was introduced [57], where Deep Recurrent Neural Network was used for automation. This solution resulted in very high (94.1%) success rate. In 2022, Johns Hopkins University published their work on first autonomous anastomosis in gastrointestinal surgery by Smart Tissue Autonomous Robot (STAR) on porcine. Nevertheless, the robotic anastomosis outperformed the human operators in terms of suture quality. However, this solution proposed high-level automation on soft tissues; it was not based on AI [74].

6.5 RAMIS Instrument Semantic Segmentation

Surgical tool segmentation is one of the most well-studied research domains in RAMIS, and while it does not directly relate to robotic task execution, it is a critical component for intelligent robotic approaches. Robotic surgical tool semantic segmentation and the knowledge of the position of the instruments are essential steps in RAMIS automation, navigation, autonomous decision-making support, workflow analysis, and autonomous skill assessment. Neural networks and deep learning methods are hot topics in AI-based image processing since the image features are not determined by a human but selected autonomously by the network [75]. It is well known that deep neural network (DNN)-based solutions' large amount of (sometimes labeled) image data is crucial for training. Furthermore, tool segmentation must deal with very different surgical tools, changing in light, environment, blood, smoke, reflections, etc. while avoiding overfitting.

Most of the RAMIS tool segmentation methods have been validated on the MICCAI dataset. Mohammed et al. proposed a hybrid deep CNN-RNN auto encoder-decoder method for tool segmentation and resulted 93.3% accuracy on this dataset [49]. ToolNet is a DNN-based semantic segmentation approach, which was the first convolutional network architecture trained end to end for real-time semantic segmentation of robotic surgical tools [50]. RASNet tracked surgical instruments using Refined Attention Segmentation Network and achieved the state of the art with 94.65% mean Dice score [51]. Beyond DNN, other machine learning approaches provided promising results in robotic surgical tool segmentation, such as boosted decision trees, random forests, image data combined with kinematic data, and optical flow-based solutions [76].

While hundreds of scientific papers provide very promising solutions for RAMIS tool segmentation, DL-based approaches work typically well on known environment. Since the surgical environments can be very diverse, their adaptivity to different environments means a significant problem (just as for self-driving cars [15]). Since almost every tool segmentation is validated on the same dataset, these results can easily be compared, and the accuracy can be proven (against automation, which cannot be benchmarked easily [19]), but they have the same limitations as every other supervised learning approaches.

6.6 RAMIS Skill Assessment and Workflow Segmentation

To work with RAMIS (and MIS in general) is a hard task, which requires extensive training from surgeons. RAMIS skills involve not just technical skills (knowing the instruments, use the proper forces, depth perception, etc.) but non-technical skills (decision-making, situation awareness, dealing with stress, etc.) as well. Nowadays, in the clinical practice, surgical skill assessment is mainly based on expert-rating techniques, where a group of expert surgeons analyzes the procedure and gives assessment scores based on specific criteria. Automating the assessment of surgical skills can help the understanding of the key human factors and can be important in quality assurance and personalized training. The wide employment of RAMIS systems supports the research of automated skill assessment since kinematic (and video) data are available; the motion of the surgeon can be analyzed easier [38].

Following AI-based endoscopic image segmentation, RAMIS video and kinematic data analysis with learning algorithms are the most studied area. These studies mainly focus on surgical skill classification (expert/novice or expert/intermediate/novice) based on the JIGSAWS dataset, with kinematic and/or video data [77, 78]. Kinematic data-based skill classification in RAMIS reached 100% accuracy in some cases; however, this high accuracy can be a challenge for 2D/3D endoscopic image-based approaches [54]. Most popular kinematic data-based solutions employ convolutional neural network (CNN) [79], principal component analysis (PCA) [53], k-nearest neighbors (k-NN) [53], logistic regression (LR) [46], and fully convolutional network (FCN) [80], while video-based solutions based on 3D CNN have also been presented [52, 76]. A work by Lajkó et al. [54] compared the accuracy of 2D optical flow-based skill classification with residual neural network (ResNet), CNN, LSTM, convolutional autoencoder, and frequency domain transformations with support vector machine (SVM), where the highest performing method was ResNet with 81.89%, 84.23%, and 83.54% accuracy for suturing, needle passing, and knot-tying, respectively.

As it was presented in Sect. 2, surgical tasks are built of surgical gestures (surgemes). Autonomous surgical gesture segmentation and analysis can lead to deeper skill understanding, surgeme-level skill scoring, and real personalized skill training. For gesture and maneuver recognition, supervised and unsupervised techniques were also used: Autoencoder [56], RNN [55], LSTM [55], clustering [47], PCA [47], temporal clustering [48], Gaussian mixture models (GMM) [48], k-NN, and SVM [81] have been reported.

6.7 Future Trends in AI × Robotic Surgery

Artificial intelligence's rebirth revolutionized modern science and technology [82]. Learning and reasoning from data can be a very promising alternative to classical, deterministic algorithms. The goal of AI-based surgical robotics is to improve patient outcome: to evaluate all relevant sensory inputs and to access a database detailing how to achieve the surgical goal safely [1]. DNN, which is a dominating technique, can define the key features of the data autonomously. Nevertheless, AI needs data in quality and quantity and, in some cases, labeled data. Robotic surgical data, such as images and kinematic and tactile data, serve as input for such techniques, but since the medical market domain is very conservative, AI has not been introduced widely yet, mostly only in research projects and product concepts [83–88].

First, the technological added value will be validated; patient outcome and practicality are crucial in medical device developments. As a possible future trend, AI might be used instead of deterministic methods for advanced surgical planning, execution, evaluation and proper decision-making, and error handling. One main added value for robotic surgery can be the autonomy [5, 25, 89]. As it was presented, there are commercialized systems, which can reach medium and high autonomy, but full autonomy is still an open challenge largely because of the complexity of managing adverse medical events. Additional benefits can be precision, repeatability, and speed. Autonomous surgical skill assessment and gesture segmentation during procedures can lead to personalized training and assessment [87]. In the non-technical skill domain, AI-based approaches can support decision-making and situation awareness and can decrease the workload on the surgeon. In the future, autonomous subtasks and camera handling, pre-operative planning, motion compensation for image-guided techniques, and intelligent decision-making possibly via autonomous phase recognition can be parts of the clinical practice. On the other hand, technological challenges are still unsolved: since data-driven techniques rely on data, these data should be proper and as general as possible for adaptivity. However, ethical, legal, and cost considerations can be significant challenges, even if the technical solutions are capable for surgical automation/support [90].

Safety is critical in this research domain, but none of the currently accepted methods focus directly on the autonomous capabilities of the robot, as a primary source of hazard. AI for medical systems requires well-defined criteria for validation. According to the data-driven research framework for TAI (DaRe4TAI) [91], a trustworthy AI will have the following properties:

- Beneficence.
- Non-maleficence.
- Autonomy.
- Justice.
- Explicability.

AI ethics should also be considered in autonomous surgical robotic functions, such as the FAST Track Principles (Fairness, Accountability, Sustainability, and Transparency) [92]. From the regulatory point of view, MDR already requires the manufacturers to store and disclose their datasets employed with their AI-based solutions.

The recently introduced *Surgery 4.0* concept means *the seamless integration of medical decision support systems, imaging, and automated execution* [18]. Focusing on this topic, Verb Surgical (Mountain View, CA), the 2015 joint venture of Verily/Alphabet Inc. (Mountain View, CA) and Johnson & Johnson (New Brunswick, NJ), firstly claimed to develop a Surgery 4.0 compatible robotic system, which employs advanced vision and robotic tools with machine learning. However, the system has never been introduced publicly. Recently, Vicarious Surgical (Waltham, MA) also introduced AI algorithms and Extended Reality capabilities into the surgical workflow [93], and other competitors are on the horizon [20]. It is also worth mentioning

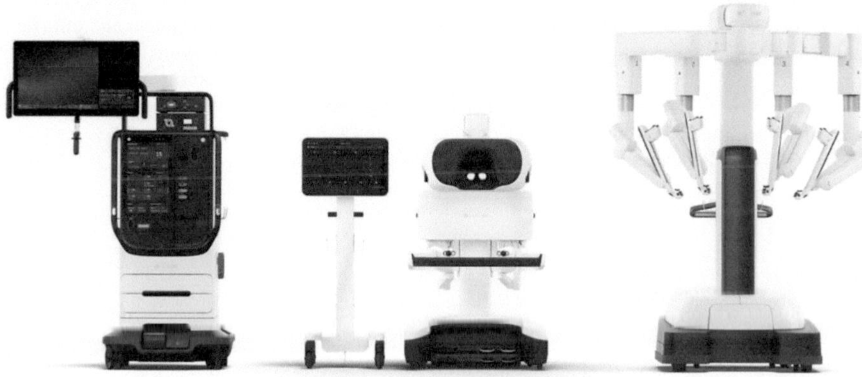

Fig. 4 The 2024 version, generation 5 of the da Vinci surgical system. It features improved accuracy and precision, advanced force sensing, expanded computing power and advanced data capabilities, complete workflow support, and greater surgeon comfort. (Image: courtesy of Intuitive)

that the latest generation of the dVSS, the da Vinci 5 features 10,000 times more computational capacity on board than the da Vinci Xi, primarily to run its enhanced simulator and to accommodate AI-based decision-support systems (Fig. 4).

Nevertheless, recent surveys found that even in less technology-dependent societies, the prevalence of robot surgery is advancing, and there is a growing trust in AI-driven healthcare [94, 95].

7 Conclusion

AI has become an integral part of many research projects and commercialized products. However, in the medical domain, it has not been applied at significant measure yet, mainly because of the ethical and legal issues, but the narrowing technological gaps have remained limiting factors as well. In surgical robotics, most successful products leave the human in the control loop or provide functions at lower levels of autonomy. Nevertheless, high level of autonomy has already been introduced in radiosurgery, yet full autonomy is still out of reach. AI methods have proven to be powerful tools in robotic surgical research (such as in subtask automation, surgical skill assessment, gesture segmentation, phase recognition, and mainly image processing), but these techniques have not been generally introduced to the market yet. In the future, AI-based pre-operative planning, autonomous execution, patient motion compensation, decision-making support, and autonomous evaluation will become parts of the clinical practice, which can significantly improve the patient outcome and decrease the workload of the surgeon, but apart from technical advancement, this also requires great standardization effort from the community.

Acknowledgments This research was performed as part of project no. 2019-1.3.1-KK-2019-00007 that has been implemented with the support of the National Research, Development and Innovation Fund of Hungary, financed under the 2019-1.3.1-KK funding scheme. This work has been partially supported by ACMIT (Austrian Center for Medical Innovation and Technology), which is funded within the scope of the COMET (Competence Centers for Excellent Technologies) program of the Austrian Government. T. Haidegger is a Consolidator Researcher, receiving financial support from the Distinguished Researcher program of Óbuda University [96].

References

1. Al-Salihi MM, Al-Jebur MS, Goto T. Artificial Intelligence and the internet of things in the neurosurgical operating theater. In: Al-Salihi MM, Tubbs RS, Ayyad A, Goto T, Maarouf M, editors. Introduction to robotics in minimally invasive neurosurgery. Cham: Springer; 2022. p. 77–99.
2. Takacs A, Nagy DA, Rudas I, Haidegger T. Origins of surgical robotics: from space to the operating room. Acta Polytech Hungar. 2016;13(1):13–30.
3. Taylor RH, Menciassi A, Fichtinger G, Fiorini P, Dario P. Medical robotics and computer-integrated surgery. In: Siciliano B, Khatib O, editors. Springer hand book of robotics. Cham: Springer; 2016. p. 1657–84.
4. Fichtinger G, Troccaz J, Haidegger T. Image-guided interventional robotics: lost in translation? Proc IEEE. 2022;110(7):932–50.
5. Haidegger T. Autonomy for surgical robots: concepts and paradigms. IEEE Trans Med Robot Bionic. 2019;l(2):65–76.
6. Tsui EYA. Application of Artificial Intelligence (AI) in Surgery; 2020. [Online]. https://www.imperial.ac.uk/news/200673/application-artificial-intelligence-ai-surgery/. Accessed 5 June 2022.
7. Takács K, Haidegger T. Eye gaze tracking in robot-assisted minimally invasive surgery: a systematic review of recent advances and applications. Acta Polytech Hungar. 2024;21(10)
8. Móga K, Hölgyesi Á, Zrubka Z, Péntek M, Haidegger T. Augmented or mixed reality enhanced head-mounted display navigation for in vivo spine surgery: a systematic review of clinical outcomes. J Clin Med. 2023;12(11):3788.
9. Artificial Intelligence (AI) definition; 2020. [Online]. https://www.britannica.com/technology/artificial-intelligence. Accessed 5 June 2022.
10. Habuza T, Navaz AN, Hashim F, Alnajjar F, Zaki N, Serhani MA, et al. AI applications in robotics, diagnostic image analysis and precision medicine: current limitations, future trends, guidelines on CAD Systems for Medicine. Inform Med Unlocked. 2021;24.
11. Ashraf H, Rafiq F. Harnessing power of Artificial Intelligence in surgery. Arch Surg Res. 2021;2(4).
12. Bellini V, Valente M, Rio PD, Bignami E. Artificial Intelligence in thoracic surgery: a narrative review. J Thorac Dis. 2021;13(12):6963–75.
13. Dagli MM, Rajesh A, Asaad M, Butler CE. The use of Artificial Intelligence and machine learning in surgery: a comprehensive literature review. Am Surg. 2021.
14. Goldenberg SL, Nir G, Salcudean SE. A new era: artificial Intelligence and machine learning in prostate cancer. Nat Rev Urol. 2019 Jul;16(7):391–403.
15. Drexler DA, Takacs A, Nagy TD, Haidegger T. Handover process of autonomous vehicles-technology and application challenges. Acta Polytech Hungar. 2019;16(9):235–55.
16. Attanasio A, Scaglioni B, De Momi E, Fiorini P, Valdastri P. Autonomy in surgical robotics. Annu Rev Contr Robot Autonom Syst. 2021;4(1):651–79.
17. Nagy TD, Haidegger T. Autonomous surgical robotics at task and subtask levels. In: Advanced robotics and intelligent automation in manufacturing; 2020. p. 296–319.

18. Nagy TD, Haidegger T. A DVRK-based framework for surgical subtask automation. Acta Polytechn Hungar. 2019:61–78.
19. Nagy TD, Haidegger T. Performance and capability assessment in surgical subtask automation. Sensors. 2022;22(7):2501.
20. Haidegger T, Speidel S, Stoyanov D, Satava R. Robot-assisted minimally invasive surgery-surgical robotics in the data age. Proc IEEE. 2022;110(7):835–46.
21. Péntek M, Haidegger T, Czere JT, Kovács L, Zrubka Z, Gulácsi L. EQ-5D studies in robotic surgery: a mini-review. In: 2023 IEEE 17th international symposium on applied computational Intelligence and informatics (SACI); 2023. p. 519–24.
22. Franz AM, Haidegger T, Birkfellner W, Cleary K, Peters TM, Maier-Hein L. Electromagnetic tracking in medicine-a review of technology, validation, and applications. IEEE Trans Med Imaging. 2014;33(8):1702–25.
23. Maier-Hein L, Eisenmann M, Sarikaya D, Marz K, Collins T, Malpani A, et al. Surgical data science—from concepts toward clinical translation. Med Image Anal. 2022 Feb;76.
24. Schleer P, Drobinsky S, de la Fuente M, Radermacher K. Toward versatile cooperative surgical robotics: a review and future challenges. Int J Comput Assist Radiol Surg. 2019;14(10):1673–86.
25. Dupont PE, Nelson BJ, Goldfarb M, Hannaford B, Menciassi A, O'Malley MK, et al. A decade retrospective of medical robotics research from 2010 to 2020. Sci Robot. 2021;6(60):eabi8017.
26. Mapara S, Patravale V. Medical capsule robots: a renaissance for diagnostics, drug delivery and surgical treatment. J Control Release. 2017 Jul;261.
27. Nelson B, Kaliakatsos I, Abbott J. Microrobots for minimally invasive medicine. Annu Rev Biomed Eng. 2010;12:55–85.
28. Ceylan H, Yasa IC, Kilic U, Hu W, Sitti M. Translational prospects of untethered medical microrobots. Progr Biomed Eng. 2019;1(1):012002.
29. Simaan N, Yasin RM, Wang L. Medical technologies and challenges of robot assisted minimally invasive intervention and diagnostics, vol. ID 3330456. Rochester, NY: Social Science Research Network; 2018.
30. Ullrich F, Bergeles C, Pokki J, Ergeneman O, Erni S, Chatzipirpiridis G, et al. Mobility experiments with microrobots for minimally invasive intraocular surgery. Invest Ophthalmol Vis Sci. 2013;54(4):2853–63.
31. Aziz A, Pane S, Iacovacci V, Koukourakis N, Czarske J, Menciassi A, et al. Medical imaging of microrobots: toward in vivo applications. ACS Nano. 2020;14(9):10865–93.
32. Burgner-Kahrs J, Rucker DC, Choset H. Continuum robots for medical applications: a survey. IEEE Trans Robot. 2015 Dec;31(6):1261–80.
33. da Veiga T, Chandler JH, Lloyd P, Pittiglio G, Wilkinson NJ, Hoshiar AK, et al. Challenges of continuum robots in clinical context: a review. Progr Biomed Eng. 2020;2(3).
34. Haidegger T. Taxonomy and standards in robotics. In: Ang MH, Khatib O, Siciliano B, editors. Encyclopedia of robotics; 2022. https://doi.org/10.1007/978-3-642-41610-1_190-1.
35. Mai V, Vanderborght B, Haidegger T, Khamis A, Bhargava N, Boes DB, et al. The role of robotics in achieving the United Nations sustainable development goals-the experts' meeting at the 2021 IEEE/RSJ IROS workshop [industry activities]. IEEE Robot Automat Magaz. 2022;29(1):92–107.
36. Haidegger T, Mai V, Mörch CM, Boesl DO, Jacobs A, Khamis A, Lach L, Vanderborght B. Robotics: enabler and inhibitor of the sustainable development goals. Sustain Product Consump. 2023;1(43):422–34.
37. Kader R, Baggaley RF, Hussein M, Ahmad OF, Patel N, Corbett G, et al. Sur vey on the perceptions of UK gastroenterologists and endoscopists to Artificial Intelligence. Frontline Gastroenterol. 2022.
38. Nagyne Elek R, Haidegger T. Non-technical skill assessment and mental load evaluation in robot-assisted minimally invasive surgery. Sensors. 2021 Jan;21(8):2666.
39. Litjens G, Kooi T, Bejnordi BE, Setio AAA, Ciompi F, Ghafoorian M, et al. A survey on deep learning in medical image analysis. Med Image Anal. 2017;42:60–88.

40. Lu ZX, Qian P, Bi D, Ye ZW, He X, Zhao YH, et al. Application of AI and IoT in clinical medicine: summary and challenges. Curr Med Sci. 2021;41(6):1134–50.
41. Pati S, Baid U, Zenk M, Edwards B, Sheller M, Reina GA, et al. The Federated Tumor Segmentation (FeTS) challenge. arXiv. 2021;210505874 preprint.
42. Ribli D, Horvath A, Unger Z, Pollner P, Csabai I. Detecting and classifying lesions in mammograms with deep learning. Sci Rep. 2018 Mar;8(1):4165.
43. Shah RM, Wong C, Arpey NC, Patel AA, Divi SN. A surgeon's guide to understanding artificial intelligence and machine learning studies in Orthopaedic surgery. Curr Rev Musculoskelet Med. 2022;l5:121–32.
44. Topol EJ. High-performance medicine: the convergence of human and Artificial Intelligence. Nat Med. 2019;25(1):44–56.
45. Pakhomov D, Shen W, Navab N. Towards unsupervised learning for instrument segmentation in robotic surgery with cycle-consistent adversarial net works. In: 2020 IEEE/RSJ International Conference on Intelligent Robots and Systems (IROS); 2020. p. 8499–504.
46. Fard MJ, Ameri S, Darin Ellis R, Chinnam RB, Pandya AK, Klein MD. Automated robot-assisted surgical skill evaluation: predictive analytics approach. Int J Med Robot Comput Assist Surg. 2018;14(1):el850. El850 RCS-16-0174.R4.
47. Fard MJ, Ameri S, Chinnam RB, Ellis RD. Soft boundary approach for unsupervised gesture segmentation in robotic-assisted surgery. IEEE Robot Automat Lett. 2017;2(1):171–8.
48. Zia A, Zhang C, Xiong X, Jarc AM. Temporal clustering of surgical activities in robot-assisted surgery. Int J Comput Assist Radiol Surg. 2017;l2(7):1171–8.
49. Mohammed A, Hossny M, Nahavandi S, Asadi H. Surgical tool segmentation using a hybrid deep CNN-RNN auto encoder-decoder. In: 2017 IEEE International Conference on Systems, Man, and Cybernetics (SMC); 2017.
50. Garcia-Peraza-Herrera LC, Li W, Fidon L, Gruijthuijsen C, Devreker A, Attilakos G, et al. ToolNet: holistically-nested real-time segmentation of robotic surgical tools. In: 2017 IEEE/RSJ international conference on intelligent robots and systems (IROS); 2017. p. 5717–22.
51. Ni ZL, Bian GB, Xie XL, Hou ZG, Zhou XH, Zhou YJ. RASNet: segmentation for tracking surgical instruments in surgical videos using refined attention segmentation network. In: 2019 41st annual international conference of the IEEE engineering in Medicine &Biology Society (EMBC); 2019. p. 5735–8.
52. Funke I, Mees ST, Weitz J, Speidel S. Video-based surgical skill assessment using 3D convolutional neural networks. Int J Comput Assist Radiol Surg. 2019;14(7):1217–25.
53. Zia A, Essa I. Automated surgical skill assessment in RMIS training. Int J Comput Assist Radiol Surg. 2018;13(5):731–9.
54. Lajkó G, Nagyne Elek R, Haidegger T. Endoscopic image-based skill assessment in robot-assisted minimally invasive surgery. Sensors. 2021 Jan;21(16):5412.
55. DiPietro R, Ahmidi N, Malpani A, Waldram M, Lee GI, Lee MR, et al. Segmenting and classifying activities in robot-assisted surgery with recurrent neural net works. Int J Comput Assist Radiol Surg. 2019;14(11):2005–20.
56. Khalid S, Goldenberg M, Grantcharov T, Taati B, Rudzicz F. Evaluation of deep learning models for identifying surgical actions and measuring performance. JAMA Netw Open. 2020 Mar;3(3):e201664.
57. Hwang M, Thananjeyan B, Seita D, Ichnowski J, Paradis S, Fer D, et al. Superhuman surgical peg transfer using depth-sensing and deep recurrent neural networks. arXiv. 2020;201212844 preprint.
58. Marban A, Srinivasan V, Samek W, Fernandez J, Casals A. Estimation of inter action forces in robotic surgery using a semi-supervised deep neural network model. In: 2018 IEEE/RSJ International Conference on Intelligent Robots and Systems (IROS); 2018. p. 761–8.
59. Osa T, Harada K, Sugita N, Mitsuishi M. Trajectory planning under different initial conditions for surgical task automation by learning from demonstration. In: 2014 IEEE International Conference on Robotics and Automation (ICRA); 2014. p. 6507–13.

60. Shin C, Ferguson PW, Pedram SA, Ma J, Dutson EP, Rosen J. Autonomous tissue manipulation via surgical robot using learning based model predictive control. In: 2019 International Conference on Robotics and Automation (ICRA); 2019. p. 3875–81.
61. Murali A, Sen S, Kehoe B, Garg A, McFarland S, Patil S, et al. Learning by observation for surgical subtasks: multilateral cutting of 3D viscoelastic and 2D orthotropic tissue phantoms. In: 2015 IEEE International Conference on Robotics and Automation (ICRA); 2015. p. 1202–9.
62. Nguyen ND, Nguyen T, Nahavandi S, Bhatti A, Guest G. Manipulating soft tissues by deep reinforcement learning for autonomous robotic surgery. In: 2019 IEEE International Systems Conference (SysCon); 2019. p. 1–7.
63. Su YH, Huang K, Hannaford B. Multicamera 3D viewpoint adjustment for robotic surgery via deep reinforcement learning. J Med Robot Res. 2021 Mar;06(01&02):214–30.
64. Tan X, Chng CB, Su Y, Lim KB, Chui CK. Robot-assisted training in laparoscopy using deep reinforcement learning. IEEE Robot Automat Lett. 2019;4(2):485–92.
65. Gao X, Jin Y, Dou Q, Heng PA. Automatic gesture recognition in robot-assisted surgery with reinforcement learning and tree search. In: 2020 IEEE International Conference on Robotics and Automation (ICRA); 2020. p. 8440–6.
66. D'Ettorre C, Mariani A, Stilli A, Baena FR, Valdastri P, Deguet A, et al. Accelerating surgical robotics research: a review of 10 years with the Da Vinci research kit. IEEE Robot Automat Magaz. 2021;28(4):56–78.
67. Laina I, Rieke N, Rupprecht C, Vizcaino JP, Eslami A, Tombari F, et al. Con current segmentation and localization for tracking of surgical instruments. In: Descoteaux M, Maier-Hein L, Franz A, Jannin P, Collins DL, Duchesne S, editors. Medical image computing and computer-assisted intervention—MICCAI 2017. Cham: Springer; 2017. p. 664–72.
68. Colleoni E, Edwards P, Stoyanov D. Synthetic and real inputs for tool segmentation in robotic surgery. In: Martel AL, Abolmaesumi P, Stoyanov D, Mateus D, Zuluaga MA, Zhou SK, et al., editors. Medical image computing and computer assisted intervention—MICCAI 2020. Cham: Springer; 2020. p. 700–10.
69. Gao Y, Vedula SS, Reiley CE, Ahmidi N, Varadarajan B, Lin HC, et al. JHU ISI gesture and skill assessment working set (JIGSAWS): a surgical activity dataset for human motion modeling. MICCAI workshop. 2014;3:10.
70. Kehoe B, Kahn G, Mahler J, Kim J, Lee A, Lee A, et al. Autonomous multilateral debridement with the raven surgical robot. In: 2014 IEEE International Conference on Robotics and Automation (ICRA); 2014. p. 1432–9.
71. McKinley S, Garg A, Sen S, Gealy DV, McKinley JP, Jen Y, et al. Autonomous multilateral surgical tumor resection with interchangeable instrument mounts and fluid injection device. In: 2016 IEEE International Conference on Robotics and Automation; 2015.
72. Elek R, Nagy TD, Nagy DA, Garamvolgyi T, Takacs B, Galambos P, et al. Towards surgical subtask automation—blunt dissection. In: 2017 IEEE 21st International Conference on Intelligent Engineering Systems (INES); 2017. p. 253–8.
73. Nagy TD, Takacs M, Rudas IJ, Haidegger T. Surgical subtask automation—soft tissue retraction. In: 2018 IEEE 16th world symposium on applied machine Intelligence and informatics (SAMI); 2018. p. 55–60.
74. Saeidi H, Opfermann J, Kam M, Wei S, Leonard S, Hsieh M, et al. Autonomous robotic laparoscopic surgery for intestinal anastomosis. Sci Robot. 2022;7(62).
75. Esteva A, Robicquet A, Ramsundar B, Kuleshov V, DePristo M, Chou K, et al. A guide to deep learning in healthcare. Nat Med. 2019;25(1):24–9.
76. Moglia A, Georgiou K, Georgiou E, Satava RM, Cuschieri A. A systematic re view on artificial Intelligence in robot-assisted surgery. Int J Surg. 2021;95:106151.
77. Lam K, Chen J, Wang Z, Iqbal FM, Darzi A, Lo B, et al. Machine learning for technical skill assessment in surgery: a systematic review. Digit Med. 2022;5(1).
78. Nagyne Elek R, Haidegger T. Robot-assisted minimally invasive surgical skill assessment-manual and automated platforms. Acta Polytech Hungar. 2019;16(8):141–69.

79. Wang Z, Majewicz FA. Deep learning with convolutional neural network for objective skill evaluation in robot-assisted surgery. Int J Comput Assist Radiol Surg. 2018;13(12):1959–70.
80. Ismail Fawaz H, Forestier G, Weber J, Idoumghar L, Muller PA. Accurate and interpretable evaluation of surgical skills from kinematic data using fully convolutional neural networks. Int J Comput Assist Radiol Surg. 2019;14(9):1611–7.
81. Despinoy F, Bouget D, Forestier G, Penet C, Zemiti N, Poignet P, et al. Unsupervised trajectory segmentation for surgical gesture recognition in robotic training. IEEE Trans Biomed Eng. 2016;63(6):1280–91.
82. Ahuja AS. The impact of artificial intelligence in medicine on the future role of the physician. PeerJ. 2019.
83. Giansanti D, Di Basilio F. The Artificial Intelligence in digital radiology: part 1: the challenges, acceptance and consensus. Healthcare. 2022;10(3).
84. Kurmis AP, Ianunzio JR. Artificial Intelligence in orthopedic surgery: evolution, current state and future directions. Arthroplasty. 2022;4(1).
85. Wong SY, Soh MY, Wong JM. Internet of medical things: brief overview and the future. In: 2021 IEEE 19th Student Conference on Research and Development (SCOReD); 2021. p. 427–32.
86. Orosz G, Szabó RZ, Ungi T, Barr C, Yeung C, Fichtinger G, Gál J, Haidegger T. Lung ultrasound imaging and image processing with artificial intelligence methods for bedside diagnostic examinations. Acta Polytech Hungar. 2023;20(8).
87. Lukács E, Levendovics R, Haidegger T. Enhancing skill assessment of autonomous robot-assisted minimally invasive surgery: a comprehensive analysis of global and gesture-level techniques applied on the JIGSAWS dataset. Acta Polytech Hungar. 2023;20(8):133–53.
88. Pentek M, Zrubka Z, Gulacsi L, Weszl M, Czere JT, Haidegger T. 10 pragmatic points to consider when performing a systematic literature review of clinical evidence on digital medical devices. Acta Polytech Hung. 2023;20:110–28.
89. Nagy TD, Haidegger T. Autonomous peg transfer—a gateway to surgery 4.0. In: 2022 IEEE 10th Jubilee International conference on computational cybernetics and cyber-medical systems (ICCC). IEEE; 2022. p. 69–76.
90. Mistry P. The new frontiers of AI in medicine. In: Lidstromer N, Ashrafian H, editors. Artificial Intelligence in medicine. Cham: Springer; 2022. p. 115–27.
91. Thiebes S, Lins S, Sunyaev A. Trustworthy Artificial Intelligence. Electron Mark. 2021;31(2):447–64.
92. Wodlin NB, Nilsson L. The development of fast-track principles in gynecological surgery. Acta Obstet Gynecol Scand. 2013;92(1):17–27.
93. Gorpas D, Phipps J, Bee J, Ma D, Dochow S, Yankelevich D, et al. Autofluorescence lifetime augmented reality as a means for real-time robotic surgery guidance in human patients. Sci Rep. 2019;9(1).
94. Hölgyesi Á, Zrubka Z, Gulácsi L, Baji P, Haidegger T, Kozlovszky M, Weszl M, Kovács L, Péntek M. Robot-assisted surgery and artificial intelligence-based tumour diagnostics: social preferences with a representative cross-sectional survey. BMC Med Inform Decis Mak. 2024;24(1):87.
95. Takács K, Lukács E, Levendovics R, Pekli D, Szijártó A, Haidegger T. Assessment of surgeons' stress levels with digital sensors during robot-assisted surgery: an experimental study. Sensors. 2024;24(9):2915.
96. Haidegger TP, Galambos P, Tar JK, Kovács LA, Kozlovszky M, Zrubka Z, Eigner G, et al. Strategies and outcomes of building a successful university research and innovation ecosystem. Acta Polytech Hungar. 2024;21(10).

Future Trend: Telemedicine Using 5G

Yuki Horise, Yuya Aoki, Yoshifumi Morihiro, and Yuji Aburakawa

Abstract The fifth-generation mobile communication system (5G) with its high speed/high capacity, ultra-low latency, and massive device connectivity characteristics has expanded worldwide. Through its innovative technologies, the 5G network contributes not only consumer services but also industrial services. A medical field is one of the important industrial areas where the 5G network is expected to be effective. Studies and activities focused on telemedicine using the 5G network have been reported from various parts of the world. In this chapter, after presenting overseas cases, we introduce our solutions including advanced telemedicine using experimental and commercial 5G networks collaborating with partners such as university hospitals and those in industry. To introduce the 5G network to telemedicine, accumulating technology toward advanced telemedicine and practical demonstrations in a commercial environment are key to success. 5G technologies will become more sophisticated, and the next generation of mobile communication systems could further enhance telemedicine in the future.

Keywords Telemedicine · 5G · Cloud · Multi-access edge computing · Smart cyber operating theater · Remote surgery support · Remote robotic surgery

Y. Horise (✉) · Y. Morihiro
Mobile Innovation Tech Department, NTT DOCOMO, INC.,
Yokosuka-shi, Kanagawa, Japan
e-mail: yuki.horise.hy@nttdocomo.com; morihiro@nttdocomo.com

Y. Aoki
Radio Access Network Design Department, NTT DOCOMO, INC.,
Tokyo, Japan
e-mail: yuya.aoki.rx@nttdocomo.com

Y. Aburakawa
Platform Technology Services Division, NEC Corporation,
Kanagawa, Japan
e-mail: yuji-aburakawa@nec.com

K. Masamune et al. (eds.), *Artificial Intelligence in Surgery*,
https://doi.org/10.1007/978-981-96-6635-5_15

1 Fifth-Generation Mobile Communication System

The fifth-generation mobile communication system (5G) is the latest wireless communication system following the third- and fourth-generation mobile communication systems (3G/4G). 5G has characteristics such as high speed/high capacity represented by enhanced mobile broadband, ultra-low latency represented by Ultra-Reliable and Low Latency Communications, and massive device connectivity represented by massive Machine Type Communications. The International Telecommunication Union-Radiocommunication sector discussed the vision of mobile communication systems and indicated future target requirements such as the maximum data transmission rate of 20 Gbps, multiple simultaneous connections of 1,000,000 devices/km^2, and low latency (1 ms) [1] as shown in Fig. 1.

In Japan, a commercial 5G network was launched in March 2020. 5G services for smart phones were launched in April 2019 in South Korea and in the United States [2]. As of March 2020, most countries excluding some areas such as Africa and the Middle East have invested in the 5G network, and 70 commercial 5G networks in 40 countries have been launched. About a year later, 144 commercial networks in 57 countries have been put into operation, and 5G services are available in the Americas, Europe, Asia, and Africa [3]. Although many people are still using the 4G network, it is anticipated that the use of 5G will increase in the future.

5G network technologies are expected to be applied to industry as well as consumer services. With the spread of mobile devices such as smartphones and tablets, the amount of communication data is increasing due to, for example, social network services and video streaming services. 5G technology enables the handling of a large

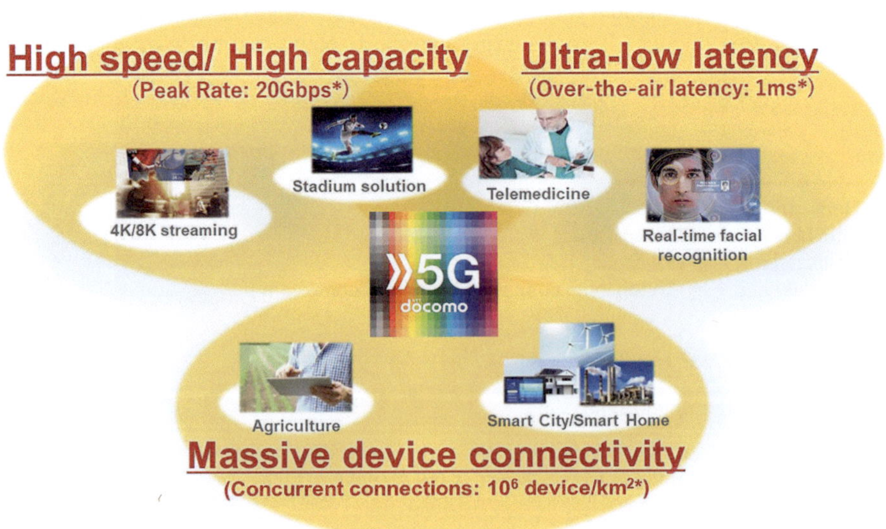

Fig. 1 5G features and future target requirements

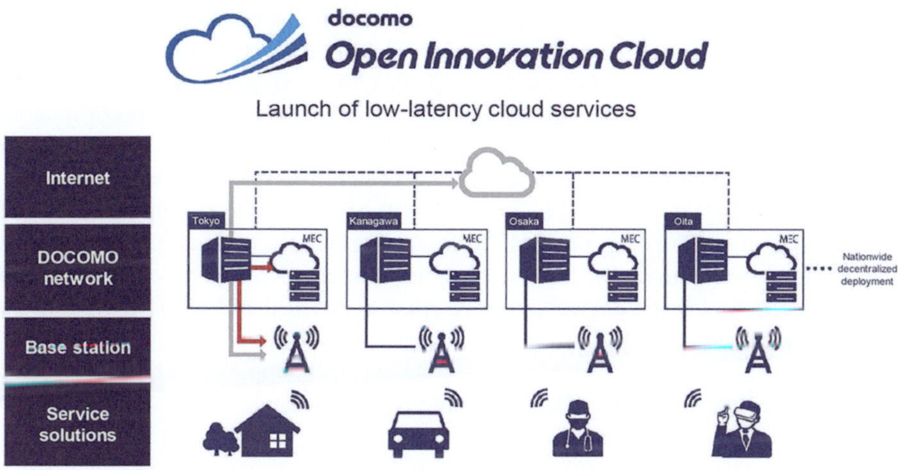

Fig. 2 NTT DOCOMO 5G cloud infrastructure

amount of data with low latency and provides a comfortable mobile communication environment for consumers. Moreover, since the 5G network offers guaranteed services compared to previous generation networks that offer best-effort services, the possibility of 5G utilization in industry has emerged. 5G technology yields new value of various types and addresses social issues. It enables industrial innovations such as the transmission of 4 K/8 K high-definition video and realistic images utilizing artificial reality/virtual reality, autonomous driving, and telemedicine.

Toward the introduction of 5G to industry, NTT DOCOMO commercialized the *docomo Open Innovation Cloud (currently docomo MEC)* shown in Fig. 2 in March 2020, which provides cloud services with low latency and high security through a cloud infrastructure within the NTT DOCOMO network employing Multi-access Edge Computing technology [4]. As an optional service, *Cloud Direct (currently MEC Direct)* was released in June 2020, which enables low-latency and high-security communication via 5G with communication-route optimization by connecting the cloud infrastructure and connected devices. Since it is a closed network separated from the Internet, cloud services in a high-security communication environment can be provided.

2 Expectations for Introducing 5G to Telemedicine

Telemedicine promotes healthcare and enables the medical practice through communication devices and services and provides medical services to people in a larger area by making effective use of limited numbers of doctors and hospitals. Especially in Japan, regional disparities in medical care are a serious issue. Depopulation and aging are problems that are accelerating, and medical resources are limited in rural areas. Meanwhile, medical facilities and doctors providing advanced medical care

are concentrated in urban areas. These issues further exacerbate problems such as the decrease in educational opportunities for young doctors in rural areas and the increase in doctor working hours in urban areas. Considering these issues, telemedicine is expected as a way to address the shortage or uneven distribution of doctors and medical facilities. Moreover, the SARS-CoV-2 or coronavirus disease 2019 (COVID-19) pandemic has been a trigger to accelerating the use of telemedicine.

Telemedicine is categorized into two main types: doctor to patient (D to P) and doctor to doctor (D to D). In the D-to-P configuration, doctors perform medical examinations on patients in a remote setting using video and voice information through communication devices. On the other hand, in the D-to-D configuration, experienced doctors or specialists collaborate with and support diagnosis or treatment of doctors in remote locations. Remote surgical support and remote surgery have received attention lately, and these are regarded as advanced cases of D to D and D to P.

For remote diagnosis and treatment, sharing of medical data such as diagnosis or surgical images and patient information between locations is essential. Recently, high-definition image equipment such as 4 K and 8 K has been introduced with the development of electronic technology, which means an increase in the amount of data traffic. Considering telemedicine with a large amount of medical data sent in real time, 5G is expected to contribute and accelerate telemedicine by leveraging its high speed/high capacity and low-latency capabilities.

To introduce 5G technology to telemedicine, system evolution and accumulation of required technology in phases toward advanced telemedicine are necessary as shown in Fig. 3. As telemedicine advances, the amount of medical information will increase, and higher technical requirements for networks must be achieved. For example, in remote diagnosis support using ultrasound, patient information, ultrasound images, and communication information including video and voice are

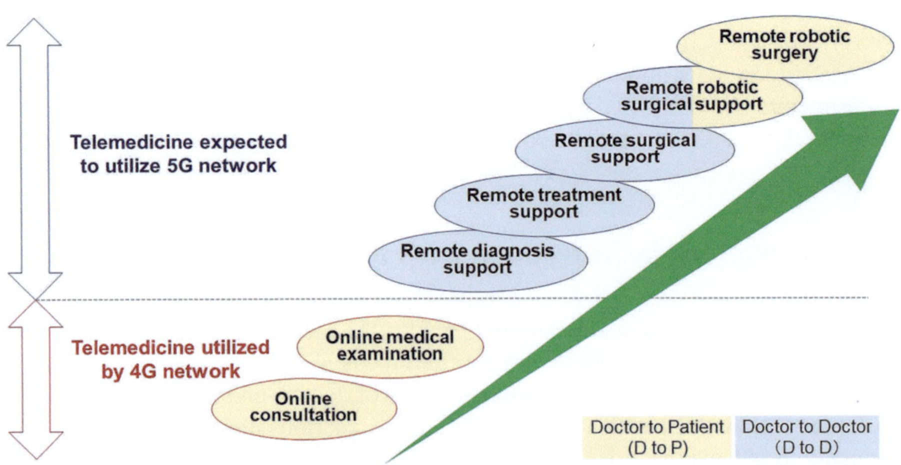

Fig. 3 Technical steps toward advanced telemedicine

needed, and a delay of a few seconds may have little influence on the diagnosis. However, in remote robotic surgery using high-definition surgical images and robotic control information, a delay of a few seconds could result in serious consequences, and large amounts of data with low latency must be transmitted.

The 5G network is flexible in addition to having high capacity, low latency, and high security. 5G is easy to handle compared to wired networks and can be utilized anywhere if there is a 5G environment. Considering the above features, 5G is also expected to be applied to medical uses in depopulated areas and in disaster scenarios.

3 Trends in Telemedicine Using 5G

Medical field activities and demonstrations using the 5G network have been reported all over the world. In Spain, Lacy et al. reported 5G-assisted telementored surgery in 2019, in which surgeons in an operating room and the mentor in a remote location communicated in real time while sharing laparoscopic images via the 5G network [5]. Telementored surgery was performed in two surgical cases of laparoscopic high anterior resection and laparoscopic low anterior resection, and the latency time was 202 ms and 146 ms, respectively. The transmission speed was approximately 100 Mbps with no significant signal loss. Based on the results, they indicated that the 5G technology enables safe and efficient complex surgical procedures using telementoring.

In China, Wu et al. conducted a pilot study of robot-assisted teleultrasound via the 5G network toward early imaging assessment during a pandemic such as COVID-19 [6]. Lung ultrasound, brief echocardiography, and blood volume assessment were performed on four patients with confirmed or suspected COVID-19. The patients were located in two different cities, and each patient was diagnosed by ultrasound specialists located in two other cities. During the procedures, the data rates of the network were 930 Mbps in the downlink and 130 Mbps in the uplink with the network latency of 23–30 ms and jitter of 1–2 ms. The doctors mentioned that the 5G network contributed to smooth scanning using the robotic arm with low risk of exposure to COVID-19. Zheng et al. reported remote laparoscopic telesurgery at a distance of nearly 3000 km using the 5G network [7]. Using a domestically produced surgical robot called MicroHand developed by Tianjin University, four laparoscopic surgeries including left nephrectomy, partial hepatectomy, cholecystectomy, and cystectomy were safely performed with the average network delay of 264 ms. They reported on the feasibility of telesurgery and provided insights on the value of 5G, especially in areas where Internet cables are difficult to lay or cannot be laid.

In the United States, the Department of Defense devised a full-scale plan for telemedicine applications using the 5G network to enable a joint medical community to sustain its long-term economic and military advantage [8]. They have worked to develop several technical areas to help augment future telemedicine and medical training applications within the 5G environment. Five technical areas regarding medical training using augmented reality (AR), telehealth, telerobotic surgery, remote integrated surgery using AR, and a mobile medic environment were initially selected. It is expected that the country-led activities will further accelerate 5G introduction into the medical field.

In the meantime, in Japan, Morohashi et al. evaluated robotic teleoperations using a domestically developed surgical robot via a commercial network [9]. Two types of robotic teleoperations were performed between hospitals 150 km apart using guaranteed-type lines (1 Gbps, 10 Mbps, and 5 Mbps) and best effort-type lines. The mean glass-to-glass times were 92 ms and 95 ms for the guaranteed-type line and best effort-type line, respectively. Although the employed network environment was different from 5G, their results indicated the importance of the implementation of telesurgery using commercial communication networks. To actualize telemedicine in an early stage, evaluations are required in an environment that is close to practical use.

4 Telemedicine Initiatives Using NTT DOCOMO 5G

NTT DOCOMO has demonstrated remote diagnosis and remote medical examinations using the 5G network in collaboration with various partners in D-to-D telemedicine since 2017. Using a 5G antenna for experimental use, we validated the effectiveness of telemedicine systems intended for clinical departments for community and emergency medicine. Furthermore, drawing on past experience, we are working on step-by-step experiments and demonstrations of advanced telemedicine systems using a commercial 5G antenna. In the following, we introduce some DOCOMO initiatives.

4.1 Telemedicine in Depopulated Areas

From 2017 to 2019, using 5G antennas for experimental use, 5G comprehensive demonstration tests led by the Ministry of Internal Affairs and Communications and demonstrations in collaboration with partners were conducted.

In Japan, the problems of depopulation and aging are progressing in rural areas, and there is a shortage of medical resources and services. To overcome these issues, we demonstrated remote medical examination between a rural clinic and an urban university hospital using an experimental 5G network in 2018.

A doctor in the clinic performed a medical examination on patients with the support from specialists in the university hospital. Five cases, including three dermatology cases, one orthopedic case, and one cardiology case, were demonstrated. According to the clinical departments, as shown in Fig. 4 medical images for diagnosis such as a 4 K image for trauma diagnosis, an ultrasound image for internal disease diagnosis, and a magnetic resonance image (MRI) were transmitted as well

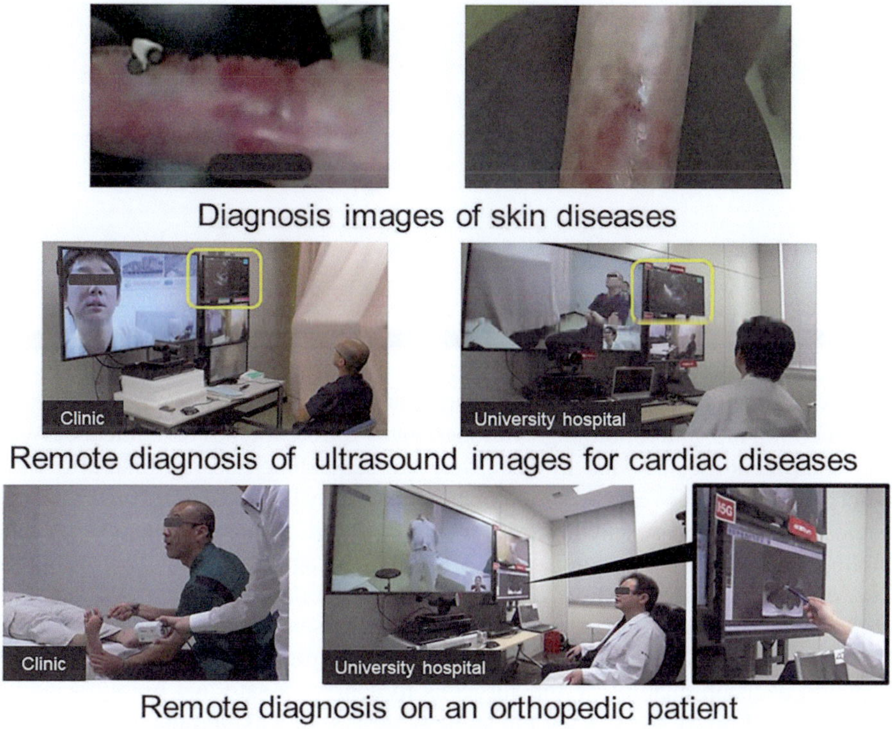

Fig. 4 5G telemedicine demonstration in a depopulated area

as voice information to the university hospital from the clinic via the 5G network. Since the 5G network enabled transmission of high-definition medical images, the specialists commented that it was easier to judge the symptoms compared to those transmitted using a conventional remote system and they could conduct the medical examinations with the feeling as if they were beside the patients. The patients commented that this method would be helpful for elderly people who often must travel more than 2 h into the city to visit the university hospital. Telemedicine in depopulated areas will contribute to reducing the burden on doctors and patients and to improve the level of medical care in rural areas.

4.2 Mobile Smart Cyber Operating Theater

Surgical technology is evolving year by year, and forms of information utilization such as the Internet of Things and Artificial Intelligence (AI) have attracted attention in recent years. Since 2019 the Tokyo Women's Medical University has led in the development of a state-of-the-art operating room (OR) called the "Smart Cyber Operating Theater (SCOT)" and has clinically applied it mainly to neurosurgery and

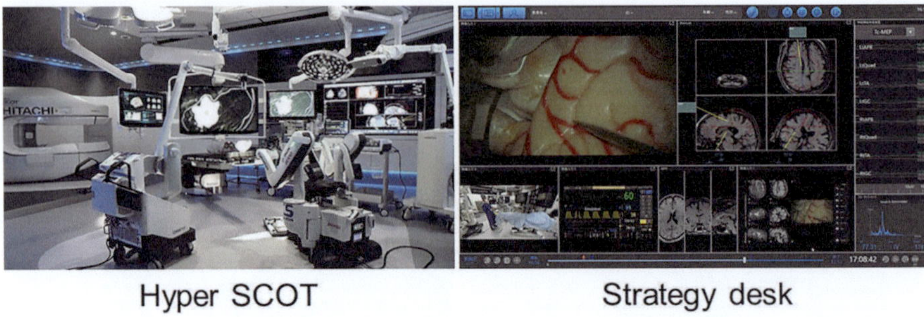

Fig. 5 Smart Cyber Operating Theater (SCOT) in Tokyo Women's Medical University

is shown in Fig. 5. The SCOT comprises four elements: packaging, networking, informationizing, and robotizing. Although many different types of medical devices and equipment are installed in ORs, they are standalone and not linked to each other, especially between different manufactures. In the SCOT, various medical devices and equipment, such as a surgical microscope, surgical navigation system, biological monitor, and intraoperative MRI, are packaged according to the clinical departments and surgical cases. These are then networked, and the digital data are collected and accumulated in time synchronization using the dedicated middleware "OPeLiNK." The intraoperative information is integrated as a strategy desk that supports decision-making by the surgeons to achieve a safe and highly accurate surgery (see Fig. 5). By sharing the strategy desk with a skilled doctor, the safety level can be further enhanced (please refer to Chapter "Deployment of Smart Cyber Operating Theater-Based Digital Operating Room to a Mobile Operating Theater" for more details on the SCOT). However, patients could not receive advanced medical care such as the SCOT without going to a hospital in an urban area.

To address this issue and to raise the level of medical care regardless of region, in collaboration with the Tokyo Women's Medical University, we proposed the concept of the "Mobile SCOT" which is a combination of the SCOT and 5G network. As shown in Fig. 6, the Mobile SCOT comprises a mobile treatment room in which the SCOT is installed in a vehicle and a mobile strategy desk that receives intraoperative information from the SCOT or the Mobile SCOT and supports the surgeon from a remote location. With the advantages of 5G, a large amount of data in the SCOT could be transmitted in real time and to provide advanced medical care anytime and anywhere.

In October 2020, we conducted the first demonstration of the Mobile SCOT and a commercial 5G network. As the first step, demonstrations of remote diagnosis support using an ultrasound system were performed in two configurations: between a medical office in the university and a location approximately 15 km away and between the medical office and a compound in the university. By using the commercial 5G network and NTT DOCOMO cloud service, the ultrasound images in the Mobile SCOT were transmitted to a second console that could control the ultrasound system remotely in the medical office, and audio data were transmitted in

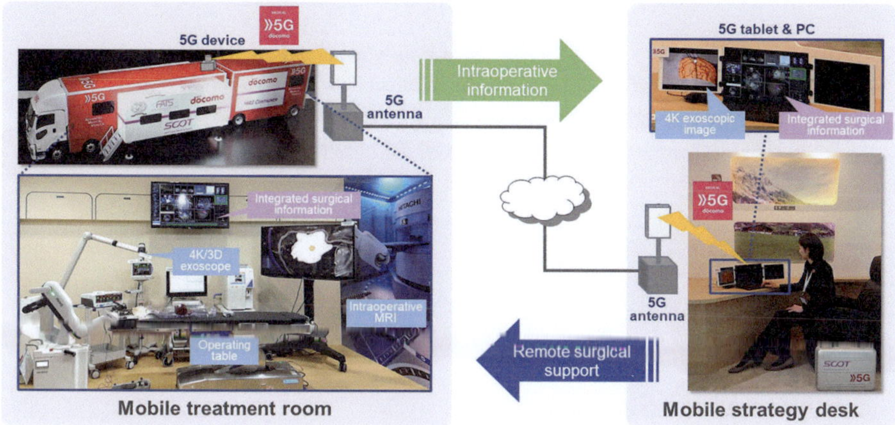

Fig. 6 Mobile SCOT concept

both directions. Evaluation results of simulated practical cases of obstetrics and cardiology demonstrated the feasibility of the Mobile SCOT and the potential for remote diagnosis support in real time.

4.3 Remote Robotic Surgical Support/Remote Robotic Surgery

Remote robotic surgery is a highly advanced technique in telemedicine. Many surgical robots have been developed thus far, and the da Vinci surgical system (Intuitive Surgical, Inc., CA, USA) is the most commonly used worldwide. The development of surgical robots has also progressed in Japan, which hosts a high level of industrial robotic technologies. In 2020, a commercial surgical robot system called hinotori™ was launched for the first time in Japan by the Medicaroid Corporation, which is a joint company between Kawasaki Heavy Industries, Ltd., and the Sysmex Corporation. The hinotori™ system comprises an operation unit with compact robotic arms similar to human arms, an ergonomically designed surgeon cockpit, and a vision unit that produces high-definition 3D images. These were developed in collaboration with Kobe University toward the actualization of precise and advanced surgeries. Although robotic surgery has become popular, it is concentrated in urban areas, and there is a large regional disparity in medical care. In association with this issue, there are concerns such as a decrease in the number of educational opportunities for young surgeons in rural areas and an increase in the working time of surgeons in urban areas. To overcome these hurdles, we have demonstrated cases of remote robotic surgery including remote support via the 5G network since 2020, under the framework of Kobe Vision for the Healthcare of Tomorrow initiative promoted by Kobe City.

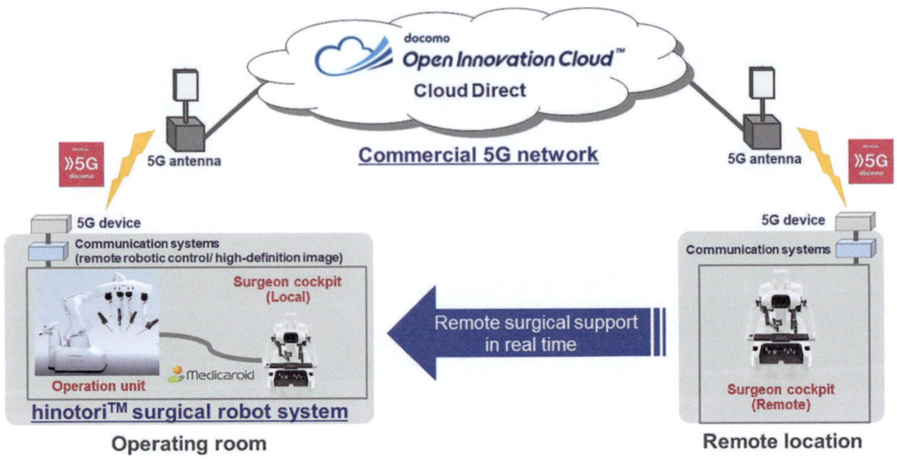

Fig. 7 Remote robotic surgical support via commercial 5G network and cloud infrastructure

In the demonstration illustrated in Fig. 7, hinotori™ was connected between two locations via a commercial 5G network and NTT DOCOMO cloud service, and a mock surgery was performed by a surgeon in the cockpit in a remote location controlling the operation unit. High-definition surgical images and robot control information were successfully transmitted in real time, and surgical operations such as blood vessel dissection, needle holding, and needle handling as well as basic operations such as grasping were achieved. We believe that this is the first demonstration of remote robotic operation with a combination of a domestic commercial surgical robot and a commercial 5G network in the world. The surgeon who is well-versed in robotic surgical techniques gave a good evaluation of the remote robotic surgical operation and said that the system using the 5G network was potentially capable of performing remote robotic surgeries. He experienced improved flexibility because of the wireless communications and expected further development toward full-scale commercialization. Remote robotic surgical support and remote robotic surgery via the 5G network could deliver advanced medical care widely and could contribute to improving the education and working styles of surgeons through efficient medical resources. This remote robotic surgery technology is also expected to contribute to easing medical problems in foreign countries especially those with expansive land areas that are facing a lack of medical resources.

5 Further Advancing Telemedicine

Toward the practical actualization of advanced telemedicine, there are still challenges such as sufficient technology development for advanced telemedicine and legal system adjustment for early social implementation. Wireless communication has characteristic challenges including the communication band, communication quality, and data communication traffic, and how to transmit medical information required for advanced telemedicine is a key point.

The sophistication of 5G technology brings various new functions such as network slicing, which provides dedicated networks with a high bandwidth or low latency by dividing the network virtually, and priority control of communication information in the application layer according to the communication situation using technologies such as AI. With these technologies, the above challenges can be solved, and advance telemedicine can be provided stably anytime and anywhere.

The mobile communication system will become more advanced in the next decade, and 5G Evolution and 6G are expected as the next technologies beyond 5G. There are mainly six target requirements for 6G technology: extremely high data rates/capacity exceeding 100 Gbps; extremely low latency of 1 ms or less; extreme coverage extension including sky, sea, and space; extremely high reliability; extremely low energy/cost; and extreme massive connectivity/sensing [10]. In the 6G era, the delay in remote robotic surgery will be improved significantly, and telemedicine sighted for cosmic space might be achieved in the future. Mobile communication technology has great potential and is expected to contribute to the further development of telemedicine.

Acknowledgments This manuscript contains some of the results of the 5G comprehensive demonstration tests undertaken by NTT DOCOMO from the Ministry of Internal Affairs and Communications.

The authors are deeply grateful to the Faculty of Advanced Techno and Surgery, Tokyo Women's Medical University, Department of Neurosurgery, Tokyo Women's Medical University, Olympus Corporation, and OPExPARK Inc. for their cooperation and support in promoting the Mobile SCOT demonstration. The authors also express their deep gratitude to the International Clinical Cancer Research Center, Kobe University, Medicaroid Corporation, and Kobe City for their cooperation and support in promoting the remote robotic surgery support/remote robotic surgery demonstrations.

References

1. ITU-R Radiocommunication Sector of ITU (Recommendation ITU-R M.2083-0). https://www.itu.int/dms_pubrec/itu-r/rec/m/R-REC-M.2083-0-201509-I!!PDF-E.pdf
2. MIC Communication White Paper 2020. https://www.soumu.go.jp/johotsusintokei/whitepaper/ja/r02/pdf/n1300000.pdf
3. GSMA The Mobile economy 2021. https://www.gsma.com/mobileeconomy/wp-content/uploads/2021/07/GSMA_MobileEconomy2021_3.pdf
4. Akashi T, Tasaki H, Koh S, Yamada M, Takashio K, Harano S, Soyano S, Yamada F. Service and solutions in 5G communications. DOCOMO Tech J. 2021;22(3):16–32. https://www.docomo.ne.jp/english/binary/pdf/corporate/technology/rd/technical_journal/bn/vol22_3/vol22_3_en_total.pdf
5. Lacy M, Bravo R, Otero-Piñeiro AM, Pena R, De Lacy FB, Menchaca R, Balibrea JM. 5G-assisted telementored surgery. BJS. 2019;106:1576–9.

6. Wu S, Wu D, Ye R, Li K, Lu Y, Xu J, Xiong L, Zhao Y, Cui A, Li Y, Peng C, Lv F. Pilot study of robot-assisted teleultrasound based on 5G network: a new feasible strategy for early imaging assessment during COVID-19 pandemic. IEEE Trans Ultrason Ferroelectr Freq Control. 2020;67(11):2241–8.
7. Zheng J, Wang Y, Zhang J, Guo W, Yang X, Luo L, Jiao W, Hu X, Yu Z, Wang C, Zhu L, Yang Z, Zhang M, Xie F, Jia Y, Li B, Li Z, Dong Q, Niu H. 5G ultra-remote robot-assisted laparoscopic surgery in Chinca. Surg Endosc. 2020;34:5172–80.
8. U.S. Department of Defense, 5G Telemedicine & Medical Training. https://media.defense.gov/2021/Apr/28/2002629569/-1/-1/1/5G%20TELEMEDICINE%20TRADE%20ARTICLE%2012-10-20.PDF
9. Morohashi H, Hakamada K, Kanno T, Kawashima K, Akasaka H, Ebihara Y, Oki E, Hirano S, Mori M. Social implementation of a remote surgery system in Japan: a field experiment using a newly developed surgical robot via a commercial network. Surg Today. 2021;52(4):705–14.
10. NTT DOCOMO White Paper "5G Evolution and 6G". https://www.docomo.ne.jp/english/binary/pdf/corporate/technology/whitepaper_6g/DOCOMO_6G_White_PaperEN_v4.0.pdf

Future Trend: AI × XR (VR, AR)

Yuichiro Hayashi and Kensaku Mori

Abstract This chapter describes surgical assistance using artificial intelligence (AI) and extended reality (XR). AI technology can now analyze various data and is gaining ground in the medical field. XR technology enables the integration of virtual environments with the real world. Computer-aided surgery (CAS) systems can be enhanced by combining these technologies. A surgical navigation system is a typical CAS system using AI and XR. This system provides surgical assistance information about the anatomical structures in the operative field by fusing the real and virtual environments. In this chapter, we focus on surgical navigation systems using AI and XR and present our surgical navigation systems based on virtual endoscopy systems and their clinical applications.

Keywords Virtual reality · Augmented reality · Deep learning · Machine learning Visualization · Segmentation · Registration · Virtual endoscopy · Surgical navigation · Laparoscopic surgery

1 Introduction

AI technology, such as deep learning, has made remarkable progress and is used in various fields. It is also expected to make headway in the medical field. AI technology can analyze various data produced in the hospital and automatically generate

---

Y. Hayashi (✉)
Graduate School of Informatics, Nagoya University, Nagoya, Japan
e-mail: yhayashi@mori.m.is.nagoya-u.ac.jp

K. Mori
Graduate School of Informatics, Nagoya University, Nagoya, Japan

Information Technology Center, Nagoya University, Nagoya, Japan

Research Center for Medical Bigdata, National Institute of Informatics, Tokyo, Japan

K. Masamune et al. (eds.), *Artificial Intelligence in Surgery*,
https://doi.org/10.1007/978-981-96-6635-5_16

valuable information from these data. Therefore, computer-aided surgery (CAS) systems using AI technology have been studied for assisting surgeons during surgery. AI technology is useful for generating surgical assistance information in these CAS systems. It is also important for the CAS system to present the assistance information in an easily understandable way. Extended reality or cross reality (XR) technology, a collective term for VR (virtual reality), AR (augmented reality), MR (mixed reality), and other related technologies, has also been attracting attention. These technologies allow us to experience a realistic virtual environment constructed on a computer. Furthermore, these technologies can augment information in the real world by combining the virtual environment and the real environment, as seen in the entertainment field in game applications. They are expected to enhance human machine interaction and extend human capabilities in many areas. XR technology has also been introduced into CAS systems to more effectively present surgical assistance information.

The location and shape of anatomical structures in the human body differ for each patient. Understanding a patient's specific anatomical structures is vital for surgeons when planning and performing surgery, and, thus, the ability of CAS systems to assist in understanding patient-specific anatomical structures has been studied. To obtain patient-specific anatomical information, various kinds of medical images are utilized. Imaging scanners such as X-ray computed tomography (CT) or magnetic resonance imaging (MRI) machines can capture three-dimensional (3D) internal anatomical structures in the human body. These medical images can be considered a virtualized human body (VHB) constructed on a computer that corresponds to an individual patient in the real world [1]. Therefore, medical images (VHB) can be used to generate the virtual environment in XR. XR technology enables observation and manipulation of medical images in the virtual environment. AI technology can thus provide a wealth of surgical assistance information from the huge amount of information in the medical images. AI technology can be also analyzed surgical scenes in the real environment captured by surgical microscopes or endoscopes, such as during laparoscopic surgery. Combining these AI and XR technologies substantially enhances the CAS system. Observation and analysis of the medical images (VHB) lead to preoperative diagnosis and surgical planning. In addition, surgical simulation can be performed by adding deformations to the medical images. Furthermore, surgical navigation can be performed by combining the medical images with the real human body during surgery.

In this chapter, we describe how AI and XR technologies provide surgical assistance based on medical images. A typical CAS system using these technologies acts as a surgical navigation system. Various image processing techniques, dramatically improved by AI and XR, are used to construct surgical navigation systems. In this chapter, we explain the fundamentals, discuss recent research on surgical navigation systems, and show several examples and their clinical applications.

2 Surgical Navigation System

2.1 *System Configuration*

A surgical navigation system provides surgical assistance information synchronized with the operative field during surgery. To combine the virtual environment constructed from the medical images with the real world, this system mainly consists of three processes: (a) measurements of the surgical instrument position, (b) patient-to-image registration, and (c) presentation of the surgical assistance image. The system first measures the positions of the surgical instruments using a positional tracker and then generates surgical assistance images based on the obtained positional information and the medical images, such as CT or MRI images. To synchronize the generation of the assistance images with the operative field, it is necessary to know the position of the surgical instruments on the medical image. Therefore, a registration process that aligns the coordinate systems between the positional tracker and the medical images is performed before generating the surgical assistance images.

2.2 *Measurements of Surgical Instrument Position*

Real-time measurement of the 3D position and orientation of surgical instruments is necessary for performing surgical navigation. A 3D positional tracker is commonly used for this purpose. There are two types of position tracking methods, optical tracking and electromagnetic tracking, one of which is selected depending on the characteristics of each measurement method and type of surgery. Vision-based tracking methods that calculate the position of surgical instruments from endoscopic images have also been studied.

2.2.1 Optical Tracking Method

The optical tracking method uses two or more infrared (IR) cameras, and spherical markers reflecting IR light to track. Using multiple cameras, the 3D positions of the spherical makers are computed. The position and orientation of the surgical instruments are measured by attaching three or more markers to them. Since it is often difficult to attach the markers directly to the tip of the instruments, they are attached to appropriate locations on the surgical instruments. The position of the tip can be calculated using the positional relationship between the markers and the tip. This type of positional tracker provides wireless tracking and more precise measurement than the other tracking methods. However, if there is an obstruction between the IR cameras and the markers, the optical tracker cannot be measured.

2.2.2 Electromagnetic Tracking Method

The electromagnetic tracking method can obtain the position and orientation of an electromagnetic (EM) sensor in the EM field by the EM field generator. Advantages of this method over the optical tracking method are that the size of the sensor is smaller and measurement is possible even with obstructions. Therefore, the position of a flexible endoscopic tip inside the body can be directly measured by attaching a small EM sensor to the tip. Furthermore, by attaching multiple sensors, the shape of the flexible endoscope can be estimated. However, the presence of metal causes measurement errors, and the sensor and EM field generator must be connected to the system control unit with a cable.

2.2.3 Vision-Based Tracking Method

Endoscopic and microscopic images are also used to obtain positional information. By directly calculating the camera position from these images, surgical navigation can be performed without the external positional tracker described above. Therefore, various vision-based camera tracking methods have been studied. A simultaneous localization and mapping (SLAM) framework is often used to compute the camera position and orientation [2, 3]. This method can estimate not only the camera positions but also the 3D shape of the organ in the images. The 3D organ shape can be used for the patient-to-image registration as follows. By aligning the 3D organ shapes reconstructed from the real endoscopic image and the medical images, we can obtain the position of the endoscope in the image coordinate system. Therefore, 3D reconstruction of the organ shape or depth estimation from the endoscopic images [4, 5] and 3D pose estimation methods for surgical instruments in the endoscopic images [6] have also been studied. Scene recognition is also utilized to obtain roughly positional information from the endoscopic images. A recognition method of the surgical areas currently observed by surgeons using the laparoscope has been proposed [7]. The surgical navigation system can generate assistance information using the recognition results of the surgical areas without calculating the camera's position.

2.3 Patient-to-Image Registration

To generate surgical assistance images corresponding to the position of surgical instruments, patient-to-image registration, which aligns the coordinate systems between the positional tracker and the medical image, is needed in the surgical navigation system. This process computes a transformation from the positional tracker coordinate system to the medical image coordinate system. Rigid transformation consisting of translation and rotation is typically used. The surgical navigation system computes the positions of the surgical instruments on the medical images from their positions measured by the positional tracker using the transformation computed by the registration process. Two types of registration methods can be used: point-based registration, which uses point correspondences, and surface-based registration, which uses the surface shape.

2.3.1 Point-Based Registration

In point-based registration, multiple fiducial points are used for the registration. Artificial markers that are clearly visible on CT or MRI images or anatomical landmarks that are distinct body points such as a bone process are used as the fiducials. The positions of the fiducials are measured in both the positional tracker and image coordinate systems, and the transformation matrix is calculated using their correspondences. Let $\boldsymbol{p}_i$ be the position of the i-th fiducials in the positional tracker coordinate system and $\boldsymbol{q}_i$ be the position of the i-th fiducials in the medical image coordinate system. The point-based registration computes the rigid transformation matrix $\mathbf{T}^*$ by

$$\mathbf{T}^* = \arg\min_{\mathbf{T}} \sum_{i=1}^{N} \left|\mathbf{T}\boldsymbol{p}_i - \boldsymbol{q}_i\right|^2,$$

where N is the number of fiducials [8].

2.3.2 Surface-Based Registration

In surface-based registration, the organ shapes are used for the registration. The rigid transformation matrix is usually computed from these shapes using the iterative closest point (ICP) algorithm [8]. Here, we assume that the surface shape of the organ is represented by a point set. Let $P = \{\boldsymbol{p}_i | i = 1, \cdots, M\}$ be the point set of the organ surface measured by the positional tracker and $Q = \{\boldsymbol{q}_j | j = 1, \ldots, N\}$ be the point set of the organ surface measured on the medical image. The ICP algorithm iteratively aligns the two point sets. For each point in point set P, the closest point in point set Q is obtained as the corresponding point. Using the obtained correspondences, the rigid transformation matrix $\mathbf{T}$ is computed using the point-based registration method. Point set P then transforms using the rigid transformation matrix $\mathbf{T}$, and the distance between the transformed point set P and point set Q is calculated. This registration process is repeated until the distance is smaller than the predefined thresholding.

2.3.3 Intraoperative Registration

The registration process is important to perform accurate surgical navigation. In the surgical navigation of soft tissues, tissue deformation increases registration error. Anatomical landmarks on the body surface are often used as the fiducials. Registration error can occur due to differences in the patient's posture between the image scan and surgery [9]. Furthermore, organ deformations due to surgical operations reduce the accuracy of surgical navigation during surgery. Therefore, several registration methods to reduce registration error using the internal anatomical structures during surgery have been considered [10–14]. These methods use the position of the blood vessels or landmarks on the organs as the fiducials in point-based registration [10, 11] and organ surfaces for surface-based registration [12–14]. A registration error compensation method has been proposed that analyzes the positional information of the fiducials, the guidance targets, and registration result in prior surgeries [15]. In addition, intraoperative imaging systems such as intraoperative MRI, C-arm, and ultrasound are used to capture the organ deformation during surgery in the surgical navigation system [16–19]. Since the medical images captured by these intraoperative scanners are reflected tissue deformations during surgery, more accurate surgical navigation can be achieved by updating the medical images and registration based on the intraoperative images.

2.3.4 Vision-Based Registration

Vision-based registration methods without positional trackers have also been studied. These methods directly align optical images, such as endoscopic images, and 3D medical images, such as CT images. Surgical navigation systems using a tablet PC perform the registration using the positions of the fiducial markers or the anatomical landmarks in both the camera images and CT images [3, 20]. The information of the 3D organ shapes is also used for registration in the surgical navigation system for laparoscopic surgery [21–24]. There are studies on 2D-3D registration that aligns 3D organ shapes reconstructed from the CT images with the organ regions in 2D laparoscopic images [21, 22]. Registration methods using 3D point clouds reconstructed from the laparoscopic images and CT images have also been proposed [23, 24].

2.4 Presentation of Surgical Assistance Information

The surgical navigation system outputs patient-specific anatomical structures or surgical plans generated from the medical images as surgical assistance information. The conventional surgical navigation system often displays the positions of the surgical instruments on the axial, sagittal, and coronal images of the CT or MRI images. A 3D medical image visualization process is needed to observe the 3D anatomical structures in these images. The medical images and other information are further analyzed to generate surgical assistance information. This information is usually a monitor in the surgical navigation system. XR devices are sometimes used to make the surgical assistance information more comprehensible.

2.4.1 Visualization of Medical Images

Visualization of the medical images is performed to generate surgical assistance information to aid in the understanding of patient-specific 3D anatomical structures. Computer graphics techniques such as surface rendering or volume rendering methods are usually used to visualize the 3D medical images [1]. The surface rendering method renders the organ surface represented by triangular patches and so on. These triangular patches are generated from organ regions extracted from the medical images using the marching cubes algorithm. On the other hand, the volume rendering method assigns a color and opacity to each voxel in the medical images and performs ray-casting to visualize them. A virtual endoscopy system can generate virtual endoscopic views that depict the VHB from an arbitrary viewpoint in the virtual environment using these visualization methods [25]. This system is often used to generate surgical assistance images in the surgical navigation system for laparoscopic and other endoscopic surgeries.

2.4.2 Generation of Surgical Assistance Information

To enhance the important anatomical structures for surgery in the surgical assistance images for visualization, these anatomical structures should be extracted from the medical images. Since manual segmentation of anatomical structures is time-consuming and labor intensive, automated segmentation methods for extracting various anatomical structures from the medical images have been proposed. Multiple organs can be automatically extracted from CT images with high accuracy using deep learning [26, 27]. Fully convolutional networks (FCNs), such as U-Net or its variants, are commonly used for segmentation. In addition to the organ segmentation, methods for assigning extracted blood vessels or bronchial branches to anatomical names have also been considered [28, 29]. The extracted anatomical structures can be displayed in different colors in the rendered images.

Other information, such as surgical plans, is displayed in the surgical navigation system. For example, a surgical navigation system using the optimal port placement planning method has been studied for determining port locations in laparoscopic surgery [30]. A brain risk area creation method has been introduced for decision-making using surgical navigation [31]. These methods select the optimal port placement or brain risk area by analyzing data obtained during previous surgeries using the surgical navigation system. Information such as surgical instrument motion from the surgical navigation system is also utilized for analyzing surgical procedures [32].

2.4.3 Display of Surgical Assistance Image

Surgical assistance images can be displayed in a variety of ways. They are usually displayed on a monitor in the surgical navigation system. For endoscopic surgery, the important anatomical structures derived from the medical images are overlaid on the endoscopic images [11–13]. A surgical navigation system has been used to overlay the surgical assistant images on stereo images obtained from a stereo endoscope and display them on a 3D monitor [33]. Surgical navigation systems that superimpose the anatomical structures on the camera images of a tablet PC have also been developed [3, 20]. In addition, surgical assistance images have been projected onto the body surface using a projector [34, 35]. XR devices, such as a head mounted display (HMD), are also used to observe the surgical assistance information [36, 37]. Optical see-through HMDs and video see-through HMDs can display the surgical assistance images overlaid onto a patient's body in the real space.

3 Examples of Surgical Navigation Systems for Laparoscopic Surgery

3.1 Laparoscopic Surgery

Examples of surgical navigation for laparoscopic surgery are shown in this section. Minimally invasive surgery (MIS) such as laparoscopic surgery is widely performed because of its patient benefits. In laparoscopic surgery, a laparoscope and surgical instruments are inserted into the abdominal cavity through small incisions in the abdominal wall. Surgeons control these instruments while watching the laparoscopic view displayed on a monitor. The limited field of view or limited workspace in MIS, however, makes MIS more difficult than conventional surgery. Patient anatomy beyond the limited view cannot be observed. Furthermore, important anatomical structures often cannot be directly observed because they are obscured by other organs or tissues such as adipose tissue at the beginning of the surgery. Even if the important anatomical structures are visible, they may be difficult to recognize in the operative field because their surface textures are similar to the surrounding tissues. It is vital to comprehend the patient-specific anatomical structures around the operative field during MIS. Therefore, a surgical navigation system can help surgeons understand patient-specific anatomical structures during laparoscopic surgery.

3.2 Surgical Navigation System Based on Positional Tracker and Virtual Endoscopy System

3.2.1 System Overview

A virtual endoscopy system generates virtual endoscopic views from medical images such as CT and MRI images. By combining a surgical navigation system with a virtual endoscopy system, the virtual laparoscopic views corresponding to the operative field observed using a real laparoscope can be generated for surgical assistance information. This surgical navigation system consists of a 3D positional tracker and computer that runs a virtual endoscopy system [9]. Optical positional tracker markers or electromagnetic positional tracker sensors are attached to the laparoscope. The positional relationship between the markers and the laparoscopic tip is then measured to obtain the laparoscopic tip's positional information. Before the surgical navigation, registration is performed to obtain a transformation matrix transformed from the coordinate system of the positional tracker to that of the medical image. Using the transformation matrix, the position and orientation of the laparoscopic tip measured by the positional tracker are transformed into the position and orientation in the medical images. The virtual laparoscopic images corresponding to the position of the laparoscopic tip are generated using the virtual endoscope system based on the transformed positional information and the medical image. The position of the surgical tools can also be displayed in the virtual endoscope image in the same way.

3.2.2 Surgical Navigation in Laparoscopic Gastrectomy

Surgical navigation was performed in laparoscopic gastrectomy for gastric cancer using this system [9]. The Polaris Spectra optical tracking system (NDI, Waterloo, Ontario, Canada) was used as the 3D positional tracker. The infrared camera of the Polaris system was mounted on an arm attached to the ceiling of the operating room (Fig. 1a). Reflective marker spheres were attached to the laparoscope (Fig. 1b), and the monitor for displaying the surgical assistance images was installed alongside the laparoscope monitor. We performed point-based registration to compute the rigid transformation using six anatomical landmarks as the fiducials. These landmarks were the xiphoid process, the umbilicus, about 50 mm ~ 100 mm right and left of the umbilicus, and the right and left anterior superior iliac spine palpated through the body surface. The landmark positions in the image coordinate system were specified while observing a volume-rendered image of the CT images. The positions of the corresponding landmarks in the positional tracker coordinate system were measured by the tracked pointer. We converted the positional information of the laparoscopic tip from the Polaris system using the transformation matrix computed in the registration process. The surgical navigation system generated the

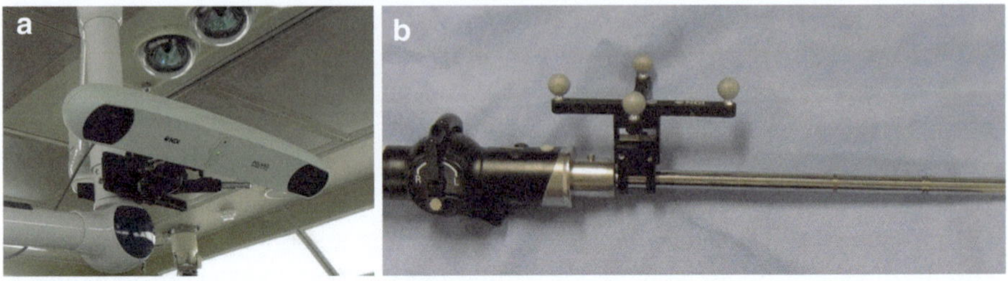

Fig. 1 Example of optical tracking system. (**a**) Infrared camera. (**b**) Spherical markers attached to laparoscope

virtual laparoscopic views in synchronization with the laparoscope position in real time using the virtual endoscopy system from preoperative CT images and the transformed positional information.

In laparoscopic gastrectomy for gastric cancer, the blood vessels around the stomach need to be cut before resecting the stomach including the cancer. Since the branching patterns of the blood vessels differ from patient to patient, the branching patterns and positional relationship between the blood vessels and surrounding organs are important. Therefore, the artery, portal vein, liver, spleen, gallbladder, stomach, and pancreas were extracted from the arterial and portal venous phase contrast-enhanced CT images. Then, the extracted regions and CT images were rendered by a volume rendering method using a virtual endoscopy system. In the virtual laparoscopic views, the extracted anatomical structures were displayed in different colors.

Figure 2 shows the surgical navigation scene. In this figure, the laparoscope view from the real laparoscope is displayed on the right monitor, and the virtual laparoscopic view generated by the surgical navigation system is displayed on the left monitor. The red, blue, brown, dark brown, white, and yellow regions indicate the artery, portal vein, liver, spleen, gallbladder, and pancreas, respectively. The registration error was evaluated using the fiducial registration error (FRE), which is the root mean square of the distance between the corresponding fiducials after registration. Average and standard deviation of the FRE in 23 cases was 14.0 ± 5.6 mm. Although there were some registration errors, the surgical navigation system was able to present the virtual laparoscopic views corresponding to the position of the laparoscope as a surgical assistance image. The surgeons were able to intuitively identify the anatomical structures around the operative field by observing the virtual laparoscopic views synchronized with the laparoscope's position. They confirmed the usefulness of the virtual laparoscopic views generated by the surgical navigation system.

3.2.3 Surgical Navigation in Laparoscopic Hepatectomy

The surgical navigation system was also used in a laparoscopic hepatectomy [38]. The Aurora electromagnetic tracking system (NDI, Waterloo, Ontario, Canada) was used in this surgical navigation. The electromagnetic field generator was placed

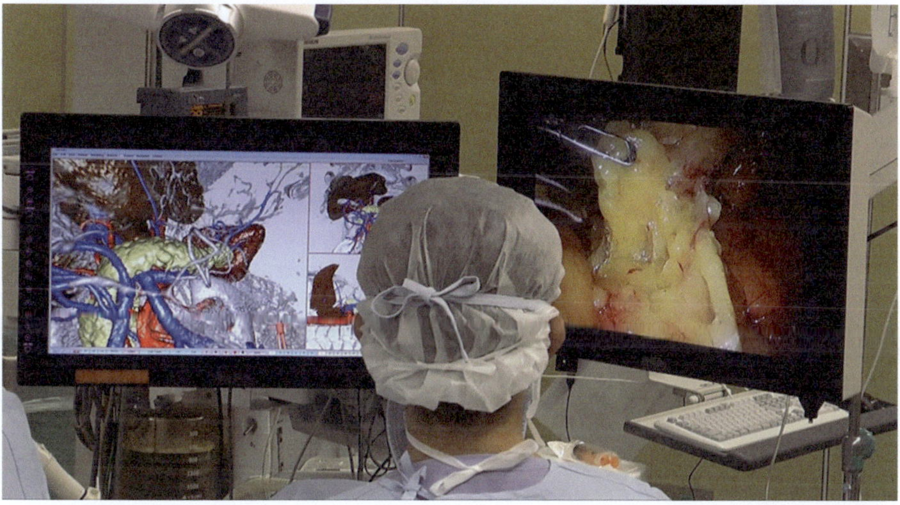

Fig. 2 Surgical navigation during laparoscopic gastrectomy for gastric cancer. The right and left monitors display the laparoscopic image from the laparoscope and surgical assistance image from the surgical navigation system, respectively. The red, blue, brown, dark brown, white, and yellow regions in the surgical assistance image indicate the artery, portal vein, liver, spleen, gallbladder, and pancreas, respectively

above the operating table, and magnetic sensors were attached to the laparoscope and forceps to measure their position and orientation. A monitor for displaying the surgical assistance images was installed alongside the laparoscope monitor. In this surgical navigation system, crosshair-shaped skin-affixed markers, which were clearly depicted in the CT images, were attached on the body surface as the fiducials, and point-based rigid registration was performed using these fiducials. The virtual laparoscopic views were generated using the positional information from the Aurora system and the transformation matrix from the registration process. When resecting a tumor in the liver, the positional relationship between the tumor and surrounding blood vessels is important. Therefore, the liver, tumor, hepatic artery, portal vein, and hepatic vein were extracted from the arterial and portal venous phase contrast-enhanced CT images for generating the virtual laparoscopic views. The surgical navigation scene is shown in Fig. 3. The right monitor shows the virtual laparoscopic view, and the left monitor shows the real laparoscopic view. In this figure, the brown, yellow, purple, and blue regions in the virtual laparoscopic views indicate the liver, tumor, portal vein, and hepatic vein, respectively. The surgical navigation system was used to confirm the location of the tumor and the surrounding blood vessels. Since the surgical navigation system can generate virtual laparoscopic views synchronized with the laparoscope's motion, this system could help surgeons understand the positional relationships between anatomical structures.

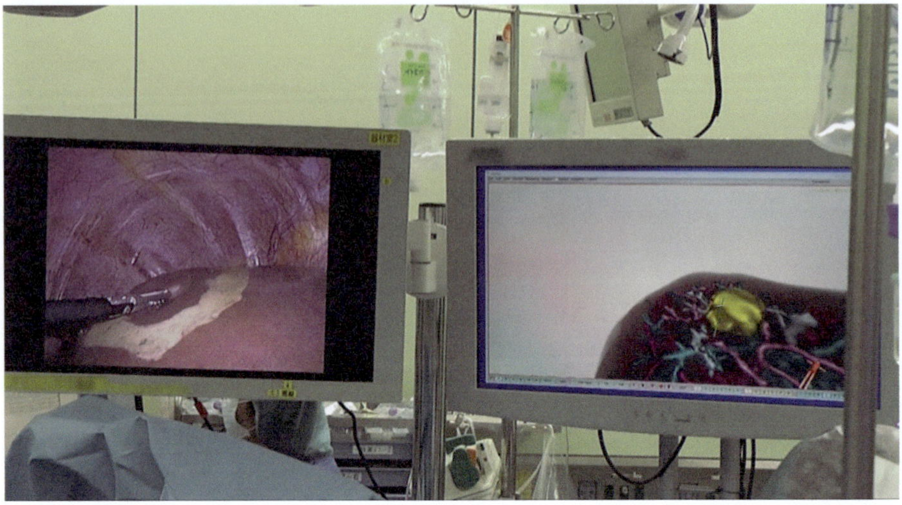

Fig. 3 Surgical navigation during laparoscopic hepatectomy. The right and left monitors display the surgical assistance image from the surgical navigation system and laparoscopic image from the laparoscope, respectively. The brown, yellow, purple, and blue regions in the surgical assistance image indicate the liver, tumor, portal vein, and hepatic vein, respectively

3.3 Surgical Navigation System Based on Scene Recognition of Laparoscopic Videos

3.3.1 System Overview

A surgical navigation system usually uses the laparoscope's positional information to present the surgical assistance information around the operative fields. If the surgical area being operated on can be recognized from the laparoscopic view during surgery, the surgical navigation system could generate surgical assistance images around the operative fields without the positional tracker. Therefore, a surgical navigation system based on laparoscopic image recognition has been studied. As mentioned above, in laparoscopic gastrectomy for gastric cancer, since the blood vessels around the stomach are dissected, understanding of the blood vessel structures is vital. Therefore, the surgical navigation system generates information on the structure of the blood vessels based on the blood vessel currently being processed during surgery. This system recognizes the surgical areas from the laparoscopic views in real time and presents the surgical assistance images according to the recognition results. The surgical area recognition method is based on an image classification method using deep learning [7]. This method classifies each image extracted from laparoscopic videos into the following seven scenes: (1) the left gastroepiploic artery (LGEA) or the left gastroepiploic vein (LGEV) is observed, (2) the right gastroepiploic artery (RGEA) or the right gastroepiploic vein (RGEV) is observed,

(3) the right gastric artery (RGA) is observed, (4) the left gastric artery (LGA) or the left gastric vein (LGV) is observed, (5) the abdominal cavity is observed, (6) the laparoscope is inside the trocar, and (7) the laparoscope is outside the body. We selected DenseNet for the laparoscopic image classification and trained it using laparoscopic images and their annotations for the seven scenes. During the surgical navigation, the system classifies the laparoscopic images captured by the laparoscope into the seven scenes using the trained DenseNet. The surgical assistance images corresponding to each scene are generated in advance by visualizing the blood vessels and surrounding organs extracted from the contrast-enhanced CT images using the virtual endoscopy system. The surgical navigation system presents these surgical assistance images according to the image classification results during surgery.

3.3.2 Surgical Navigation for Laparoscopic Gastrectomy

The surgical navigation system based on laparoscopic image recognition was used during laparoscopic gastrectomy for gastric cancer. Figure 4 shows the surgical navigation in action. In this figure, the left monitor shows the surgical navigation system's screen. The left side of the screen in the surgical navigation system shows the laparoscopic image captured from the laparoscope and its scene classification

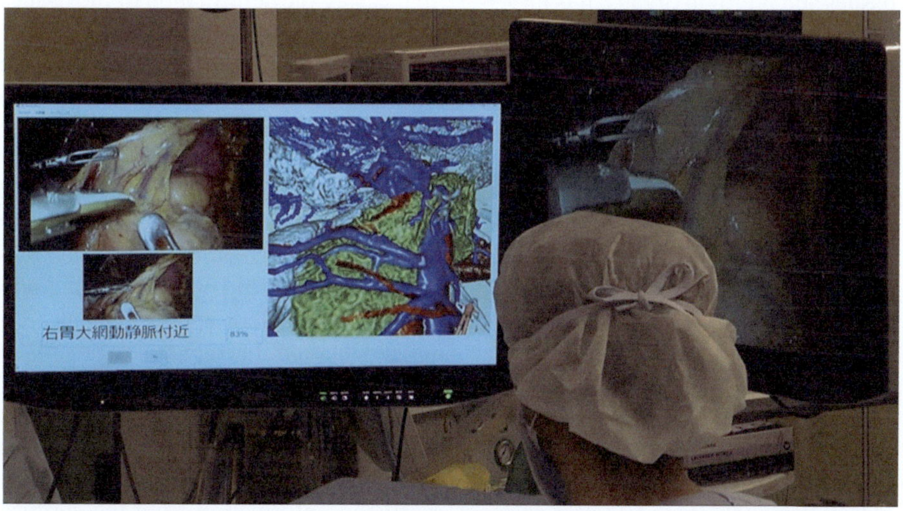

Fig. 4 Surgical navigation using laparoscopic image recognition. The left monitor shows the surgical navigation system screen. The left side of the screen shows the laparoscopic view from the laparoscope and its recognition result. This image is classified as a scene observing RGEA or RGEV. The right side of the screen is the surgical assistance image. The red, blue, dark brown, and yellow regions in the surgical assistance image indicate the artery, portal vein, spleen, and pancreas, respectively

result. The right side of the screen shows the virtual laparoscopic image generated based on the classification results. This system can provide surgical assistance images corresponding to the blood vessels being currently processed in the operative field without a positional tracker by recognizing the surgical area from the laparoscopic image. By observing the virtual laparoscopic image in this system, surgeons can obtain information about the anatomical structures around the operative fields such as blood vessel branching patterns.

4 Conclusions

This chapter described future trends for assisting surgery using AI and XR technologies. We introduced the surgical navigation system, which is a typical computer-aided surgery (CAS) system using AI and XR technologies. The surgical navigation system displays surgical assistance images generated from the medical images around the operative field. As shown in several examples, this system is useful for surgeons to comprehend patient-specific anatomical structures during surgery.

A challenge for the surgical navigation systems is dealing with tissue deformation during surgery. Accurate surgical navigation has been achieved for the rigid organs. However, for soft tissue surgical navigation, deformation reduces the accuracy of the surgical navigation. To achieve accurate surgical navigation for the soft tissues and nonrigid organs, it is necessary to measure the deformation of the tissues and organs during surgery and update the registration and surgical assistance information. Currently, to improve the accuracy of the surgical navigation, intraoperative images are taken during surgery, or registration is performed using information from inside the body. In the future, more accurate surgical navigation would be performed by estimating the tissues and organ deformations from the surgical videos. The estimated deformations could be used to align endoscopic images with the preoperative medical images or generate surgical assistance images simulating the intraoperative deformation. Furthermore, if the surgical navigation system can recognize surgical situations by analyzing the surgical videos and other information in the operating room, the system will be able to present more appropriate surgical assistance information according to the surgical situation. Further developments in AI and XR technologies will improve the surgical navigation systems.

In the operating room, surgery is performed using many surgical devices. Robotic surgical systems have also been introduced in various surgical procedures. Analyzing the data from these devices in addition to the image analysis in the surgical navigation system will provide better surgical assistance. Information from the surgical navigation system will also be useful in controlling the robotic surgical system. We can therefore expect that new computer-aided surgery systems combining surgical navigation systems and surgical devices will be developed in the future.

Acknowledgments The authors thank their colleagues for their suggestions and advice. This work was supported in part by JST CREST Grant No. JPMJCR20D5, JSPS KAKENHI Grant Nos. JP26108006 and JP17H00867, and AMED Grant No. JP16ck0106036.

References

1. Toriwaki J, Mori K. Visualization of the human body toward the navigation diagnosis with the virtualized human body. J Vis. 1998;1:111–24.
2. Mahmoud N, Collins T, Hostettler A, Soler L, Doignon C, Montiel JMM. Live tracking and dense reconstruction for handheld monocular endoscopy. IEEE Trans Med Imaging. 2019;38(1):79–89.
3. Mahmoud N, Grasa ÓG, Nicolau SA, Doignon C, Soler L, Marescaux J, Montiel JMM. On-patient see-through augmented reality based on visual SLAM. Int J Comput Asst Radiol Surg. 2017;12(1):1–11.
4. Maier-Hein L, Mountney P, Bartoli A, Elhawary H, Elson D, Groch A, Kolb A, Rodrigues M, Sorger J, Speidel S, Stoyanov D. Optical techniques for 3D surface reconstruction in computer-assisted laparoscopic surgery. Med Image Anal. 2013;17(8):974–96.
5. Li W, Hayashi Y, Oda M, Kitasaka T, Misawa K, Mori K. Spatially variant biases considered self-supervised depth estimation based on laparoscopic videos. Comput Methods Biomech Biomed Eng Imaging Vis. 2022;10(3):274–82.
6. Hasan MK, Calvet L, Rabbani N, Bartoli A. Detection, segmentation, and 3D pose estimation of surgical tools using convolutional neural networks and algebraic geometry. Med Image Anal. 2021;70:101994.
7. Hayashi Y, Misawa K, Mori K. Surgical area recognition from laparoscopic images in laparoscopic gastrectomy for gastric cancer using label smoothing and uncertainty. In: Proceedings of SPIE 12466, Medical Imaging 2023: image-guided procedures, robotic interventions, and modeling. p. 1246624.
8. Fitzpatrick JM, Hill DLG, Maurer CR Jr. Image registration. In: Sonka M, Fitzpatrick JM, editors. Handbook of medical imaging, Medical image processing and analysis, vol. 2. Bellingham: SPIE; 2000. pp. 447–513.
9. Hayashi Y, Misawa K, Oda M, Hawkes DJ, Mori K. Clinical application of a surgical navigation system based on virtual laparoscopy in laparoscopic gastrectomy for gastric cancer. Int J Comput Assist Radiol Surg. 2016;11(5):827–36.
10. Hayashi Y, Misawa K, Hawkes DJ, Mori K. Progressive internal landmark registration for surgical navigation in laparoscopic gastrectomy for gastric cancer. Int J Comput Assist Radiol Surg. 2016;11(5):837–45.
11. Ochiai K, Kobayashi E, Tsukihara H, Nozawa H, Kawai K, Sasaki K, Murono K, Ishihara S, Sakuma I. Stereotactic navigation system for laparoscopic lateral pelvic lymph node dissection. Dis Colon Rectum. 2021;64(6):e372–7.
12. Yasuda J, Okamoto T, Onda S, Fujioka S, Yanaga K, Suzuki N, Hattori A. Application of image-guided navigation system for laparoscopic hepatobiliary surgery. Asian J Endosc Surg. 2020;13(1):39–45.
13. Ieiri S, Uemura M, Konishi K, Souzaki R, Nagao Y, Tsutsumi N, Akahoshi T, Ohuchida K, Ohdaira T, Tomikawa M, Tanoue K, Hashizume M, Taguchi T. Augmented reality navigation system for laparoscopic splenectomy in children based on preoperative CT image using optical tracking device. Pediatr Surg Int. 2012;28:341–6.
14. Morita C, Hayashi Y, Oda M, Hawkes D, Misawa K, Mori K. Intra-operative registration method using organ surface information for surgical navigation in laparoscopic gastrectomy. Int J Comput Assist Radiol Surg. 2015;10(Suppl 1):S55–6.

15. Hayashi Y, Misawa K, Mori K. Database-driven patient-specific registration error compensation method for image-guided laparoscopic surgery. Int J Comput Assist Radiol Surg. 2023;18(1):63–9.
16. Tsutsumi N, Tomikawa M, Uemura M, Akahoshi T, Nagao Y, Konishi K, Ieiri S, Hong J, Maehara Y, Hashizume M. Image-guided laparoscopic surgery in an open MRI operating theater. Surg Endosc. 2013;27(6):2178–84.
17. Okada T, Kawada K, Sumii A, Itatani Y, Hida K, Hasegawa S, Sakai Y. Stereotactic navigation for rectal surgery: comparison of 3-dimensional C-arm-based registration to paired-point registration. Dis Colon Rectum. 2020;63(5):693–700.
18. Konishi K, Nakamoto M, Kakeji Y, Tanoue K, Kawanaka H, Yamaguchi S, Ieiri S, Sato Y, Maehara Y, Tamura S, Hashizume M. A real-time navigation system for laparoscopic surgery based on three-dimensional ultrasound using magneto-optic hybrid tracking configuration. Int J Comput Assist Radiol Surg. 2007;2(1):1–10.
19. Pelanis E, Teatini A, Eigl B, Regensburger A, Alzaga A, Kumar RP, Rudolph T, Aghayan DL, Riediger C, Kvarnström N, Elle OJ, Edwin B. Evaluation of a novel navigation platform for laparoscopic liver surgery with organ deformation compensation using injected fiducials. Med Image Anal. 2021;69:101946.
20. Mochizuki Y, Hosaka A, Kamiuchi H, Nie JX, Masamune K, Hoshina K, Miyata T, Watanabe T. New simple image overlay system using a tablet PC for pinpoint identification of the appropriate site for anastomosis in peripheral arterial reconstruction. Surg Today. 2016;46(12):1387–93.
21. Koo B, Robu MR, Allam M, Pfeiffer M, Thompson S, Gurusamy K, Davidson B, Speidel S, Hawkes D, Stoyanov D, Clarkson MJ. Automatic, global registration in laparoscopic liver surgery. Int J Comput Assist Radiol Surg. 2022;17(1):167–76.
22. Labrunie M, Ribeiro M, Mourthadhoi F, Tilmant C, Le Roy B, Buc E, Bartoli A. Automatic preoperative 3D model registration in laparoscopic liver resection. Int J Comput Assist Radiol Surg. 2022;17(8):1429–36.
23. Guan P, Luo H, Guo J, Zhang Y, Jia F. Intraoperative laparoscopic liver surface registration with preoperative CT using mixing features and overlapping region masks. Int J Comput Assist Radiol Surg. 2023;18(8):1521–31.
24. Yang Z, Simon R, Linte CA. Learning feature descriptors for pre- and intra-operative point cloud matching for laparoscopic liver registration. Int J Comput Assist Radiol Surg. 2023;18(6):1025–32.
25. Mori K, Urano A, Hasegawa J, Toriwaki J, Anno H, Katada K. Virtualized endoscope system - an application of virtual reality technology to diagnostic aid. IEICE Trans Inf Syst. 1996;E79-D-6:809–19.
26. Roth HR, Oda H, Zhou X, Shimizu N, Yang Y, Hayashi Y, Oda M, Fujiwara M, Misawa K, Mori K. An application of cascaded 3D fully convolutional networks for medical image segmentation. Comput Med Imaging Graph. 2018;66:90–9.
27. Wasserthal J, Breit HC, Meyer MT, Pradella M, Hinck D, Sauter AW, Heye T, Boll DT, Cyriac J, Yang S, Bach M, Segeroth M. TotalSegmentator: robust segmentation of 104 anatomic structures in CT images. Radiol Artif Intell. 2023;5(5):e230024.
28. Mori K, Hasegawa J, Suenaga Y, Toriwaki J. Automated anatomical labeling of the bronchial branch and its application to the virtual bronchoscopy system. IEEE Trans Med Imaging. 2000;19(2):103–14.
29. Kitasaka T, Kagajo M, Nimura Y, Hayashi Y, Oda M, Misawa K, Mori K. Automatic anatomical labeling of arteries and veins using conditional random fields. Int J Comput Assist Radiol Surg. 2017;12(6):1041–8.
30. Hayashi Y, Misawa K, Mori K. Optimal port placement planning method for laparoscopic gastrectomy. Int J Comput Assist Radiol Surg. 2017;12(10):1677–84.

31. Yamaguchi T, Kuwano A, Koyama T, Okamoto J, Suzuki S, Okuda H, Saito T, Masamune K, Muragaki Y. Construction of brain area risk map for decision making using surgical navigation and motor evoked potential monitoring information. Int J Comput Assist Radiol Surg. 2023;18(2):269–78.
32. Sugino T, Nakamura R, Kuboki A, Honda O, Yamamoto M, Ohtori N. Comparative analysis of surgical processes for image-guided endoscopic sinus surgery. Int J Comput Assist Radiol Surg. 2019;14(1):93–104.
33. Okamoto T, Onda S, Yanaga K, Suzuki N, Hattori A. Clinical application of navigation surgery using augmented reality in the abdominal field. Surg Today. 2015;45(4):397–406.
34. Sugimoto M, Yasuda H, Koda K, Suzuki M, Yamazaki M, Tezuka T, Kosugi C, Higuchi R, Watayo Y, Yagawa Y, Uemura S, Tsuchiya H, Azuma T. Image overlay navigation by markerless surface registration in gastrointestinal, hepatobiliary and pancreatic surgery. J Hepatobiliary Pancreat Sci. 2010;17(5):629–36.
35. Gavaghan K, Oliveira-Santos T, Peterhans M, Reyes M, Kim H, Anderegg S, Weber S. Evaluation of a portable image overlay projector for the visualisation of surgical navigation data: phantom studies. Int J Comput Assist Radiol Surg. 2012;7(4):547–56.
36. Fotouhi J, Unberath M, Song T, Hajek J, Lee SC, Bier B, Maier A, Osgood G, Armand M, Navab N. Co-localized augmented human and X-ray observers in collaborative surgical ecosystem. Int J Comput Assist Radiol Surg. 2019;14(9):1553–63.
37. Saito Y, Sugimoto M, Imura S, Morine Y, Ikemoto T, Iwahashi S, Yamada S, Shimada M. Intraoperative 3D hologram support with mixed reality techniques in liver surgery. Ann Surg. 2020;271(1):e4–7.
38. Igami T, Hayashi Y, Yokyama Y, Mori K, Ebata T. Development of real-time navigation system for laparoscopic hepatectomy using magnetic micro sensor. Minim Invasive Ther Allied Technol. 2024;33(3):129–39.

MIX
Papier aus verantwortungsvollen Quellen
Paper from responsible sources
FSC® C105338

If you have any concerns about our products,
you can contact us on
ProductSafety@springernature.com

In case Publisher is established outside the EU,
the EU authorized representative is:
Springer Nature Customer Service Center GmbH
Europaplatz 3, 69115 Heidelberg, Germany

Printed by Libri Plureos GmbH
in Hamburg, Germany